FETAL NUTRITION, METABOLISM, AND IMMUNOLOGY

The Role of the Placenta

TROPHOBLAST RESEARCH

Series Editors

Richard K. Miller and Henry A. Thiede

University of Rochester Medical Center
Rochester, New York

Volume 1 FETAL NUTRITION, METABOLISM, AND IMMUNOLOGY
The Role of the Placenta
Edited by Richard K. Miller and Henry A. Thiede

A Continuation Order Plan is available for this series. A continuation order will bring delivery of each new volume immediately upon publication. Volumes are billed only upon actual shipment. For further information please contact the publisher.

FETAL NUTRITION, METABOLISM, AND IMMUNOLOGY

The Role of the Placenta

Edited by

Richard K. Miller and
Henry A. Thiede

University of Rochester Medical Center
Rochester, New York

PLENUM MEDICAL BOOK COMPANY
New York and London

Library of Congress Cataloging in Publication Data

Rochester Trophoblast Conference (9th: 1983)
Fetal nutrition, metabolism, and immunology.

(Trophoblast research; v. 1)
"Derived from the Ninth Rochester Trophoblast Conference, held October 3–5, 1983, in Rochester, New York"–T.p. verso.
Includes bibliographical references and index.
1. Fetus–Nutrition–Congresses. 2. Fetus–Metabolism–Congresses. 3. Miscarriage–Immunological aspects–Congresses. 4. Placenta–Congresses. I. Miller, Richard K. II. Thiede, Henry A. III. Title. IV. Series. [DNLM: 1. Fetus–Metabolism–Congresses. 2. Nutrition–In pregnancy–Congresses. 3. Placenta–Metabolism–Congresses. 4. Maternal-fetal exchange–Congresses. 5. Immunity, Maternally-acquired–Congresses. W1 TR877 v.1/WQ 210.5 R676 1983f]
RG615.R63 1983 618.3′4 84-3419

ISBN-13: 978-1-4684-1193-5 e-ISBN-13: 978-1-4684-1191-1
DOI: 10.1007/978-1-4684-1191-1

Derived from the 9th Rochester Trophoblast Conference field
October 3–5, 1983, in Rochester, New York

Plenum Medical Book Company is an imprint of Plenum Publishing Corporation
233 Spring Street, New York, N.Y. 10013

TROPHOBLAST RESEARCH

Trophoblast Research publishes contributions concerning the placenta and the extraembryonic membranes as they relate to embryonic and fetal development and to trophoblastic neoplasia. Original articles, reviews and reports are published in single bound volumes. All articles are peer-reviewed.

Editorial Office for *Trophoblast Research*

Department of Obstetrics and Gynecology
University of Rochester, School of Medicine and Dentistry
601 Elmwood Avenue, Rochester, New York, USA 14642

PAST ROCHESTER TROPHOBLAST CONFERENCES

MODERATORS

First Conference 1961	Arthur T. Hertig Ernest Witebsky
Second Conference 1963	Rupert Billingham Jack Davies
Third Conference 1965	Donald H. Barron Claude A. Villee
Fourth Conference 1967	Roy Hertz Ralph M. Wynn
Fifth Conference 1969	E. J. Quilligan Kenneth Ryan
Sixth Conference 1971	Donald L. Hutchinson Frederick P. Zuspan
Seventh Conference 1977	Griff Ross Ralph M. Wynn

STATE OF THE ART SPEAKERS

Eighth Conference 1980	W. Page Faulk Maurice Panigel
Ninth Conference 1982	Arnold Klopper Claude A. Villee Myron Winick

PREFACE

Each year since 1961, the Rochester Trophoblast Conference has grown in the diversity of its approaches to trophoblast research. At the Ninth Conference, Professors Klopper, Villee and Winick molded the conference with their state of the art addresses on Endocrinology, Metabolism and Nutrition of the Trophoblast.

The Conference was favored with a multitude of creative studies and with warm, sunny, autumn weather to discuss these results. In October of 1982, one hundred and five investigators from 12 countries and 21 states discussed 42 different presentations at the Holiday Inn in Rochester, New York. The Ninth Conference introduced workshops on Metabolism, Nutrition, Endocrinology and Trophoblastic Neoplasia. The chairmen of these workshops were: Metabolism - Villee and Miller; Nutrition - Winick and Maulik; Endocrinology - Klopper and Muechler; and Trophoblastic Neoplasia - Szulman and Helmkamp. These two-hour, intimate discussion groups were well-received by all who attended.

As with the Eighth Conference, the University of Rochester will no longer produce a transcript of the Conference. Beginning with the Ninth Conference, Plenum Press in association with the University, will publish a peer-reviewed series entitled Trophoblast Research. An international editorial advisory board has been named to assure the direction of the series. The editorial board and the organizing committee will develop the future meetings of the Rochester Trophoblast Conference. Trophoblast Research will be published as single bound volumes with original contributions and editorial reports of presentations from the Conference.

The editors wish to express their gratitude to Hilary Evans and Leslie Schmidt of Plenum Press for their advice and support in this undertaking. Without the financial support of the March of Dimes Birth Defects Foundation, which sponsored Arnold Klopper's state of the art address; of the American Cancer Society and the Upjohn Pharmaceutical Company, which sponsored Claude Villee's state of the art address; of Ross Laboratories and the Hoffmann-LaRoche Company, which sponsored Myron Winick's state of the art address, and of Wampole Laboratories, Xerox Corporation and the Department of Obstetrics and Gynecology of the University of Rochester, this conference would not have been possible.

We also acknowledge sincerely the efforts of the Organizing Committee: Virginia Anderson, Raymond B. Baggs, B. Frederick Helmkamp, Debabrata Maulik, Eberhard K. Muechler, Wendy W. Ng; the assistance of Kenneth Case, Ellen Henry, Rogelio Perez and Roy Simmons; the expert wordprocessing of Elaine Acresti and Eileen Williams; and especially the dedication of our conference secretaries, Paula Waite and Jacqulyn White.

We hope that this volume will stimulate the reader to initiate studies which are left unresolved by the Ninth Conference and to join us in October of 1985 for the Tenth Rochester Trophoblast Conference.

CONTENTS

History of the Rochester Trophoblast Conferences 1
R. M. Wynn

NUTRITION

Nutrition, Intrauterine Growth Retardation and the Placenta 7
M. Winick

The Ultrastructural Basis of the Nutritional Transfer: Evidence of Different Patterns in the Plasma Membranes of the Multilayered Placental Barrier 15
M. Sideri, G.de Virgiliis, R. Rainoldi and *G. Remotti*

Human Placental Amino Acid Transfer and Metabolism in Oxygenated and Anoxic Conditions 27
P. Penfold, N. P. Illsley, P. Purkiss and P. Jennings

Bidirectional Transfer of α-Aminoisobutyric Acid by the Perfused Human Placental Lobule 37
P. J. Wier, R. K. Miller, D. Maulik and P. A. di Sant'Agnese

The Effects of Anoxia on Human Placental Metabolism and Fetal Substrate Profile Investigated by an In Vitro Placental Perfusion Technique 55
N. P. Illsley, P. Penfold, S. E. Bardsley, B. M. Tracey and J. G. Aarnoudse

Clearance of α-Aminoisobutyric Acid during In Situ Perfusion of the Guinea Pig Placenta 71
B. J. Kelman and M. R. Sikov

Factors Affecting the Uptake of α-Amino Acids by Human Placental Villus: Acetylcholine, Phospholipid Methylation, Ca^{++}, and Cytoskeletal Organization 81
B. V. R. Sastry, S. L. Barnwell and *R. D. Moore*

Depression of Amino Acid Uptake in Human Placental Villus by Cocaine, Morphine and Nicotine 101
S. L. Barnwell and B. V. R. Sastry

Transport of Nutrients in the Early Human Placenta: Amino Acid, Creatine, Vitamin B_{12} 121
W. W. Ng and R. K. Miller

Studies on the Placental Hydrolysis and Transfer of Lipids to the Fetal Guinea Pig 135
C. R. Thomas, C. Lowy, R.J. St. Hillaire and J.D. Brunzell

Doppler Assessment of Fetoplacental Circulatory Dynamics 149
D. Maulik, V. D. Saini and N. C. Nanda

Fine Structure of the Human Chorion Laeve 159
T. Wang and D. H. A. Maas

Nutrition Reports 167

METABOLISM

Enzymes, Receptors, Metabolism and Placental Function 175
C. A. Villee

cAMP-Dependent Protein Kinase and cAMP, cGMP and Calcium Stimulated Phosphorylation in Human Placenta: Comparison of Cytosol and Membrane Fractions 185
J. J. Moore, J. V. Baker and J. A. Whitsett

Interaction between Membrane Function and Protein Synthesis in the Human Placenta In Vitro 197
O. Genbacev, B. Cemerikic and M. Cvetkovic

Metabolic Changes in Human Placental Tissue in Diabetes Mellitus 209
Y. Z. Diamant and R. Kissilevitz

Steroid and Protein Metabolism by the Trophoblast 223
A. Klopper

In Vivo and In Vitro Studies of the Dehydroepiandosterone Sulfate Metabolism in Cases of Impaired Estrogen Secretion 237
E. Alsat, M. Bedin, G. Tanguy, H. Thoumsin and L. Cedard

The Placenta as a Target Tissue for Steroids 249
C. B. Coulam and T. C. Spelsberg

The Placental Secretion of SP_1: A Comparison of Concentrations in Retroplacental and Peripheral Blood 271
A. G. M. Ahmed, D. Goodwin and A. Klopper

Storage and Release of Renin and hCG in Trophoblast from Human Chorion Laeve 279
A.M. Poisner, H.-C. Cheng, G. W. Wood and R. Poisner

The Arachidonic Acid Pathway and the Secretion of Chorionic Gonadotropin (hCG) and Progesterone by the Cultured Human Choriocarcinoma JEG-3 Cell 289
J. Ilekis and R. Benveniste

Metabolism Reports 301

IMMUNOLOGY

Antibody-Induced Abortion in pp Women in Three Different Studies 307
P. Levine

A Cell-Mediated Immune Defect in Recurrent Spontaneous Abortions 315
J. A. McIntyre and W. P. Faulk

Pregnancy-Associated Plasma Protein-A (PAPP-A) is a Specific Inhibitor of the Third Component of Human Complement 323
P. Bischof and A. Geinoz

The Embryopathologic Effects of Teratogenic Yolk Sac Antiserum 335
R. L. Brent, D. A. Beckman, M. Jensen, T. R. Koszalka, and I. Damjanov

Analysis of Sera from Monkeys with Histories of Fetal Wastage and the Identification of Teratogenicity in Sera from Human Chronic Spontaneous Aborters using Rat Embryo Cultures 347
S. W. Carey, N. W. Klein, W. T. Fredrickson, G. P. Sackett, R. M. Greenstein, P. Sehgal and M. Elliott

Prolonged Survival of Human Decidual Grafts in a Xenogeneic Host 361
H. Arab, J. A. McCoshen, M.K. Leith, A. Wodzicki and J. E. Tyson

Immunology Reports 371

List of Contributors 375

Index 383

Trophoblast Research 1: 1-4, 1983

HISTORY OF THE ROCHESTER TROPHOBLAST CONFERENCES

Ralph M. Wynn

Ravenswood Hospital Medical Center
& Department of Obstetrics and Gynecology
Rush Medical College, Chicago, Illinois, U.S.A.

For more than twenty years the Rochester Trophoblast Conferences have provided a forum for exchange of the newest information relating to the structure and function of the placenta and in particular its chorionic epithelium, or trophoblast. Since November 13, 1961, scientists at these conferences discussed, often for the first time in public, new data and hypotheses relevant to interdisciplinary investigation of the placenta. I believe that immunobiology of the placenta first attracted widespread attention in the United States as a result of the initial Rochester Trophoblast Conference.

Very few of the 41 participants in the original conference imagined that well over twenty years later these interdisciplinary symposia would remain a major stimulus to trophoblastic research throughout the United States and, more recently, throughout the world. In the first and subsequent conferences work in progress was discussed, hypotheses were developed and refined, and concepts were formulated through an exchange of ideas among world-famous authorities and scientific neophytes.

In light of the significance of these conferences, it was a highly acceptable honor for me to have been asked to prepare the introduction to the Ninth Conference. My primary qualification for this assignment is longevity, inasmuch as I am the only member of the original conference who has had the good fortune to attend all the subsequent conferences. The first meeting in Rochester strongly influenced the subsequent fifteen years of my career. The moderators in 1961, Arthur Hertig and the late Ernest Witebsky, used their great knowledge and wit to stimulate, cajole, and challenge the other participants. The immunologists recognized the necessity of learning the anatomic details of the tissues they were studying, and the morphologists were stimulated to reinterpret the implications of their findings. The principle of constructive criticism of work in progress has been maintained, fortunately, throughout most of the conferences.

Major accomplishments of that First Conference included the introduction of several young investigators to the disciplines of electron microscopy and tissue culture. At that meeting the biologic enigma of the evolution of the syncytium and the concept of the placenta as an allograft were stressed. Henry Thiede served most capably as convener, and Curtis Lund and he were editors of the first three conferences. The Second Conference, in 1963, again comprised an interdisciplinary group, who emphasized the correlation of placental morphology and immunology.

Significant papers dealing with the ultrastructure of normal trophoblast and choriocarcinoma were presented along with several concerned with current concepts in immunology. The stimulating moderators of the 1963 meeting were Jack Davies and Rupert Billingham, and the number of participants had almost doubled. The Third Conference, in 1965, deviated somewhat from the immunobiologic path of its predecessors. Under the chairmanship of Donald Barron and Claude Villee, the emphasis switched to placental circulation, physiology, biochemistry, and transport. The Fourth Conference, in 1967, under the chairmanship of Ralph Wynn, Roy Hertz, and John Vaughan, having reverted to immunology and morphology, was highly focused. Choriocarcinoma and its immunologic and endocrine implications figured prominently in the interdisciplinary discussions throughout both days of the conference.

The Fourth, Fifth, and Sixth Trophoblast Conferences were convened and edited by John Choate and Curtis Lund, during Henry Thiede's tenure in Mississippi. The fifth meeting, in 1969, was under the chairmanship of Kenneth Ryan, Ernest Page, and Edward Quilligan. Important new information on steroid metabolism, enzymology, and biochemistry of the placenta were presented along with new techniques of placental perfusion. Papers dealing with chorionic gonadotropin and its subunits were featured in the program. The Sixth Trophoblast Conference, in 1971, marked the end of the predictable biennial sequence. The moderators at that time were Ralph Wynn, Donald Hutchinson, and Frederick Zuspan, and the emphasis switched to the amnion. Although ultracytochemistry of the fetal membranes and paraplacental transfer were discussed, several of the papers dealt with clinical applications and failed to meet the scientific standards of the earlier conferences.

After the 1971 meeting many of the original group feared that the Trophoblast Conferences might disappear permanently; but with Henry Thiede's return to Rochester, the phoenix arose, after six years, as the Seventh Trophoblast Conference. In 1977, Griff Ross and Ralph Wynn moderated the Seventh Conference, which was devoted largely to the chemistry, physiology, and biochemistry of placental peptide hormones, particularly human placental lactogen (human chorionic somatomammotropin). Furthermore, we returned during this conference to the immunology of the fetoplacental unit. For those who were at the First Conference, sixteen years earlier, the veritable explosion of knowledge in this field was impressive. The group in 1977 was small, but the exchange of information among the participants was invaluable. Again, immunologists and morphologists learned from one another, as witnessed by the appearance of several major publications shortly thereafter. This meeting marked Richard Miller's first association with the organization and publication of the Trophoblast Conferences, an association that fortunately has continued. The transcript of the seventh meeting is only a summary of the conference, without illustrative material. In 1977, I had the privilege of reviewing the major accomplishments of the Rochester Conferences to date. At the Seventh Conference the various concepts invoked to explain the immunologic protection of the placenta were scrutinized. Immunopathology of the placenta and the immunologic implications of preeclampsia in particular were discussed. In the ensuing discussion it became clear that the riddle of preeclampsia-eclampsia was not likely to be solved simplistically. It is now six years since the Seventh Conference and we are hardly closer to a unified etiologic concept of preeclampsia, although in the interim a great many facts and figures have accumulated. Stimulating concepts, faulty hypotheses, and preposterous suggestions have all appeared in print. It is likely that some of the least impressive reports would never have been published had they first been subjected to the scientific criticism of the interdisciplinary investigators at Rochester.

Three years elapsed between the Seventh and Eighth Trophoblast Conferences. For the Eighth Conference, in 1980, Richard Miller had joined Henry Thiede as coeditor. In the interval between the Seventh and Eighth Conferences Curtis Lund, who was Chairman of the Department of Obstetrics and Gynecology at Rochester during the early years of the conferences, had died; the eighth volume was dedicated appropriately to his memory. One hundred and twenty-six investigators attended the Eighth Conference (*Placenta: Receptors, Pathology, and Toxicology*), which assumed an international flavor. Although more papers on more topics were discussed, the conference lost a degree of intimacy, as the time for informal exchange of information was limited. This was the first meeting at which "state of the art" lectures were included as part of the program. Page Faulk and Maurice Panigel introduced the discussions of placental immunobiology and toxicology, respectively. Faulk's comprehensive and stimulating summary provided the background for the detailed immunologic discussions encompassed by the nineteen papers in that session. Again, hormonal production by neoplastic trophoblast received considerable attention and an interesting chemically induced neoplasm of the placenta of the patas monkey was demonstrated. This conference was published as a supplement to the new journal Placenta, which was founded by Harold Fox and Page Faulk. It seems likely that the impetus to creation of this interdisciplinary journal devoted to studies of the placenta was the Rochester Trophoblast Conferences.

Serious students of the placenta should be pleased to learn that the distinguished firm of Plenum Press has agreed to publish the Ninth (1982) and subsequent Conferences, as a series entitled *Trophoblast Research*. At this critical juncture in the history of the Trophoblast Conferences, several stimulating possibilities are under serious consideration. First, a European study group similar in format to the Rochester Conferences but somewhat broader in scope has had its first meeting. As I write these words, I am discussing the relation of the two groups with Peter Kaufmann from Hamburg, who catalyzed the formation of the European group. The two organizations may affiliate informally through an exchange of information about dates of meetings and topics, or they may move even more closely together. Current plans do not include formation of a society with dues-paying members on either side of the Atlantic. The relation of the journal Placenta to one or both of these groups is another significant issue to be addressed in the immediate future.

The scientific community dealing with the placenta is now larger and closer than ever before. It is my personal hope that the Rochester group remain identified with and active in the organization and publication of conferences. Inasmuch as the participation in Rochester by European colleagues has been increasingly visible during the last few years, it might be appropriate to maintain a schedule of biennial meetings, alternating between Rochester and a convenient location in Europe. We would thus return to Rochester at four-year intervals. Alternatively, we could maintain biennial meetings on both sides of the Atlantic, with a joint meeting perhaps every four years. Two annual conferences seem excessive, but intervals of greater than two years could decrease the cohesiveness of these international groups, whose members share an interest in the most fascinating of biological models, the mammalian placenta.

I look forward to the Tenth Rochester Trophoblast Conference in 1985; to the First European meeting, which is already scheduled for 1984; and to a long-range plan that will ensure the continuation of a tradition that has been of inestimable value to the development of modern reproductive biology.

NUTRITION

Trophoblast Research 1:7-14, 1983

NUTRITION, INTRAUTERINE GROWTH RETARDATION AND THE PLACENTA
- A Review-

Myron Winick

Institute of Human Nutrition
College of Physicians and Surgeons
Columbia University
701 West 168th Street
New York, New York 10032, U.S.A.

Fetal malnutrition may be viewed as any condition which will reduce the final quantity of nutrients reaching the fetus. Theoretically, the fetus may be malnourished because not enough nutrients are available in the maternal blood, because the placenta is not adequately supplied with maternal blood, or because the placenta is unable to extract and transport nutrients from the maternal circulation.

Historically, the mother, particularly the human mother, has been viewed as carrying sufficient nutrient reserves within her body to supply her fetus regardless of whether or not she herself was adequately nourished. Certainly simple calculations relating maternal body composition to fetal body composition even at term would suggest this is true. Yet the evidence that fetal growth is retarded when the mother is undernourished during pregnancy is overwhelming. This evidence comes from animal experiments in various species demonstrating that restriction of maternal caloric intake will lead to reduced fetal growth (Zamenhof et al., 1968) and from human studies demonstrating that reduced food intake will result in a decrease in birth weight (Stein et al., 1975). In addition, studies in which undernourished pregnant women were supplemented with extra food have demonstrated that birth weight can be increased if caloric intake is substantially increased. (Lechtig et al., 1975).

Thus the evidence suggests a paradox. The mother is capable of supplying nutrients to the fetus even if she herself is undernourished, and yet for some reason the fetus is not getting those nutrients. Recent studies are beginning to explain how this may occur (Rosso and Cramoy, 1979). During pregnancy, all mammals undergo an adaptive response which involves an expansion in maternal blood volume, an increase in maternal cardiac output and an increase in uterine blood flow which reflects not only the increased vascularity of the uterus itself but also the growth of the highly vascular placenta. Maternal undernutrition will curtail this adaptive response and result in a placenta with reduced blood flow. This will in turn result in a retarded placental growth and in a reduced overall capacity of the placenta to transport nutrients to the fetus. Thus fetal malnutrition in the undernourished mother is not from lack of nutrients in the maternal blood but rather from an inability of the placenta to deliver those nutrients to the fetus. The result is a symmetrical growth failure which is characterized by a decrease in the rate of cell division in all of the fetal organs. The fetal brain is affected to the same extent as the other organs. By

16 days of gestation in the rat, all of the areas of fetal brain examined showed a reduced number of cells. In addition, myelination is reduced and the concentration of gangliosides and of N-acetylneuraminic acid is also reduced. Finally, animals undernourished during pregnancy gave birth to pups that show behavioral abnormalities which persist into adult life (Levitsky and Barnes, 1972).

By contrast, if the placental blood flow is allowed to develop normally and then acutely restricted, a different type of fetal malnutrition will ensue. Ligation of the uterine artery in a 17 day pregnant rat will result in fetal growth failure. However, unlike the situation in which the mother has been malnourished throughout pregnancy, this is an asymmetrical type of growth failure. The liver has 50percent of the expected number of cells at birth and is completely devoid of glycogen. The brain is not affected at all (Rosso and Winick, 1974). This is because of vasodilation of the fetal carotid artery secondary to the acute hypoxia caused by the ligation. This reflex dilation keeps the brain adequately supplied with blood at the expense of the other organs. Although these animals are small at birth and are susceptible to hypoglycemia, their brains are normal in size, contain normal quantities of myelin and gangliosides, and the pups show no behavioral abnormalities. Thus in the rat there are two distinct types of fetal malnutrition, both caused by an inadequate blood supply to the fetus. The first is due to maternal undernutrition which results in an incomplete vascularization of the placenta secondary to a curtailment of the normal increase in uterine blood flow during pregnancy. The resulting fetal abnormality is symmetrical growth failure which will affect the fetal brain. The second is due to an acute vascular insult late in pregnancy which will result in fetal growth failure but which will spare the fetal brain.

If we examine the placentae themselves in these two different types of intrauterine growth retardation, we find that they are quite different. With maternal malnutrition, placental weight is reduced often to a greater extent than fetal weight. This weight reduction can be entirely attributed to a reduced number of cells. By contrast, the placentae from animals that underwent uterine ligation, although also smaller, had a normal number of cells but a reduction in cell size. Thus the cellular characteristics of the growth failure within the placenta can be used to predict the nature and timing of the stimulus which produced the growth failure.

Clinically both types of fetal malnutrition are evident; the symmetrically growth retarded infant and the growth retarded infant who appears to have a large head for his body. In developing countries where maternal malnutrition is frequent the former is more common. In developed countries the latter seems to predominate. In all studies which examine the outcome of "fetal malnutrition" the type of growth retardation should be clearly delineated and the placenta carefully examined.

The human placenta increases in weight until shortly before term. By contrast, the total number of cells (DNA content) reaches a maximum at around 34 weeks gestation (Winick et al., 1967). Any stimulus which retards fetal growth before 34 weeks should result in a smaller placenta with fewer cells. Any stimulus beginning after 34 weeks should result in a smaller placenta with smaller cells. And any stimulus beginning early and lasting throughout pregnancy would be expected to result in a placenta with both reduced cell number and reduced cell size.

Several studies have shown that women who were undernourished both before and during pregnancy bore placentae which contained a reduced number of cells (Winick, 1967; Laga et al., 1972 a, b). Moreover, in one study, supplementation of 20,000 extra calories or more throughout the entire pregnancy produced infants of normal birth weight and placentae of normal weight containing a normal number of cells. Although the evidence in the human is so far not complete, what is available strongly suggests that maternal malnutrition produced fetal growth failure indirectly by curtailing the normal expansion in uterine blood flow, which in turn leads to inadequate placental blood flow and impaired placental growth. The growth failure of the placenta is associated with a reduced number of cells.

The opposite effect can be seen during gestational diabetes. Presumably due to the chronic hyperglycemia the placenta, like the fetus, is heavier. This increase in weight is a true hyperplasia resulting in a placenta with an increased number of cells (Winick and Noble, 1967). Thus the growth of placenta and the cellular characteristics of that growth can tell us about the nature and the timing of a stimulus in the human. Not enough advantage has been taken of the placental changes in the classification of human intrauterine growth retardation. The growth retardation associated with maternal smoking is a good example of this (Bassi et al., 1982). In rats subjected to chronic exposure to cigarette smoke, profound growth failure in the fetus can be induced. The growth failure has some of the characteristics of the type induced by maternal malnutrition, some of the characteristics of late placental vascular insufficiency, and some characteristics not seen in either. The brain is reduced in size but considerably less than the other fetal organs. In addition, the lungs are much more markedly affected than in either maternal malnutrition or acute vascular insufficiency. The placenta is also markedly reduced in size and the number and size of the placental cells is reduced. So far, there are no good studies delineating the growth of the placenta in human pregnancies complicated by maternal smoking.

All of the stimuli so far discussed have affected placental growth qualitatively in the same way as fetal growth. If fetal growth is curtailed, the same is true of placental growth. If fetal growth is accelerated, so is placental growth. Recently we have examined a situation in which there appears to be a paradoxical response between the fetus and the placenta.

It is now well established that consumption of large amounts of alcohol during pregnancy can result in a constellation of abnormalities including abnormal brain development. More recent evidence suggests that more moderate amounts of alcohol consumed during pregnancy may retard fetal growth and produce behavioral abnormalities. Studies in our own laboratory during the last few years have shown that consumption of relatively small amounts of alcohol (too small to affect fetal growth) by pregnant rats will result in abnormalities of placental growth (Gordon et al., 1982). The placentae are larger, contain more cells, and yet transport of nutrients per gram of tissue or per cell is reduced. The entire placenta, however, transports normal quantities of nutrients. It would appear that the placenta, when exposed to small amounts of alcohol, will undergo hyperplasia in order to keep overall nutrient transport within normal limits. Whether this is a very early response of placenta to other growth retarding stimuli, i.e., maternal malnutrition or smoking, which has so far been overlooked because of the severity of the stimulus used, or whether this is a response unique to alcohol is not known.

Of course the fetus can be affected directly without any observable effect on the placenta. For example, experiments in our laboratory have shown that both regular coffee and decaffeinated coffee fed to rats throughout pregnancy will lead to behavioral abnormalities in the offspring (Groisser et al., 1982). In the case of the decaffeinated coffee there is mild asymmetrical growth retardation with no effect on brain, and a marked reduction of liver weight. The placenta, as far as we can tell, is entirely normal.

In summary, the placenta is an organ that has been neglected in studies of intrauterine growth failure. Those studies which have been carried out suggest that changes in placenta induced by maternal malnutrition and other stimuli can give us a clue both to the nature of the stimulus and to some of the mechanisms by which the growth retardation is produced.

REFERENCES

Bassi, J.A., Rosso, P., Noessinger, A. and James, S.L. (1982) Fetal growth retardation due to maternal tobacco smoke exposure in the rat. *Fed. Proc.* 41, 285 (Abstract No. 97).

Gordon, B.H.J., Durandin, R.M., Rosso, P. and Winick, M. (1982) Placental amino acid transport in alcohol fed rats. *Fed. Proc.* 41, 947 (Abstract No. 3956).

Groisser, D.S., Rosso, P. and Winick, M. (1982) Coffee consumption during pregnancy: Subsequent behavioral abnormalities of the offspring. *J. Nutri.* 112, 829-832.

Laga, E.M., Driscoll, S.G., Munro, H.N. (1972a) Comparison of placentas from two socioeconomic groups. I. Morphometry. *Pediatrics* 50, 24-32.

Laga, E.M., Driscoll, S.G. and Munro, H.N. (1972b) Comparison of placentas from two socioeconomic groups. I. Biochemical characteristics. *Pediatrics* 50, 33-39.

Lechtig, A., Habicht, J.P., Delgado, H., Klein, R.E., Yarborough, C. and Martorell, R. (1975) Effect of food supplementation during pregnancy on birthweight. *Pediatrics* 56, 508-520.

Levitsky, D.A. and Barnes, R.H. (1972) Nutritional and environmental interactions in the behavioral development of the rat: long term effects. *Science* 176, 68-71.

Rosso, P. and Winick, M. (1974) Intrauterine growth retardation. A new systematic approach based on the clinical and biochemical characteristics of this condition. *J. Perinat. Med.* 2, 147-160.

Rosso, P. and Cramoy, C. (1979) Nutrition and pregnancy. In *Human Nutrition: A Comprehensive Treatise, Vol. 1, Nutrition: Pre-and Postnatal Development* (ed.), Winick, M., pp. 133-228, New York: Plenum.

Stein, Z., Susser, M., Saenger, G. and Marolla, F. (1975) *Famine and Human Development, The Dutch Hunger Winter of 1944-45.* New York: Oxford University Press, pp. 284.

Winick, M. (1967) Cellular growth of the human placenta. III. Intrauterine growth failure. *J. Ped.* 71, 390-395.

Winick, M. and Noble, A. (1967) Cellular growth in human placenta, II. Diabetes Mellitus. *J. Ped.* 71, 216-219.

Winick, M., Coscia, A. and Noble, A. (1967) Cellular growth in human placenta. I. Normal placental growth. *Pediatrics* 39, 248-251.
Zamenhof, S., Van Marthens, F. and Margolis, F.L. (1968) DNA (cell number) and protein in neonatal brain: Alteration by maternal dietary protein restriction, *Science* 60, 322-323.

DISCUSSION

BISCHOF (Geneva): The growth of the placenta is also dependent upon hormones. If the number of implantations at day 7 in the rat are reduced, an increase in the size of the remaining placentae is observed. If there is a reduction in the number of corpora lutea on day 7, exactly the same response occurs to the placentae. If these two procedures are combined, placentae can be obtained in the rat which are approximately 1 gram in weight or about twice the size of a normal placenta. This increased weight in the placenta can be reversed by injecting progesterone. This is a dose related response to progesterone. Thus, it appears that progesterone is important early in pregnancy in the growth of the placenta (Bischof et al., 1976, *J. Physiol.* 72, 36A).

WINICK (New York): It is certainly conceivable that hormones are involved in the malnutrition story; however, in the postnatal world, where hormones were a very attractive mechanism by which malnutrition affected growth as related to growth hormone, somatomatin and others, for the present it appears we are unable to identify a hormonal relationship. But this is not to say that a strong relationship could not occur between prenatal growth and hormones.

KLOPPER (Aberdeen): To continue this line of discussion concerning hormones, at 34 weeks besides what you describe as a change over between the growth type of placenta, there is an abrupt change in the production of estriol. Perhaps progesterone is part of a message that influences the placenta. Does the switch from hyperplasia to hypertrophy at 34 weeks relate to the rapidly increasing production of estriol.

WINICK (New York): That is an attractive hypothesis. I am not aware of any report that has evaluated the relationship between estriol production and the cessation of cell division.

SANYAL (New Haven): Estriol is a weak estrogen; however, it has been shown by Clark et al. (1977, *Endocrinol.* 100, 91) quite conclusively that if estriol is administered continuously, it can be a potent estrogen as estradiol. This is because the estriol reaches the nucleus of the estrogen sensitive tissue (e.g., rat uterus). It induces protein synthesis similar to estradiol. If we consider the endometrium as an analogous tissue to the placenta, estrogen has a mitotic effect and progesterone has a hypertrophic effect during the secretory phase, perhaps there is some analogy between the effects of estrogen and progesterone in the uterus and the cell multiplication and hyperplasia seen in the trophoblast.

WINICK (New York): You raise an interesting point; however, in the placenta one has seen the reverse effect. As estriol increases, hyperplasia is stopped. I believe it is difficult to explain it in terms of the analogy to the uterus.

GENBACEV (Zemun): We have been studying the effect of alcohol on the placenta under in vitro conditions using tissue slices. We have noted some paradoxical responses. We noted a decrease in oxygen consumption but an increase in glucose consumption and lactate production as well as an increase in human placental lactogen synthesis. These reactions were dose-dependent and were much more pronounced in the first and second trimester placentae than in term tissue. At least under these acute in vitro exposure conditions there appears to be the possibility of some direct effect of alcohol. I do not know how alcohol may be affecting the placenta in vivo. In your text, you indicated that the effect of alcohol is most likely indirect.

WINICK (New York): Your paradoxical effects are apparent following acute exposure to alcohol. It is certainly possible that alcohol could have a direct effect on the placenta not mediated through the fetus. The experiments I have described exposed animals to alcohol for a six week period. In fact, we cannot produce these changes at all if we simply give the alcohol during pregnancy. The animal has to be pretreated before pregnancy with alcohol. You may say it has to be habituated to the alcohol. We may be looking at two different mechanisms, I do not know, but your data sound most interesting.

ANDERSON (Staten Island): How would you categorize the placenta of the smoking mother? Have you any observations concerning exposure to cigarette smoke?

WINICK (New York): Pedro Rosso, a colleague at Columbia, has noted profound growth failure in rat fetuses where the mothers have been exposed via a smoking machine (Bassi et al., *Fed. Proc.* 41, 947 1982). They have also noted that the placenta is profoundly affected by a reduction in weight as well as a reduction in DNA content. It appears that this placental growth retardation is from a hyperplastic viewpoint.

ANDERSON (Staten Island): Have you observed placental hyperplasia during either fetal or maternal anemia?

WINICK (New York): We have not observed placentae from patients with anemia. We have looked at placentae from diabetic mothers who had macrosomic fetuses. As you well know, the placentae are large with increased numbers of cells. Thus, a hyperplasia is seen here; however, I have no data for anemia.

KLEIN (Storrs): I am interested in your measurement of total DNA. Many big embryos can have exencephaly and other serious abnormalities. In this case, total DNA can be very misleading. I suggest that it is the function of the DNA, the expression of the DNA, that is crucial in developmental abnormalities.

WINICK (New York): There is no question that you are correct. The only appropriate use of DNA here is as a way of counting cells without histological evaluation. Thus, we have a biochemical tool for counting cells, and it has been most useful in terms of asking questions about how many cells there are at any given time.

BRENT (Philadelphia): In relationship to estrogens and estriol, it may be worthwhile to reinvestigate the data resulting from the prenatal exposure to diethylstilbestrol. During the 1950's and 60's, massive doses of this estrogen-like compound were administered. Dosages have been reported as high as 125,000 mg of DES during pregnancy were administered. I would suspect there are multiple thousands of placental weights in growth data that are available for investigation. As a pediatric intern in Boston, I remember how the White's would show us how succulent, beautiful and healthy the placentae from these patients did look. There may in fact be some data related to hyperplasia as well. These drugs were given quite early in pregnancy for normal pregnancies, diabetic pregnancies and threatened abortions.

A second issue is that hyperplasia cannot be uniformly applied throughout pregnancy. At Columbia, Dr. Robert Rugh demonstrated that radiation can kill cells during early organogensis but that a similar exposure during the early fetal period would result in much smaller adults than from those following the earlier exposure to radiation. Thus, when malformations are produced is not necessarily the time when growth retardation is produced. Are there any data to determine whether malnutrition in different parts of the hyperplastic phases can account for differential cell loss?

WINICK (New York): Yes, that has been done both by us *(Experimental Neurology,* 1970) and by John Dobbing and his group in Manchester (*Arch. of Dis. Child.*, 1973) in the brain. In the rat, hyperplasia can at one time be neuronal and in another area of the brain, hyperplasia can be glial. If one imposes a stimulus at the time of neuronal hyperplasia, one can change the neuronal to glial ratio. Thus, the outcome will be a qualitatively different brain than if one imposes the malnutrition at a different time. Thus, it is possible to alter such development; however, not with the precision that one could do with radiation.

BRENT (Philadelphia): We have been developing a malnutrition model where the embryo can be malnurished. It appears that the embryos lethality or destructive processes in this model can affect the placenta. (Brent et al., this volume).

Trophoblast Research 1:15-26, 1983

THE ULTRASTRUCTURAL BASIS OF THE NUTRITIONAL TRANSFER: EVIDENCE OF DIFFERENT PATTERNS IN THE PLASMA MEMBRANES OF THE MULTILAYERED PLACENTAL BARRIER

Mario Sideri, Giuseppe de Virgiliis, Roberto Rainoldi and Gianni Remotti

First Clinic of Obstetrics and Gynecology, Section of Obstetrical and Gynecological Pathology, and CNR Center of Cytopharmacology
University of Milan, Milan, Italy

INTRODUCTION

Fetal growth and development are promoted by an active nutritional transfer involving a variety of mechanisms ('carriers', 'pumps', receptors) observed in the placental plasma membranes (Whitsett and Brownscheidle, 1979). From the anatomical point of view, the series of plasma membranes interposed between mother and fetus are formed by 1) the syncytial plasma membrane in contact with the maternal blood (SPM-m), 2) the syncytial plasma membrane in contact with the cytotrophoblast or the trophoblastic basement membrane (SPM-f), 3) the different cytotrophoblastic plasma membranes (CPM), and 4) the endothelial plasma membranes of the fetal capillary.

Microvillous and non-microvillous membrane fractions have been isolated and characterized. Most of the reported data on the composition, receptor activity and amino acid uptake were obtained from the microvillous membrane fraction (Smith et al., 1977; Ruzycki et al., 1978; Loh et al., 1980), while the non microvillous membrane fraction remains a heterogeneous entity whose activities could not be localized at precise subcellular levels (Whitsett, 1980).

The freeze fracture technique easily allows the investigation of 1) large surfaces of the placental membranes, 2) membrane associated structures, such as junctional devices, and 3) membrane involving events, such as membrane fusion, endocytotic and pinocytotic processes. In particular, the freeze fracture technique offers the possibility of investigating the protein components of the plasma membranes, which are formed by a lipid bilayer in which proteins are embedded in an iceberg-like fashion (Robertson, 1981). The frozen biological membranes tend to fracture centrally, and the fractured replicated surfaces display particles (IMP) 50-100 Å in diameter, that are associated with proteins in membranes.

This study reports the results of freeze fracture investigations conducted with early and term human placentae.

MATERIALS AND METHODS

Ten early (10-13 weeks) human placentae, obtained from voluntary interruptions of pregnancy performed by dilatation and curettage, and ten term human placentae, obtained by vaginal deliveries, were examined.

Fragments of terminal villi, biopsied under stereoscopic control, were processed for freeze fracture examination. Samples were fixed in cold 2% glutaraldehyde in 0.1 M cacodylate buffer, pH 7.3, and then infiltrated with 10-30% glycerol in the same buffer. They were subsequently frozen in freon 22, cooled at -150°C in liquid nitrogen, and finally freeze fractured and replicated according to Moor and Muhlethaler (1963) in a Balzers freeze etching device (Balzers AG, Balzers, Liechtenstein). The fracturing temperature was -110°C. Thickness of platinum-carbon deposited films was regulated by a quartz crystal thin-film monitor (Balzers AG, Balzers, Liechtenstein). Platinum-carbon replicas were washed in sodium hypochlorite solution, to remove organic material, then in distilled water, recovered on 200 mesh copper grids, and finally examined with a Philips EM 200 electron microscope. The fractured faces were designated as P and E faces according to Branton et al. (1975). P face indicates the fractured side of the membrane contacting the intracellular compartment, and E face indicates the fractured side of the membrane contacting the extracellular compartment. Illustrations show the platinum-carbon shadowing directed approximately from the bottom to the top.

IMP counting was performed in SMP-m, SMP-f and CPM in three early placentae, and in SPM-m and SPM-f in three term placentae. Micrographs showing flat exposed surfaces and the pits of the complementary face were selected. In every placenta, five to ten satisfactory micrographs were taken at the same original magnification (75,000 x) for each fractured face of the studied membranes. Counting was performed on three areas of 0.04 μ^2 for each micrograph (magnified 150,000 x), so that a total of 630 areas were evaluated. In every single placenta, the mean value ($\pm$ SD) of the IMP number/0.04 μ^2, is calculated from each fractured face (E or P) of the five considered plasma membranes (SPM-m, SPM-f and CPM for early ones, SPM-m and SPM-f for term placentae). Each mean value is converted into IMP number/μ^2.

The significance of IMP density differences has been determined by Student's-t-test on original data obtained from the 0.04 μ^2 areas.

RESULTS

Tight junctions (t.j.) were observed as maculae or fasciae occludentes on the SPM-m (Figure 1), between SPM-f and CPM (Figure 2), and between two adjacent cytotrophoblastic cells; tight junctions were also observed, as rows of IMPs or very short strands, between the adjacent endothelial cells of the fetal capillary (Figure 3). Gap junctions (g.j.) were rarely seen in the trophoblastic epithelium and were more frequently found in the early than in the term placentae: they were located between the syncytium and the cytotrophoblast and were always associated with t.j. (Figure 4).

Table I
Numerical density of intramembranous particles (IMPs) per square micrometer. First trimester placentae

Fracture face	Plasma membrane	Mean value ± SD
P	SPM-m	1462 ± 37 (*)
P	SPM-f	1929 ± 187 (*)
P	CPM	1888 ± 79
E	SPM-m	799 ± 43 (**)
E	SPM-f	1242 ± 61 (**)
E	CPM	1211 ± 69

(*) (**) The difference between the similar marked values is statistically, highly significant ($p<0.001$).

Table II
Numerical density of intramembranous particles (IMPs) per square micrometer. Term placentae

Fracture face	Plasma membrane	Mean value ± SD
P	SPM-m	2265 ± 619 (*)
P	SPM-f	3445 ± 396 (*)
E	SPM-m	1859 ± 66
E	SPM-f	799 ± 43

(*) The difference between the similar marked values is statistically, highly significant ($p<0.001$).

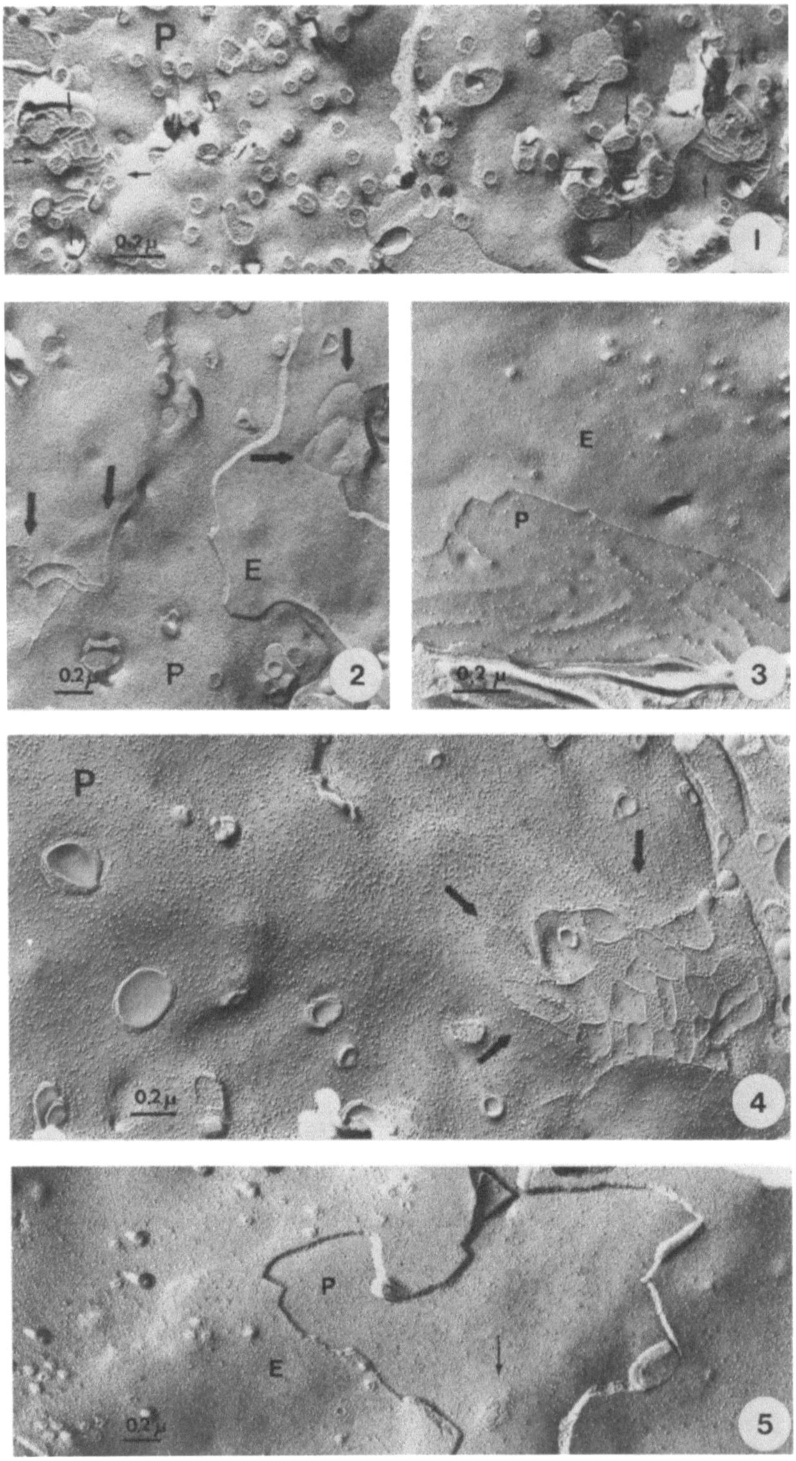
P
0.2 μ
1
E
P
0.2 μ
2
E
P
0.2 μ
3
P
0.2 μ
4
P
E
0.2 μ
5

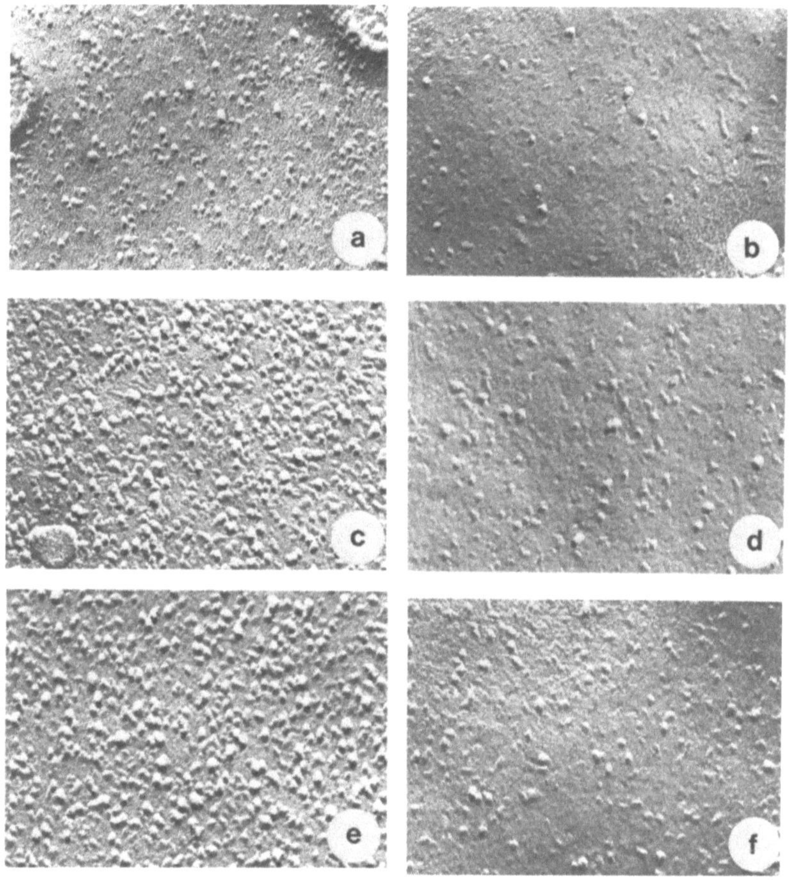

Figures 6a-f. Density of intramembranous particles (IMPs) in early placenta. P faces are shown on the left side, and E faces on the right one. Figures a and b (top) show the syncytial plasma membrane in contact with the maternal blood (SPM-m). Figures c and d (2nd row) show the syncytial plasma membrane in contact with the cytotrophoblast (SPM-f). Figures e and f (bottom) show the cytotrophoblastic plasma membrane (CPM). Note the different IMP density between SPM-m and SPM-f, and the similarity between SPM-f and CPM on both the fractured faces. In all figures, X = 100,000.

Figures 1-5. Trophoblastic junctions. Figure 1 (top) shows tight junctions as maculae or fasciae occludentes (arrows) on the syncytial plasma membrane in contact with maternal blood. Figure 2 (2nd row, left) shows tight junctions as maculae occludentes (arrows) between the syncytium and the cytotrophoblast. Figure 3 (2nd row, right) shows tight junctions between adjacent endothelial cells of the fetal capillary. Figure 4 (3rd row) shows numerous gap junctions (arrows) between syncytium and cytotrophoblast: note their association with tight junctional strands. Figure 5 (bottom) shows a gap junction (arrow) between adjacent cells of the fetal capillary. E = E fractured face; P = P fractured face.

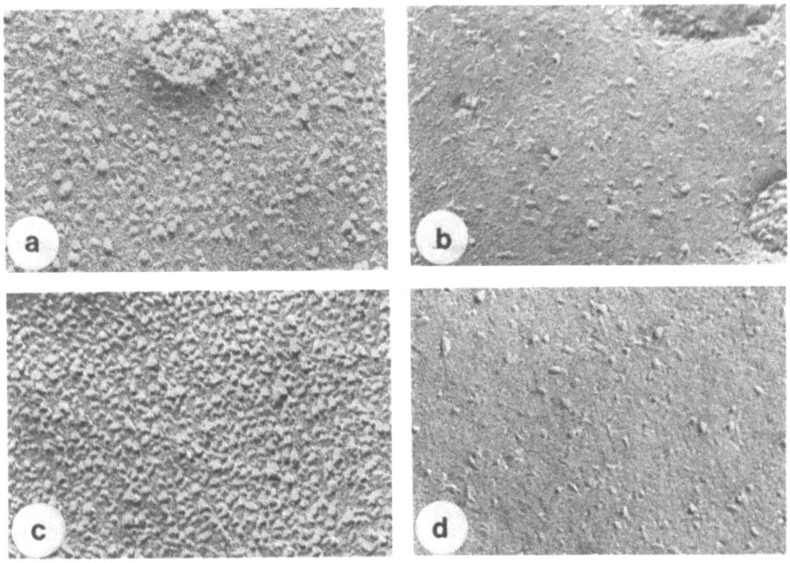

Figures 7 a-d. Density of intramembranous particles (IMPs) in term placenta. P faces are shown on the left side and E faces on the right. Figures a and b (top) show the syncytial plasma membrane in contact with the maternal blood (SPM-m). Figures c and d (bottom) show the syncytial plasma membrane in contact with the cytotrophoblast SMP-f. Note the different IMP density between the P fractured faces and the similarity between the E fractured faces.

In the fetal capillary, gap junctions were frequently observed between two adjacent endothelial cells (Figure 5).

IMPs were homogeneously distributed on all the trophoblastic plasma membranes. In the early placentae, a different IMP density was observed between the SMP-m and the SMP-f, either on the E or the P fractured faces, and a similar IMP density was observed between the SPM-f and the CPM (Figures 6a to 6f). IMP counting showed that the differences were statistically, highly significant ($p < 0.001$) (Table I). In the term placentae, a difference in IMP density was observed between the SPM-m and SPM- f only on the P fractured faces, while on the E fractured faces a similar density was found (Figures 7a to 7d). IMP counting also showed that the difference was statistically, highly significant ($p < 0.001$) (Table 2).

In the trophoblastic epithelium, openings of endocytotic vesicles in membrane faces were rarely seen: on the SPM-m, they were more frequently observed at the bases of microvilli (Figure 8), while on the SPM-f and on the CPM they were randomly distributed (Figure 9). Their aspects varied from very little hemispherical pits to caveolae. On the contrary, in the fetal capillary, the fractured faces of the endothelial cells showed numerous pinocytotic openings; different from the openings observed in the trophoblastic epithelium, they were uniform in size and diameter, and showed a characteristic flat floor (Figure 10).

DISCUSSION

In our results, SPM-m and SPM-f appear to be the most important plasma membranes involved in the nutritional transfer: in fact, we confirm that no subcompartimentalization is present between syncytium and cytotrophoblast (De Virgiliis et al., 1982), and we give evidence that the fetal capillary is a highly permeable structure. Thus, the SPM-f is the second and last membrane barrier in the way of the fetal capillary.

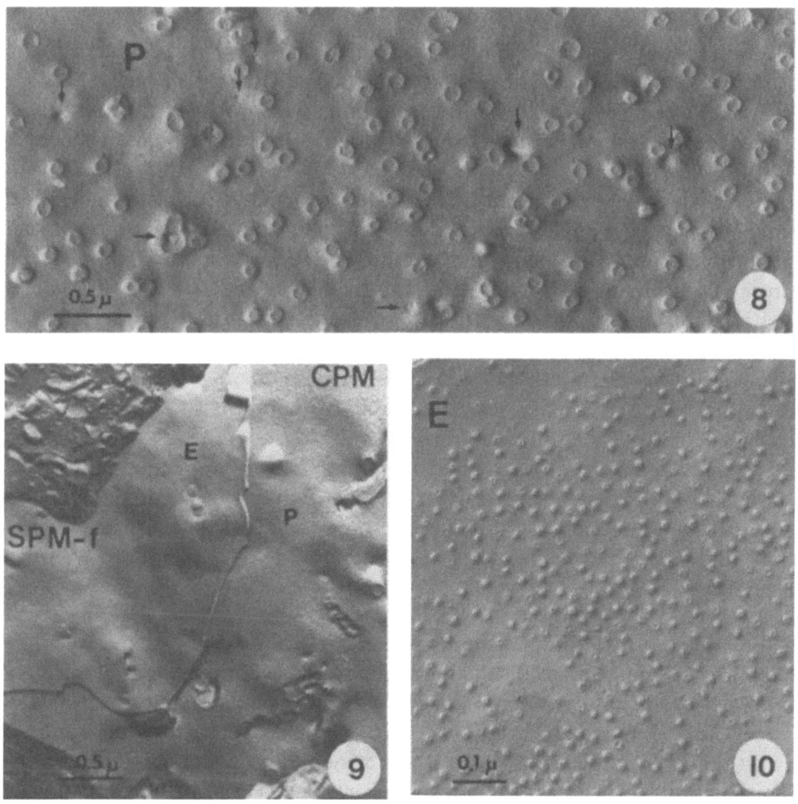

Figures 8-10. Endocytotic and pinocytotic vesicles in the trophoblast. Figure 8 shows openings of endocytotic vesicles varying from little hemispherical pits to caveolae (arrows) on the syncytial plasma membrane in contact with the maternal blood (SPM-m); the sectioned basis of microvilli are very evident. Figure 9 shows openings of endocytotic vesicles, as caveolae, on the syncytial plasma membrane in contact with the cytotrophoblast (SMP-f) and on the cytotrophoblastic plasma membrane (CPM). Figure 10 shows numerous pinocytotic openings uniform in size and diameter, and characterized by a flat floor.

The basis of these statements are the following: a) t.j. were observed between SMP-f and CPM as maculae or fasciae occludentes, while zonulae occludentes were never found; b) t.j. observed between the endothelial cells of the fetal capillary are similar to those described between the endothelial cells of regenerating rat liver (Yee and Revel, 1975). According to these observations, it is unlikely that these junctions play a role in preventing the passage of material between the endothelial cells, while it is possible that they represent regions of cell recognition and anchors for holding the cells together in a loose endothelial sheet. Consequently, t.j. of the fetal endothelium may allow the passage of substances directed to the fetus. The presence of IgG molecules in the interendothelial space of the fetal capillary, demonstrated by Lin (1980), adds further evidence to this hypothesis. However, we have to mention the possibility that the above described endothelial junctional pattern is a stage of a disassembling process induced by blood flow interruption occurring after the clamping of the umbilical cord.

Moreover, our results demonstrate that the two syncytial plasma membranes are not only the most important elements of the multilayered barrier, but also they have different composition. These differences could be observed on the two hemi-membranes (i.e., E and P fractured faces) obtained by the freeze fracture technique.

In fact, in the early placenta, IMP counting showed a different IMP density between SMP-m and SPM-f in both the hemi-membranes. This observation is in agreement with our previous cytochemical study demonstrating a different ruthenium red staining pattern between the SPM-m and the SPM-f (Sideri et al., 1982). Both, different IMP density and different ruthenium red staining pattern, support the idea that SPM-m and SPM-f perform two different levels of selection and, possibly, two different functional activities. In the term placentae, IMP counting showed a different IMP density between the SPM-m and the SPM-f on only one (the P fractured face) of the two hemi-membranes, so that an asymmetry of the two syncytial plasma membranes is realized. This asymmetry is of particular interest in the dynamics of the maternal-fetal transfer. In fact, it may represent the morphological basis of the asymmetric distribution of some nutrient substances between the maternal and the fetal compartment (Miller and Berndt, 1975; Whitsett and Brownscheidle, 1979).

The different IMP distribution between early and term placenta, suggests that a remodeling of the syncytial plasma membrane occurs during pregnancy. It is commonly believed that syncytium growth occurs by fusion of cytotrophoblastic cells with syncytium (Boyd and Hamilton, 1975). Our observations of a similar IMP density on the SPM-f and CPM, even if performed only in the early placenta, on one hand, confirms our previous cytochemical report (Sideri et al., 1982), and on the other, supports the opinion that SPM-f originates from CPM by fusion of other cytotrophoblastic cells in the synctium (Reale et al., 1980). Moreover it is suggested that the gap junctions which have been observed in this study may be related to the fusion process. This hypothesis is based on the following considerations: a) the presence of gap junctions has been demonstrated in an experimental model of membrane fusion (Fumagalli et al., 1981); b) gap junctions have been observed at the moment at which the cytotrophoblast fuses into the syncytium of the guinea pig placenta (Firth et al., 1979); c) in the human placenta gap junctions have been observed only between syncytium and cytotrophoblast (De Virgiliis et al., 1982), and also on few occasions, as demonstrated by the fact that they have not been reported in previous freeze fracture studies (Metz and Weihe, 1980; Reale et al., 1980). Thus their presence may be related to the modulation of the fusion process, or to the metabolic coupling occurring before fusion (Kalderon and Gilula, 1979).

The differences between the luminal maternal (SPM-m) and the basal fetal (SPM-f) side of the syncytium, demonstrated in this current work, strongly suggest that syncytium is a highly polarized cell. In fact, SPM-m and SPM-f are likely to represent the two plasma membrane domains characterizing any epithelial polar cell: the luminal and the baso-lateral respectively (Louvard, 1980). Consequently, placental syncytium and other polarized epithelia may be similar. The only difference is the series of lateral plasma membranes that are absent in the syncytium and present in the multicellular epithelia.

Thus, the presence of t.j. on the SPM-m may be related to the polarity of the syncytium. In fact, t.j. characterizing the polarized multicellular epithelia, generally appear as zonulae occludentes, having three functions (Meldolesi et al., 1978; Louvard, 1980): a) to prevent lateral diffusion of macromolecules between the luminal and lateral extracellular space; b) to prevent lateral diffusion of proteins from one surface domain of the membrane to the other; c) to be the site of insertion of apical membrane proteins. Functions a) and b), which require the integrity of zonulae occludentes, are excluded by the nature of the syncytium. Then, it is possible that t.j. observed as maculae on the SPM-m, mark limited areas of the membrane involved in the insertion of proteins (De Virgiliis et al., 1982). This suggestion, more easily than others (Metz et al., 1980; Reale et al., 1980), explains the presence of 'junctions' on a surface that is in contact only with the maternal blood.

Finally, the endocytotic processes observed by us at both sides of the syncytium, can be subjected to its polarity. They appear very different from the pinocytotic process occurring in the fetal capillaries, but further studies are necessary to evaluate the relevance of these phenomena in the placental transfer.

SUMMARY

The plasma membranes between mother and fetus were studied in early and term human placentae by the freeze fracture technique. Detailed information was obtained on tight junctions, gap junctions, intramembraneous particles (IMP), endocytotic and pinocytotic vesicles. The most important finding in this study is that the two syncytial plasma membranes, maternal (i.e., in contact with the maternal blood) and fetal (i.e., in contact with the cytotrophoblast or the trophoblastic basement membrane) respectively, had different intramembranous particle densities, thus demonstrating a different structure. The analysis of data obtained suggests that: a) the two syncytial plasma membranes are the most important membrane barriers involved in maternal-fetal transfer; b) the structural difference between the two syncytial plasma membranes is present both in early and late pregnancy, and in the course of gestation the maternal syncytial membrane undergoes some structural modification; c) the syncytium appears to be similar to other polarized epithelia, e.g., exocrine glands.

ACKNOWLEDGMENTS

The authors are very grateful to Dr. Dino Fesce for his skillful help in evaluating IMP counting data, to Drs. Maurizio Bini and Sergio Beolchi for their technical assistance, and to Dr. Mimi Younes for her linguistic assistance and advice.

REFERENCES

Boyd, J.D. and Hamilton, W.J. (1975) *The human placenta*, London: Macmillan.

Branton, D., Bullivant, S., Gilula, N.B., Karnovsky, M.J., Moor, H., Muhlethaler, K., Northcote, D.H., Packer, L., Satir, B., Satir, P., Speth, V., Staehelin, L.A., Steere, R., and Weinstein, R.S. (1975) Freeze etching nomenclature. *Science* 190, 54-56.

De Virgiliis, G., Sideri, M., Fumagalli, G. and Remotti, G. (1982) The junctional pattern of the human villous trophoblast. A freeze fracture study. *Gynecol. Obstet. Invest.* 14, 263-272.

Firth, A., Bauman, K. and Farr, A. (1979) Intercellular junctions in guinea pig development. *J. Anat.* 129, 862.

Fumagalli, G. Brigonzi, A., Tachikawa, T. and Clementi, F. (1981) Rat myoblast fusion: morphological study of membrane apposition, fusion and fission during controlled myogenesis in vitro. *J. Ultrastruct. Res.* 75, 112-125.

Kalderon, N. and Gilula, N.B. (1979) Membrane events involved in myoblast fusion. *J. Cell. Biol.* 81, 411-425.

Lin, Chin-Tarng (1980) Immunoelectron microscopic localization of immunoglobin G in human placenta. *J. Histochem. Cytochem.* 28, 339-346.

Loh, T.T., Higuchi, D.A., van Bockxmeer, F.M., Smith, C.H. and Brown, E.B. (1980) Transferrin receptors on the human placental microvillous membrane. *J. Clin. Invest.* 65, 1182-1191.

Louvard, D. (1980) Apical membrane amniopeptidase appears at site of cell-cell contact in cultured kidney epithelial cells. *Proc. Nat. Acad. Sci. USA* 77, 4132-4136.

Meldolesi, J., Castiglioni, G., Parma, R., Nassivera, N. and De Camilli, P. (1978) Ca^{++} dependent disassembly and reassembly of occluding junction in guinea pig pancreatic acinar cells. *J. Cell. Biol.* 79, 156-172.

Metz, J. , Weihe, E. and Heinrich, D. (1980) Intercellular junctions in the full term human placenta. I syncytiotrophoblast layer. *Anat. Emb.* 158, 41-50.

Metz, J. and Weihe, E. (1980) Intercellular junctions in the full term human placenta. *Anat. Embr.* 158, 167-178.

Miller, R.K. and Berndt, W.O. (1975) Mechanisms of transport across the placenta: An in vitro approach. *Life Sci.* 16, 7-30.

Moor, H. and Muhlethaler, K. (1963) Fine structure in frozen-etched yeast cells. *J. Cell Biol.* 17, 69- 628.

Reale, E, Wang, T., Zaccheo, D., Maganza, G. and Pescetto, G. (1980) Junctions on the maternal blood surface of the human placental syncytium. *Placenta* 1, 245-258.

Robertson, J.D. (1981) Membrane structure. *J. Cell. Biol.* 91, pt. 2, 189s-204s.

Ruzycki, S.M., Kelley, L.K. and Smith, C.H. (1978) Placental amino acids uptake. IV. Transport by microvillous membrane vesicles. *Amer. J. Physiol.* 234, C27-C35.

Sideri, M., de Virgiliis, G., Rainoldi, R. and Remotti, G. (1982) Peculiar Ruthenium Red staining pattern of the human early trophoblast. *Experientia* 38, 847-848.

Smith, C.H., Nelson, D.M., King, B.F., Donohue, T.M., Ruzycki, S.M. and Kelley, L.K. (1977) Characterization of microvillous membrane preparation from human tissue syncytiotrophoblast: A morphologic, biochemical, and physiologic study. *Amer. J. Obstet. Gynec.* 128, 190-196.

Yee, A.G. and Revel, J.P. (1975) Endothelial cell junctions. *J. Cell. Biol.* 6, 200-204.

Whitsett, J.A. and Brownscheidle, C.M. (1979) Aspects of placental structure and function in maternal diabetes. In *The Diabetic Pregnancy, a perinatal perspective* (Ed.) Merkatz, I.R. and Adam, P.A.J., pp. 123-143, New York: Grune and Stratton.

Whitsett, J.A. (1980) Specializations in plasma membranes of the human placenta. *J. Pediat.* 96, 600-604.

DISCUSSION

PANIGEL (Paris): In your freeze fractured preparation you have called certain structures in your replicas, intramembranous particles (IMP). What do you believe is the composition of these IMP particles?

SIDERI (Milan): IMPs are clearly associated with proteins and membranes. The number of IMPs is reduced in red cell membranes treated with proteases (*Brantonphil Trans. R. Soc. Lond. B. Biol. Sci.* 261, 133, 1971). Pure lipid bilaters do not normally contain IMPs by the addition of rhodopsin to bilayer vesicles causes the appearance of IMPs (Hong and Hubbel, *Proc. Natl. Acad. Sci. USA* 69, 2617-2621, 1972). However, it has been shown that in some biological systems (sarcoplasmic retriculum membranes), protease treatment does not effect the number of IMPs (Demer and Yamanaka, *Biophys. J.* 15, 110-111, 1975). Because of the known association for some IMPs with membrane proteins, there is a tendency to regard any IMP literally as a metal-plated protein molecule. This oversimplification is not correct because the exact nature of IMPs has not been resolved. Therefore, I have called the protein associated structures of the membrane.

Trophoblast Research 1: 27-36, 1983

HUMAN PLACENTAL AMINO ACID TRANSFER AND METABOLISM IN OXYGENATED AND ANOXIC CONDITIONS

Paul Penfold[1], Nicholas P. Illsley[1], Paul Purkiss[2] and Patricia Jennings[2]

Division of Perinatal Medicine[1] and Division of Inherited Metabolic Diseases [2]
Medical Research Council, Clinical Research Centre
Watford Road, Harrow, HA1 3UJ, Middlesex, U.K.

INTRODUCTION

The study of placental amino acid transport is an intimidating one, not only for the complexity of the transfer mechanisms (Christensen, 1981) but also because it is closely interlocked with placental amino acid metabolism. Reduction of this problem using non-metabolizable amino acids to investigate transfer has demonstrated the existence of active transport in the placenta (Dancis et al., 1968). On the other hand, the in vivo measurement of umbilical venous-arterial amino acid differences has shown the range and extent of transfer processes (Lemons et al., 1976). The use of non-metabolizable amino acids or of unphysiological levels of amino acids can be helpful in defining parameters such as individual amino acid binding constants or exchange rates. These conditions are, however, very different from those observed in vivo and may lead to distortions of transfer and metabolism by competition or inhibition (Eaton et al., 1982; Steel et al., 1982). In vivo measurements are circumscribed by the inability to define all of the possible metabolic and hormonal effects operating on the placenta which may regulate transport.

An in vitro placental perfusion model was utilized which has the advantages of simulating in vivo conditions and allows the use of the range of naturally occurring amino acids without the intervening effects of maternal and fetal metabolism. It is possible to investigate placental metabolic pathways in isolation, the peculiarities of which may then in turn be examined in a simplified and more detailed manner. Previous research in this laboratory demonstrated that the placenta was able to maintain a stable carbohydrate metabolism under anoxic conditions over a two hour perfusion period (Illsley et al., in press), suggesting that oxidative metabolism might not be necessary for the metabolic operation of the placenta. This investigation was conducted to see whether oxygen deprivation affected another important aspect of placenta function, amino acid transport. To assess the ability of the placenta to transfer amino acids, the preparation was initially perfused with identical levels of amino acids in both fetal and maternal circulations. A closed fetal circulation enabled the observation of cumulative changes over the course of the perfusion.

METHODS

The experimental technique used in this work was the in vitro dual perfusion of a placental lobule. Placentae were obtained from uncomplicated pregnancies (gestation 38-41 weeks) and perfused for a two hour period during which the perfusate flow through the umbilical capillary network was recirculated. The procedures for cannulation and clearance have been detailed elsewhere (Penfold et al., 1981; Illsley et al., in press). In all perfusions the closed fetal circulation was established using a circuit volume of 150 ml together with an open maternal circulation. At the start of the recirculation period, perfusate gas concentrations were adjusted to the required level. This was achieved by mixing 95 percent O_2/5 percent CO_2 with 95 percent N_2/5 percent CO_2 and monitoring the resultant pO_2 values using Clark-type oxygen electrodes (Rank Bros., Bottisham, Cambs) inserted into the maternal and fetal arterial and venous circulations close to the placental cannulation points. In the oxygenated experiments, maternal inflow pO_2 was maintained betwen 560 and 595 mm Hg, while the fetal inflow pO_2 was adjusted to a range of 25-50 mm Hg. In the anoxic perfusions, both circulations were gassed with 95 percent N_2/5 percent CO_2, producing an inflow pO_2 of less than 5mm Hg in both circuits.

The medium used for perfusion was a Krebs-Ringer phosphate/bicarbonate buffer containing 3 percent dextran (mol. wt. 70,000) and 0.1 percent bovine serum albumin. Twenty amino acids were added to the medium at concentrations equivalent to those measured in term maternal plasma (Table 1). These concentrations were based on findings reported by Lindblad and Baldesten (1967), Young and Prenton (1969), Cockburn et al. (1971), and Philipps et al. (1978). In all of the perfusions the medium used for fetal perfusion contained no glucose to enable the assessment of glucose transfer and accumulation. The maternal medium contained approximately 4.2 mM glucose. ^{14}-C Alanine was added to the fetal circulation of six oxygenated and three of the four anoxic perfusions (5 microcuries in 150 ml).

Throughout each experiment fetal inflow pressure was measured using a pressure transducer (Druck PDCR 10/DPI 201) located close to the fetal inflow cannulation point. Fetal arterial pressure ranged between 24 and 50 mm Hg over the experimental series with a maximum change of 7 mm Hg in any one perfusion. Oxygen electrode and pressure transducer measurements were sampled every second, using an analogue to digital converter (CIL Electronics: PCI 1001) and the data was located on an Apple II microcomputer for display. Every 30 seconds these data were stored on a floppy disk for later analysis.

Arterial and venous samples of fetal and maternal perfusates were taken at 30 minute intervals throughout the perfusion. Where samples were removed from the closed fetal circuit, the sample volume was replaced with fresh perfusate to maintain a constant volume. Perfusions in which the recirculating volume decreased were excluded from consideration here. After two hours of perfusion, the perfused lobule was excised, weighed and frozen in liquid nitrogen. Lobule weights were 28.6 $\pm$ 3.7 and 23.3 $\pm$ 3.9 g for the six oxygenated and four anoxic perfusions respectively. Maternal flow rates were 18.4 $\pm$ 0.6 and 20.0 $\pm$ 0.6 ml/min and fetal flow rates were 6.1 $\pm$ 0.1 and 6.4 $\pm$ 0.3 ml/min for the oxygenated and anoxic perfusions.

Frozen tissue was extracted by homogenization under 14 percent trichloroacetic acid and after washing, the precipitated fraction was solubilised (NCS

Table 1. Initial amino acid concentration in maternal and fetal perfusates.

Amino acid	Concentration	Amino acid	Concentration
Glutamine	300	Histidine	77
Alanine	287	Leucine	74
Threonine	135	Arginine	44
Proline	134	Isoleucine	42
Glycine	110	Phenylalanine	38
Valine	110	Tyrosine	31
Lysine	101	Tryptophan	25
Asparagine	100	Aspartate	21
Serine	94	Cysteine	17
Glutamate	90	Methionine	17

*Values expressed as μmoles per liter.

Tissue Solubiliser: Amersham) and samples were removed for liquid scintillation counting of ^{14}-C. Oxygenated and anoxic samples had comparable radiolabel quenching and so no quench correction was applied.

Samples for amino acid analysis were deproteinized with 5-sulphosalicyclic acid and norleucine was added as an internal standard. Samples were analyzed on an LKB 4400 Amino Acid Analyser as described in LKB Protein Chemistry Note PCN 12 (LKB Biochrom Ltd., Cambridge). Glutamine was measured according to the method of Lund (1974), and urea assays were conducted according to the method of Gutmann and Bergmeyer (1974). Statistical analysis was performed using one and two sample student-t-testing.

RESULTS

Oxygenated perfusions

The mean fetal amino acid concentrations measured in six oxygenated perfusions after two hours were compared to the initial perfusate concentrations (Figure 1). The final fetal perfusate contained a mean increase of 100 $\pm$ 11 μmoles of total amino acid compared to the initial, 66 percent of which was accounted for by six amino acids; asparagine, threonine, alanine, glycine, valine and lysine in order of their respective contributions. The inclusion of glutamine brings this total up to nearly 80 percent. Excluding ornithine, which was not present in the initial medium, the overall fetal to maternal ratio of amino acids at the end of the perfusion was 1.40, ranging from 0.7 for glutamate to 2.38 for aspargine.

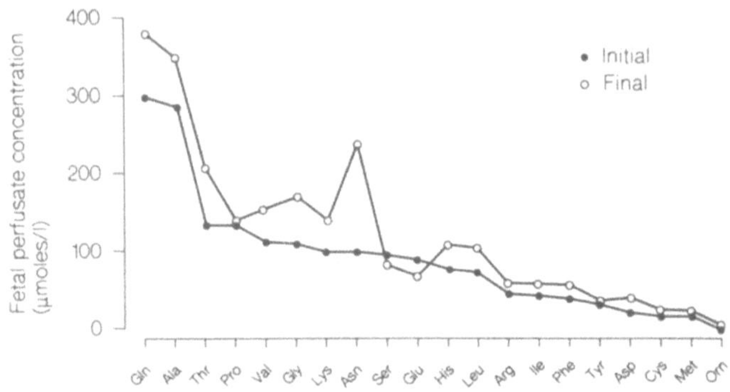

Figure 1. Fetal amino acid profile for oxygenated perfusions. Profile of the initial and mean final concentration of amino acids in the fetal samples from oxygenated perfusions. Values are taken from six experiments and are expressed as µmoles per liter. Final concentrations > initial concentrations ($P < 0.01$) except for arg ($P < 0.05$) and pro, ser and tyr (no significant difference). Final concentration of glu < initial ($P < 0.05$).

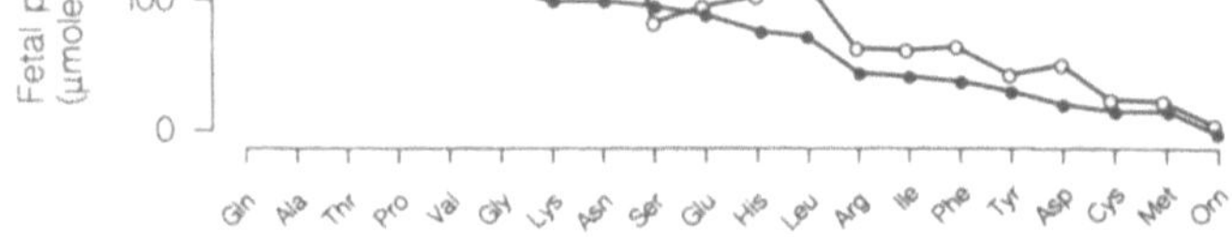

Figure 2. Fetal amino acid profile for anoxic perfusions. Profile of the initial and mean final concentration of amino acids in the anoxic fetal perfusates. Values are taken from four perfusions and expressed in µmoles per liter. Final concentrations > initial concentrations ($P < 0.05$) except for pro, ser, glu, his, arg and cys (no significant difference).

Apart from the alterations in the levels of glutamate and ornithine which will be examined in a later section, the behavior of three other amino acids, serine, proline and tyrosine was noticed to be anomalous. These amino acids showed no significant change over the course of the perfusion.

Anoxic perfusions

Four perfusions were conducted in a manner identical to that described for the oxygenated perfusions except that immediately prior to the initiation of fetal recirculation, gassing of both perfusate reservoirs was switched to 95 percent N_2/5 percent CO_2. The overall level of transfer was similar, the final fetal perfusate containing a mean of 102 ± 11 µmoles of total amino acid more than the initial. The pattern of transfer, illustrated in Figure 2, is similar to that seen for the oxygenated perfusions. The same six amino acids (asn, thr, ala, gly, lys, val) accounted for 75 percent of the change in total amino acid concentrations. As in the oxygenated perfusions, no significant change was observed in serine or proline concentrations. In addition, glutamate, histidine, arginine and cysteine showed no significant differences between initial and final fetal concentrations. The concentration of glutamine in the final anoxic perfusate decreased by 12 per cent compared to the initial concentration.

Oxygenated-anoxic differences

The percentage changes in the oxygenated and anoxic perfusions compared to the initial fetal amino acid concentrations are shown in Figure 3. Although thirteen out of twenty amino acids showed increased concentrations in the anoxic samples compared to the equivalent levels in the oxygenated samples, none of the differences between oxygenated or anoxic concentrations were significant.

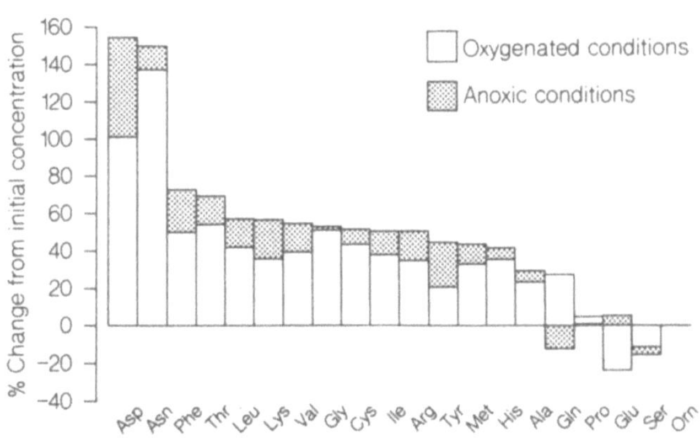

Figure 3. Oxygenated-anoxic differences. Percentage change in amino acid concentrations between initial and final fetal perfusates after six oxygenated (open) or four anoxic (hatched) perfusions. No significant differences were observed between oxygenated and anoxic perfusions.

Extraction of the frozen perfused tissue and separation of the acid soluble and acid insoluble fractions permitted measurement of the amount of ^{14}-C alanine label incorporated into protein. The level of incorporation was similar in oxygenated and anoxic tissue samples (4487 ± 426 cpm per g - oxygenated; 4380 ± 219 cpm per g - anoxic). This represents an incorporation of one per cent of the label originally added into the fetal circulation. It is impossible to quantitate the extent of protein synthesis from these data, since we cannot assess the contribution from maternal and endogenous amino acids. These data do, however, demonstrate that protein synthesis took place during the perfusions, and also that the oxygen deprivation in anoxic perfusions did not affect protein synthesis.

Urea production

Arterial and venous urea concentrations were measured in maternal and fetal samples from oxygenated perfusions at 30 minute intervals after the start of fetal recirculation. The initial perfusates contained 300 µmoles of glutamine per liter. Urea concentrations, flow rates and lobule weights (see Methods) were used to calculate the rate of urea production.

DISCUSSION

In studying placental amino acid transport and metabolism as an integrated unit, it is important to use the physiological range and concentrations of amino acids. The initial perfusate amino acid concentrations used were designed to simulate in vivo concentrations in maternal plasma. Cross-inhibition of transfer, that is, the competition between a number of amino acids for the same carrier, or trans-inhibition (Steel et al., 1982), the suppression of carrier uptake by high concentrations of amino acid substrate, probably operate in vivo as regulatory systems. Use of high concentrations of amino acids, such as those found in tissue culture media and commonly used for organ perfusion, would be likely to distort transfer and metabolic processes in the placenta. Initial amino acid concentrations were developed as an approximation of the levels found in term maternal plasma.

Maternal and fetal circulations both contained the same concentrations of amino acids prior to fetal recirculation. The pattern of increased concentrations of amino acids in the fetal circulation after two hours of oxygenated perfusion suggested the active transfer of amino acids from maternal to fetal circulations as observed by several other workers (Hill and Young, 1973; Philipps et al., 1978; Schneider et al., 1979a). The alternative to an active transport system would require that amino acids be transferred by a diffusion process (either simple or facilitated) from placental tissue into the fetal circulation. It is possible to estimate the concentration of amino acids contained in the perfused tissue using the previously determined figures for placental tissue amino acid content (Lemons, 1979). Even if all of the amino acids contained in the placental tissue were to be released into the fetal circulation, the increased concentrations would not correlate with the concentrations measured after perfusion. This evidence, combined with the specific nature of some of the changes discussed below, supports the suggestion of amino acid accumulation by active transport.

The profile of amino acid concentration increases measured in the oxygenated perfusions is difficult to reconcile with the limited data on human fetal amino acid requirements for tissue growth (Ziegler et al., 1976). A better comparison can be made with the umbilical venous-arterial differences in human fetal plasma amino acids. Hayashi et al. (1978) measured these differences in the cord blood of premature (29-36 weeks gestation) and mature (38-40 weeks gestation) infants. A parallel was found in the final concentrations in oxygenated perfusions and the umbilical venous-arterial differences observed in premature newborns. In both cases there was an increase in all the essential amino acids (lysine, leucine, valine, isoleucine, phenylalanine, histidine, threonine and methionine). There was also an increase observed for eight of the non-essential amino acids in both cases. In addition to a decrease in glutamate, Hayashi et al. (1978) found no increase in serine concentrations, findings that were echoed in our measurements and in earlier cord blood measurements by Prenton and Young (1969). There are a large number of similarities between the placental transport of amino acids in the in vitro perfusion and the venous-arterial uptake in vivo, but equally, there are several disparities such as the low uptake of asparagine or the high uptake of alanine measured in vivo.

One marker for human placental amino acid transport is the placental uptake of glutamate from the fetal circulation. This has been observed in sheep (Lemons et al., 1976), monkey (Stegnik et al., 1975) and human placentae (Schneider et al., 1979b) and is paralleled by the measurements here. The increase in cysteine in the oxygenated perfusions (52 per cent) was greater than the average amino acid concentration increase of 40 per cent, in contrast to previously published results showing a low level of transfer compared to other amino acids (Gaull et al., 1973). However, we found no increase in cysteine in the anoxic perfusions.

The concentration of amino acids measured after two hours of anoxic perfusion demonstrated that oxidative metabolism is not necessary for amino acid transport. This confirms the suggestion made by Longo et al. (1973) who observed the accumulation of α-aminoisobutyric acid by placental slices under anaerobic conditions. It also extends the hypothesis to the physiological range of metabolizable amino acids and their transfer in the intact organ. Previous research implied that oxidative metabolism was required for amino acid transport (Sybulski and Tremblay, 1967; Dancis et al., 1968). This work, however, was accomplished using metabolic poisons, such as 2,4-dinitrophenol, which may well have had effects beyond the inhibition of oxidative phosphorylation when used in cellular rather than mitochondrial fractions. Miller and Berndt (1974) demonstrated that α-aminoisobutyric acid uptake into placental tissue slices was supported by glucose in the presence of 2,4-dintrophenol or in a 100 per cent nitrogen atmosphere.

In another report we have shown that in the same series of experiments there is a 2-3 fold increase in glucose utilization under anoxic conditions (Illsley et al., 1983). It seems possible, therefore, that the amino acid transfer seen here in anoxic conditions is powered by anaerobic glycolysis. Our evidence suggests that as long as a substrate is available to satisfy the energy demands of amino acid transport, the actual method of energy production is not important. This is also true of protein synthesis since the levels of ^{14}-C alanine incorporation did not differ significantly between oxygenated and anoxic perfusions. Further work is required to establish the full extent and location of protein synthesis under these conditions.

The ability of the perfused placenta to transport amino acids from maternal to fetal circulations under anoxic conditions suggests that it is unlikely that chronic fetal hypoxia alone is a significant causative factor in problems of intrauterine growth retardation and other situations where a restricted substrate supply is suspected. The limited data on protein synthesis suggest also that placental growth would not be restricted by mild oxygen deprivation.

The rate of urea production observed in both oxygenated and anoxic perfusions was very high compared to measurements of fetal urea nitrogen excretion conducted previously by Gresham et al. (1972) for the human fetus. They estimate a fetal urea production of 2.5 µmoles/min/kg compared to the placental production observed here of 30-40 µmoles/min/kg. While deamination and oxidation of amino acids through the tricarboxylic acid cycle may have been a source of urea production, there are other possible sources which may have contributed, such as proteolysis and non-oxidative deamination. It is also conceivable that the enzyme arginase, which cleaves arginine to produce urea and ornithine, was operating at a higher rate than that observed in vivo. In the presence of a supply of arginine from both maternal and fetal circulations, the arginase could produce urea without the necessity for a metabolic nitrogen source. This would explain the presence of small amounts of ornithine found in the final fetal perfusates.

SUMMARY

1. An in vitro placental dual perfusion demonstrated the active transport of amino acids from maternal to fetal circulations. The use of a physiological range and concentrations of amino acids in placental transport experiments produced a transfer profile which paralleled the umbilical uptake profile of amino acids measured in cord blood.

2. Oxidative metabolism was not required for the placental transport of amino acids or for placental protein synthesis, as demonstrated by the continued transfer of amino acids and synthesis of protein under anoxic conditions. The energy demands of both functions were satisfied by anaerobic glycolysis.

ACKNOWLEDGMENTS

The authors gratefully acknowledge the efforts of the Northwick Park Hospital Delivery Suite staff, and especially Research Sister Mona Romney, in the work of this paper.

REFERENCES

Christensen, H.N. (1981) A biochemical point of view on placental transfer: Overview. *Placenta* Supple. 2, 195-200.

Cockburn, F., Blagden, A., Michie, E.A. and Forfar, J.O. (1971) The influence of pre-eclampsia and diabetes mellitus on plasma free amino acids in maternal, umbilical vein and infant blood. *J. Obstet. Gyna. Bri. Comwlth.* 78,215-231.

Dancis, J., Money, W.L., Springer, D. and Levitz, M. (1968) Transport of amino acids by placenta. *Amer. J. Obst. Gyn.* 101,820-829.

Eaton, B.M., Mann, G.E. and Yudilevich, D.L. (1982) Transport specificity for neutral and basic amino acids at maternal and fetal interfaces of the guinea pig placenta. *J. Physiol.* 328,245-258.

Gaull, G.E., Raiha, N.C.R., Sarikoski, S. and Sturman, J.A. (1973) Transfer of cysteine and methionine across the human placenta. *Pediat. Res.* 7,908-913.

Gresham, E.L., James, E.J., Raye, J.R., Battaglia, F.C., Makowski, E.L. and Meschia, G. (1972) Production and excretion of urea by the fetal lamb. *Pediat.* 50,372-379.

Gutmann, I. and Bergmeyer, H.U. (1974) Urea. In *Methods of Enzymatic Analysis* (ed.), Bergmeyer, H.U., pp. 1791-1794. New York: Academic Press.

Hayashi, S., Sanada, K., Sagawa, N., Yamada, N. and Kido, K. (1978) Umbilical vein-artery differences of plasma amino acids in the last trimester of human pregnancy. *Biol. Neonate*, 34,11-18.

Hill, P.M.M. and Young, M. (1973) Net placental transfer of free amino acids against varying concentrations. *J. Physiol. (London)*, 235,409-422.

Illsley, N.P., Aarnoudse, J.G., Penfold, P., Bardsley, S.E., Coade, S.B., Stacey, T.E. and Hytten, F.E. Mechanical and metabolic viability of an in vitro placental perfusion system. *Placenta* (in press).

Illsley, N.P., Penfold, P., Bardsley, S.E. and Tracey, B.M. (1983) The effects of anoxia on human placental metabolism and fetal substrate profiles investigated by an in vitro placental perfusion technique. *Trophoblast Res.* (this volume).

Lemons, J.A. (1979) Fetal-placental nitrogen metabolism. *Sem. Perinat.* 3,177-190.

Lemons, J.A., Adcock, W.E., Jones, M.D., Naughton, M.A., Meschia, G. and Battaglia, F.C. (1976) Umbilical uptake of amino acids in unstressed lambs. *J. Clin. Invest.* 58,1428-1434.

Lindblad, B.S. and Baldesten, A. (1967) The normal venous free amino acid levels of non-pregnant women and of mother and child during delivery. *Acta Pediat. Stockholm* 56,37-48.

Longo, L.D., Yuen, P. and Gusseck, D.J. (1973) Anaerobic glycogen dependent transport of amino acid by the placenta. *Nature* 243,409-411.

Lund, P. (1974) Glutamine. In *Methods of Enzymatic Analysis*. (ed.), Bergmeyer, H.U., New York: Academic Press pp. 1719-1722.

Miller, R.K., and Berndt, W.O. (1974) Characteristics of neutral amino acid accumulation by human term placental slices. *Amer. J. Physiol.* 227, 1236-1242.

Penfold, P., Drury, L., Simmonds, R.J. and Hytten, F.E. (1981) Studies of a single placental cotyledon in vitro: I. The preparation and its viability. *Placenta* 2,149-154.

Philipps, A.F., Holzman, I.R., Teng, C. and Battaglia, F.C. (1978) Tissue concentrations of free amino acids in term human placentas. *Amer. J. Obstet. Gyn.* 131, 881-87.

Prenton, M.A. and Young, M. (1969) Umbilical vein-artery and uterine aterio-venous plasma amino acid differences. *J. Obstet. Gyn. Brit. Comwlth.* 76,404- 411.
Schneider, H., Mohlen, K-H, Challier, J-C and Dancis, J. (1979a) Transfer of glutamic acid across the human placental perfused in vitro. *Brit. J. Obstet. Gyn.* 86,299-306.
Schneider, H., Mohlen, K-H. and Dancis, J. (1979b) Transfer of amino acids across the in vitro perfused human placenta. *Pediat. Res.* 13, 236-240.
Steel, R.B., Smith, C.H. and Kelley, L.K. (1982) Placental amino acid uptake. VI. Regulation by intracellular substrate. *Amer. J. Physiol.* 243,c46-c51.
Stegink, L.D., Pitkin, R.M., Reynolds, W.A., Filer, L.J., Boaz, D.P. and Brummel, M.C. (1975) Placental transfer of glutamate and its metabolites in the primate. *Amer. J. Obstet. Gyn.* 122,70-78.
Sybulski, S. and Tremblay, P.C. (1967) Uptake and incorporation into protein of radioactive glycine by human placentas in vitro. *Amer. J. Obstet. Gyn.* 97,1111-1118.
Young, M. and Prenton, M.A. (1969) Maternal and fetal amino acid concentrations during gestation and in retarded fetal growth. *J. Obstet. Gyn. Brit. Comwlth.* 76,33-334.
Ziegler, E.E., O'Donnell, A.M., Nelson, S.E. and Fomon, S.J. (1976) Body composition of the reference fetus. *Growth* 40,329-341.

Trophoblast Research 1:37-54, 1983

BIDIRECTIONAL TRANSFER OF α-AMINOISOBUTYRIC ACID BY THE PERFUSED HUMAN PLACENTAL LOBULE

Patrick J. Wier,[1,4] Richard K. Miller,[1,2,4,5] Debabrata Maulik,[1] and P. Anthony di Sant' Agnese[3]

Departments of Obstetrics and Gynecology,[1]
of Pharmacology,[2] and of Pathology,[3] , Division of Toxicology[4]
University of Rochester School of Medicine and Dentistry
Rochester, New York 14642, U.S.A.

INTRODUCTION

The role of the placenta in regulating the transport of amino acids to the conceptus is well established (reviewed by Miller et al.,1976; Young, 1981). There are two proposed mechanisms for the movement of amino acids across the placenta: active transport and passive diffusion.

For active transport several lines of evidence may be cited. First, concentrations of amino acids in fetal plasma are greater than in maternal plasma (Christensen and Streicher, 1948; Young and Prenton, 1969). Second, placental transfer of amino acids against this concentration gradient has been demonstrated in the intact pregnant animal (van Dijk and van Kreel, 1978; Hayter et al., 1964; Dancis et al., 1968), in the in situ perfused guinea-pig placenta (Hayter et al., 1964; Dancis et al., 1968; Hill and Young, 1973), and in the in vitro dually perfused placentae of man (Schneider et al., 1979) and the guinea-pig (van Dijk and van Kreel, 1978). Third, placental tissue slices and fragments actively concentrate amino acids against a concentration gradient (Dancis et al., 1968; Miller and Berndt, 1974; Schneider and Dancis, 1974; Enders et al., 1976). The active transport process for L-neutral amino acids is dependent on sodium, potassium, and the Mg^{++}-dependent, Na^+ and K^+ activated ATPase which is ouabain sensitive (Miller and Berndt, 1974).

Amino acids may also cross the placenta by passive diffusion. Schneider and coworkers (1972) showed that D-amino acids, which are not actively accumulated by the placenta, also cross the placenta; but their exchange rates are less than those of the L-isomer. Furthermore, an amino acid that has been accumulated by the guinea pig placenta appears to diffuse into both the fetal and maternal circulations in equal amounts (van Dijk and van Kreel, 1978).

These findings have led to the hypothesis (Hill and Young, 1973) that net transfer of amino acids from maternal to fetal compartments occurs against a concentration gradient. The placenta accumulates some amino acids by active transport predominantly from the maternal circulation to levels exceeding those of maternal and fetal plasma. Amino acids which have been accumulated by the placenta are believed to move by passive diffusion into the maternal and fetal circulations (van Dijk and van Kreel, 1978).

[5]To whom reprints should be addressed

Utilizing the methods of Schneider et al. (1972), perfused placental lobules have been maintained in viable condition for four to six h based on the integrity of the fetal vasculature, trophoblast metabolism, and ultrastructure. This model system was used to study the placental transport of the nonmetabolizable, neutral amino acid α-aminoisobutyric acid (AIB). AIB has been extensively used as a model substrate for amino acid transport by the placenta (Hayter et al., 1964; Dancis et al., 1968; Miller and Berndt, 1974; van Dijk and van Kreel, 1978). Enders and associates (1976) have demonstrated that AIB is transported by the human placenta by the same mechanism as for glycine, proline, alanine, serine, threonine, and glutamine known as the "A" transport system.

We have asked several questions in evaluating amino acid transfer by the perfused human placenta: 1) what transplacental gradient of AIB is established by the placenta, 2) to what degree does the human placenta accumulate AIB and what are the relative contributions of the maternal and fetal amino acid pools to the total AIB accumulated by the placenta, 3) what are the rates of placental accumulation from the maternal and fetal compartments and what are the rates of placental transfer to the maternal and fetal compartments, and finally 4) how does inhibition of the active accumulation of AIB with ouabain affect the placental transfer of this amino acid?

MATERIALS AND METHODS

Perfusion technique

The perfusion system is a modification of the isolated cotyledon perfusion method developed by Schneider et al. (1972). Term human placentae from uncomplicated pregnancies were obtained within ten minutes of delivery and examined for tears and gross lesions. A fetal artery and fetal vein on the surface of the chorionic plate serving a peripheral lobule (ca. 25 g) of the placenta were cannulated with 5 Fr. umbilical artery catheters (Sherwood Medical, St. Louis, Mo.) to establish the fetal circulation. Fetal perfusate (Krebs-Ringer's phosphate solution containing HCO_3^- (22.3 mEq/l), dextran 40 (30 g/l), glucose (1.5 g/l), Na^+ (136 mEq/l), K^+ (4.2 mEq/l), Ca^{++} (2.2 mEq/l), Mg^{++} (1.9 mEq/l), Cl^- (118 mEq/l), $SO_4^=$ (1.9 mEq/l), and heparin (25 units/ml)) was delivered through the arterial catheter at a flow rate of 3-5 ml/min by a peristaltic pump (model P3, Pharmacia, Piscataway, New Jersey). The perfused placental lobule was then secured in a plexiglass chamber as described by Schneider and associates (1972), and two catheters (5 Fr. umbilical artery catheters) representing the maternal spiral arteries were inserted into the decidual surface within the region of the fetal circulation. Maternal perfusate (a modified Krebs-Ringer's phosphate solution containing HCO_3^- (29.0 mEq/l), dextran 40 (7.5 g/l), and glucose (1.5 g/l), Na^+ (139 mEq/l), K^+ (4.2 mEq/l), Ca^{++} (2.2 mEq/l), Mg^{++} (1.9 mEq/l), Cl^- (114 mEq/l), $SO_4^=$ (1.9 mEq/l), and heparin (25 units/ml)) was pumped through the intervillous space at a flow rate of 12-15 ml/min by a Harvard Apparatus peristaltic pump. Both fetal and maternal perfusates were recirculated and gassed with 95percent O_2/5percent CO_2. The average oxygen tension in the maternal artery was 421 mm Hg (range: 350- 520 mm Hg) and 317 mm Hg (range: 214-425 mm Hg) in the fetal artery. Reservoirs in both circulations as well as the plexiglass chamber were maintained at 37°C with water baths.

The volume of perfusate in the fetal circulation (50-150 ml) was measured by a graduated scale on the fetal reservoir. Fetal arterial pressure was measured with a Grafco standard aneroid sphygmomanometer (Graham-Field, New Hyde Park, NY) Fetal perfusate flow was measured by a timed collection into a graduated syringe barrel attached to the fetal vein and was compared to the rate delivered by the pump. Flow of perfusate through the maternal circulation was measured in the same way.

The experimental conditions we considered for adequate perfusion were: (i) arterial inflow equals venous outflow in both fetal and maternal circulations, (ii) fetal arterial pressure <80 mm Hg, and (iii) maintenance of the volume of the fetal compartment with <10 ml/h volume loss.

The pH, oxygen and carbon dioxide tensions of perfusates were determined with an Instrumentation Laboratories Micro 13 pH/blood gas analyzer (Lexington, Mass.). Oxygen consumption by the tissue was calculated from arteriovenous difference in oxygen content (P_{O_2} in mm Hg), maternal perfusate flow-rate (Q in ml/min) and wet weight of the perfused region (W in kg):

$$O_2 \text{ consumption (ml/min}\cdot\text{kg)} = \frac{(P_{O_2} - 78.8) \times 0.0239}{P_B - P_{H_2O}} \times \frac{Q}{W}$$

The factor of 78.8 mm was the arteriovenous difference in oxygen tension when perfusate is circulated through the plexiglass chamber without a placenta. P_B = barometric pressure in millimeters of mercury, P_{H_2O} = water vapor pressure at 37°C in millimeters of mercury. The solubility coefficient of O_2 in milliliters of oxygen per milliliter of perfusate used was 0.0239 (Dixon, 1943). The fetal contribution (<0.5 ml/min·kg) to the oxygen consumption calculation was not included.

At the end of each experiment, the perfused area of the placenta was weighed and samples were collected for morphological evaluation and radiochemical analysis.

Measurements of ^{14}C and ^{3}H radioactivity

Perfusate samples were centrifuged at 1500xg for 10 minutes and 0.5 ml of the supernatants were mixed with 7 ml Liquiscint (National Diagnostics) radioactivity counting solution. Placental tissue samples (6-8) were blotted to remove extracellular water, weighed to the nearest 0.1 mg, and then dissolved in 0.2 ml NCS tissue solubilizer (Amersham). After neutralizing with 0.2 ml glacial acetic acid, the solubilized tissue was mixed with 10 ml Liquiscint. Radioactivity was measured with a Tracor Analytical liquid scintillation system (model 6881) with dpm quench correction.

Measurement of fetal capillary integrity

Two measurements were made to establish the integrity of the fetal capillaries: 1) volume loss from the fetal circulation and 2) inulin loss from the fetal circulation. The volume ($\pm$ 3 ml) in the fetal circulation was continuously monitored with a graduated scale on the fetal circulation reservoir. Inulin-[^{14}C] carboxylic acid (Amersham) plus unlabeled inulin were added to the fetal perfusate at a total concentration of (1×10^{-8}M; 0.007-0.02 µCi/ml). The volume change in the fetal compartment was compared to the ratio of ^{14}C-inulin (dpm/ml) in a maternal venous sample to ^{14}C-inulin (dpm/ml) in a simultaneous fetal venous sample.

α-Aminoisobutyric acid (AIB) transport studies

To study the bidirectional movement of AIB across the placenta, α-[methyl-^{3}H]-aminoisobutyric acid (New England Nuclear) plus unlabeled α-aminoisobutyric acid (Sigma Chemical) were added to the fetal circulation to a concentration of 0.761 to 1.166 mg/l (0.01-0.04 µCi/ml) and α-[1-^{14}C]-aminoisobutyric acid (New England Nuclear) plus unlabeled AIB were added to the maternal circulation to a concentration of 1.331 to 1.509 mg/l (0.01-0.02 µCi/ml). In four experiments ouabain (1.0×10^{-5}M) (Sigma Chemical, St. Louis, Mo.) was added to both maternal and fetal perfusates thirty to sixty minutes before AIB was added to the circulations.

Electron microscopy

Multiple small portions (<100 mg) of tissue were floated in Karnovsky's fixative (Karnovsky, 1965) and cut into approximately 1 mm^3 cubes. After washing in 0.1 M Sorensen's phosphate buffer (pH = 7.4), the tissue was fixed for 90 minutes at room temperature in 1percent osmium tetroxide in phosphate buffer (pH = 7.4). The tissue was then rinsed with two changes of buffer, dehydrated through a graded series of alcohols, infiltrated with Spurr epoxy resin (Spurr, 1969) and then placed in a Beem capsule for embedding. One micron sections were cut with a glass knife and stained with toluidine blue to identify the structures to be examined. The appropriate areas were cut into thin sections with a DuPont diamond knife, stained with lead citrate (Karnovsky, 1961) and uranyl acetate (Watson, 1958) and examined with a Hitachi HS-8 electron microscope.

RESULTS

Viability of the placenta during perfusion

Approximately 37percent (19/51) of the placentae available are not suitable for perfusion due to tears in the tissue or exsanguination of the blood vessels. Of fourteen perfusions maintained for 4.4 to 6.2 h under the experimental conditions given in the methods section, the average mass of the perfused lobule was 27.5 g (range: 15.1 to 45.2 g). The average fetal arterial systolic pressure increased from 33 ± 15 mm Hg to 47 ± 17 mm Hg (mean ± s.d.) during the perfusions. When ouabain was added to the maternal and fetal perfusates (1×10^{-5}M), the average fetal arterial systolic pressure increased from 32 ± 12 mm Hg to 64 ± 17 mm Hg (mean ± s.d.). The average fetal flow rate was 3.3 ± 0.1 ml/min, and the average maternal flow rate was 14.2 ± 0.2 ml/min (mean ± SEM).

The criterion for volume loss from the fetal compartment was established from the results of experiments (n = 6) in which ^{14}C- inulin was added to the fetal circulation only. The results from three such experiments are illustrated in Figure 1.

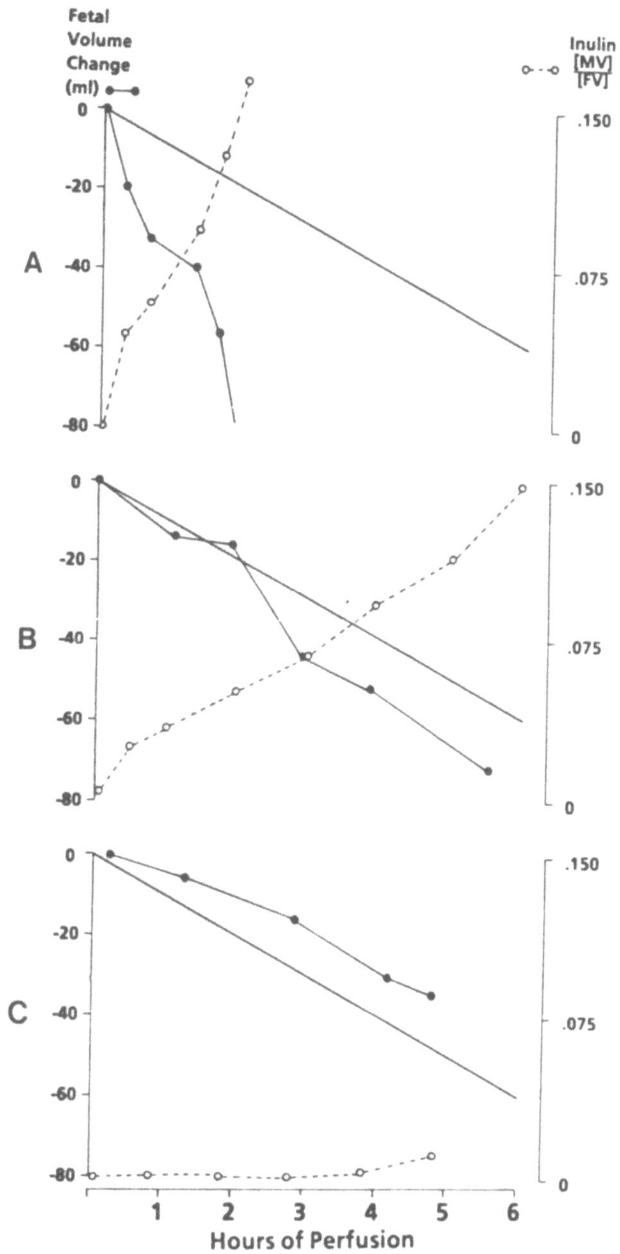

Figure 1. Volume loss from the fetal compartment and fetal to maternal movement of ^{14}C-inulin. The solid circles represent the volume in the fetal compartment; open circles indicate the ratio of inulin concentration in a maternal venous sample to a fetal venous sample simultaneously obtained. The oblique solid line is a volume loss of 10 ml/hour for reference. Each graph shows the results from a single experiment.

The experiment illustrated in panel A showed a rate of volume loss from the fetal compartment of 46 ml/h and inulin rapidly entered into the maternal compartment. Shown in panel B are the results from an experiment in which the fetal compartment lost volume at the rate of 16 ml/hour. Again there was a steady movement of inulin from the fetal to the maternal circulation. In panel C there was a volume loss of 7.4 ml/h and almost complete exclusion of inulin from the maternal compartment. Thus, fetal to maternal inulin movement was related to volume loss when volume loss exceeded 10 ml/h (panels A and B). Some volume loss may occur while fetal capillaries retain inulin (panel C). For 16 perfusions of greater than 4 h duration the average volume loss was 3.3 ± 2.4 ml/h (mean ± s.d.). The peak fetal arterial systolic pressure ranged from 24-76 mm Hg in these experiments, but volume loss was not directly related to fetal perfusion pressure over this range.

In seven experiments, the average rate of oxygen delivery by the maternal circulation was 12.03 ± 1.6 ml/min-kg and the average oxygen consumption was 3.64 ± 0.38 ml/min-kg (mean ± SEM). The average oxygen consumption measured at ca. 1.6 h perfusion was 3.35 ± 0.41 ml/min·kg and measured at ca. 4.4 h of perfusion was 3.99 ± 0.63 ml/min-kg (mean ± SEM). Thus oxygen consumption by the placenta did not decrease during 4 h in vitro.

The pH of the maternal compartment decreased by 0.046 ± 0.007 pH units/h (mean ± SEM) as a metabolic acidosis occurred. To compensate for this metabolic acidosis, 0.1 to 1.0 ml of 7.5 percent sodium bicarbonate was added to the maternal vein as necessary to maintain the pH at approximately 7.38. The pH of the fetal perfusate did not require adjustment during the perfusion.

As a further analysis of tissue viability in vitro, the perfused placenta was examined by electron microscopy. After five h of perfusion, the tissue showed no detectable degenerative changes; and the overall quality of preservation was excellent (Figure 2). The microvilli of the syncytiotrophoblast had characteristic finger-like projections into the maternal intervillous space, mitochondria of the cytotrophoblast cells were well-preserved with prominant cristae, and the ribosomes remained associated with the endoplasmic reticulum as polyribosome rosettes. Trophoblastic nuclei were intact and did not show degenerative changes such as chromatin clumping (not shown). Little vacuolization of the syncytiotrophoblast was observed. Fetal vessel endothelial cells and stromal fibroblasts were unchanged (not shown).

α-Aminoisobutyric acid (AIB) transport studies

The development of a transplacental gradient of AIB was studied in six experiments. The total AIB concentration in the maternal compartment decreased (Figure 3) due to placental accumulation of the amino acid and transfer to the fetal compartment (Figure 4). The total AIB level in the fetal compartment increased or remained approximately constant as its loss to the maternal compartment and loss to the tissue amino acid pool were balanced by AIB transferred from the maternal compartment (Figures 3 and 4). In each experiment a comparable concentration of ^{3}H-AIB was reached in the maternal compartment, but differences in the transplacental gradient of total AIB and the concentration of ^{14}C-AIB in the fetal perfusate varied in parallel.

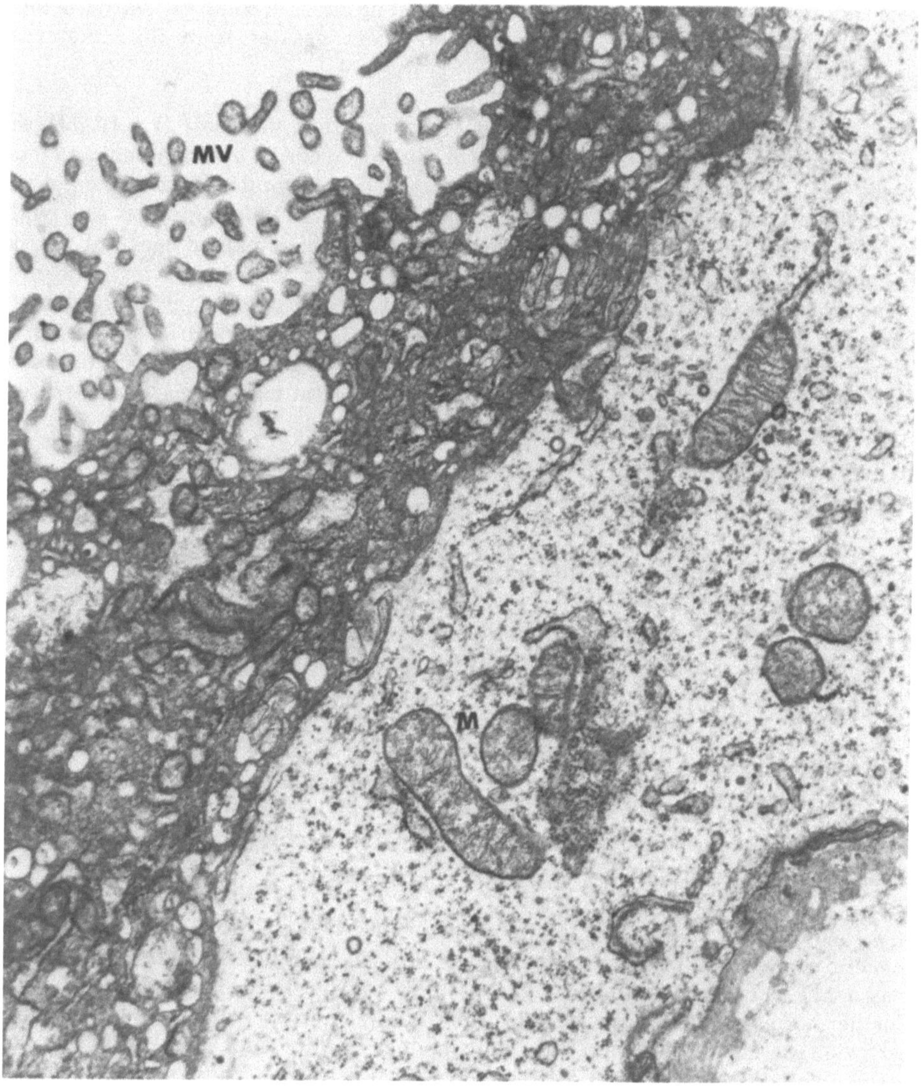

Figure 2. Electron micrograph of placenta after 5 hours of in vitro perfusion. Microvilli (MV) of syncytiotrophoblast and cytotrophoblast mitochondria (M) are well-preserved. (x30,600)

The placenta accumulated AIB against a concentration gradient in each experiment (Table 1). The average tissue AIB concentration was 2.49 ± 0.31 mg/kg of which 71 ± 3percent was ^{14}C-labeled (mean ± SEM). That most of the tissue AIB was accumulated from the maternal circulation is consistent with the decrease in AIB concentration in the maternal perfusate. The average ratio of placental to maternal total AIB concentrations was 2.79 ± 0.41, and the average ratio of placental to fetal total AIB concentrations was 2.28 ± 0.25 (mean ± SEM). The average result from these six experiments was a transplacental gradient of total AIB with the fetal concentration 1.21 ± 0.09 (mean ± SEM) times greater than the maternal concentration.

When ouabain was added to the maternal and fetal perfusate (1 x 10^{-5}M), the placenta accumulated less AIB, but some concentration of AIB over matenal and fetal levels was still evident (Table 1). The concentration of total AIB in the maternal compartment decreased from 1.24 ± 0.02 mg/l to 0.98 ± 0.11 mg/l (mean ± s.d.) while the concentration of total AIB in the fetal compartment remained constant (initial concentration = 0.95 ± 0.09 mg/l, final concentration = 0.96 ± 0.10 mg/l; mean ± s.d.). The concentration of ^{14}C-AIB in the fetal compartment, initially 0 mg/l, increased to 0.57 ± 0.17 mg/l; and the concentration of ^{3}H-AIB in the maternal compartment, also initally 0, increased to 0.15 ± 0.03 mg/l. Thus ouabain inhibited the active accumulation of AIB and the buildup of a fetal to maternal concentration gradient while bidirectional movement was still observed.

DISCUSSION

The utility of the human placental lobule perfusion technique for investigating amino acid transport was established by Schneider et al. (1979). We have further evaluated the viability of the placenta during extended (four to six hours) perfusions and applied the method to the study of AIB transport by the human placenta.

While based upon the methods of Schneider and coworkers (1972), our technique differs significantly from the original by our use of a lower flow rate (ca.3 ml/min) through the fetal vessels. In our experience fetal flow rates up to 10 ml/min can be achieved without producing arterial pressures > 60 mm Hg, but volume loss from the fetal compartment and an increasing arterial pressure are more likely to occur under that condition.

Volume losses from the fetal compartment greater than 15 ml/h occur when the fetal compartment fails to retain inulin. This rate of volume loss (0.25 ml/minute) may not be detected by simply comparing inflow and outflow rates of fetal perfusate. Furthermore, since an unacceptable volume loss may occur over the entire range of perfusion pressures (24-76 mm Hg) studied, integrity of the fetal vessels is not insured based upon this parameter alone. These observations point to the need for monitoring the total volume in the fetal compartment and establishing criteria which distinguish leaks from transcapillary movement of fluid down a hydrostatic or oncotic pressure gradient.

Challier and associates (1976) have shown that oxygen consumption by the placenta varies as a function of oxygen delivery. Because oxygen delivery may vary between experiments, the calculated oxygen consumption may best be used for comparison within each experiment. During perfusions of greater than four h in the current study, oxygen consumption did not decrease which suggests a relatively constant level of aerobic metabolism.

Table 1

Total AIB concentrations in placenta, maternal, and fetal compartments four hours after the addition of AIB.

	Perfusion Experiment (identification number)	Tissue AIB Concentration (mg/kg)	Maternal Plasma AIB Concentration (mg/l)	Fetal Plasma AIB Concentration (mg/l)	Tissue/Maternal ((mg/kg)/(mg/l))	Tissue/Fetal ((mg/kg)/(mg/l))	Fetal/Maternal ((mg/l)/(mg/l))
CONTROLS							
	30	2.67 ± 0.70[a]	1.08	1.07	2.47	2.50	0.99
	35	1.23 ± 0.19	1.06	1.10	1.16	1.12	1.04
	55	2.21 ± 0.56	0.83	0.96	2.66	2.30	1.16
	48	2.49 ± 0.40	0.91	1.03	2.73	2.41	1.13
	29	3.51 ± 0.91	0.89	1.21	3.94	2.90	1.36
	53	2.81 ± 0.37	0.74	1.16	3.80	2.42	1.57
	Mean (±SEM)	2.49 ± 0.31			2.79 ± 0.41	2.28 ± 0.25	1.21 ± 0.09
OUABAIN[b]							
	31	1.12 ± 0.02[a]	1.07	1.05	1.05	1.07	0.98
	59	0.90 ± 0.02	0.86	0.83	1.05	1.08	0.97
	65	1.32 ± 0.06	1.07	1.04	1.23	1.27	0.97
	69	1.16 ± 0.05	0.92	0.92	1.26	1.26	1.00
	Mean (±SEM)	1.13 ± 0.09[c]			1.15 ± 0.06[c]	1.17 ± 0.05[c]	0.98 ± 0.01[c]

a. Mean ± SD
b. Concentration of ouabain was 1.0 x 10^{-5} M.
c. Significantly different from controls at $P < 0.05$.

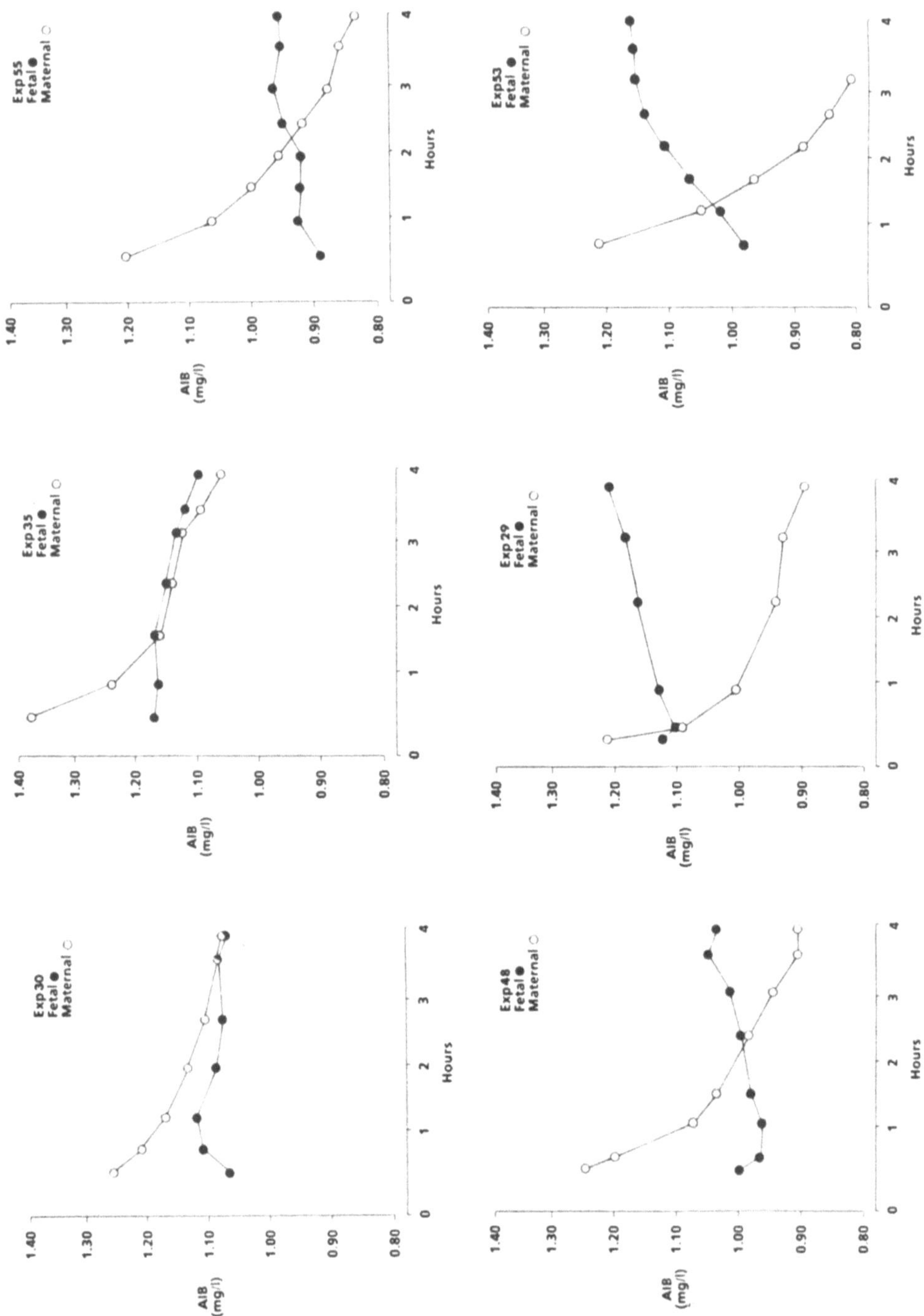
Exp 55
Fetal ●
Maternal ○
Exp 35
Fetal ●
Maternal ○
Exp 30
Fetal ●
Maternal ○
Exp 53
Fetal ●
Maternal ○
Exp 29
Fetal ●
Maternal ○
Exp 48
Fetal ●
Maternal ○
AIB (mg/l)
Hours
1.40
1.30
1.20
1.10
1.00
0.90
0.80
0
1
2
3
4

A small but consistent decrease in the pH of the maternal perfusate occurred due to a decrease in the concentration of bicarbonate. Since both perfusates were recirculated the accumulation of acidic metabolites may be the cause of the pH change. In fact, subsequent work in this laboratory has shown that the concentration of lactate in maternal perfusate increases from 0 to approximately 60 mgpercent during 4 h of perfusion (unpublished observations). Whatever the cause of the metabolic acidosis, acidic metabolites appear to be excreted into the maternal circulation preferentially as no metabolic acidosis occurred in the fetal compartment.

Ultrastructural examination of the perfused placenta provided strong evidence that neither tissue death nor significant injury occurred during these prolonged perfusions (Figure 5). Typical cellular reactions to injury (Hill and LaVia, 1980) such as dilatation of the endoplasmic reticulum, clumping of nuclear chromatin, or mitochondrial swelling were not observed. There was little syncytial vacuolization as has been reported to occur in other placental perfusions of shorter duration (Panigel, 1969 and Maulik et al.,1981).

Investigations of AIB transport across the guinea pig placenta have demonstrated a transplacental gradient of AIB in favor of the fetal circulation (Hayter et al., 1964; Dancis et al., 1968; van Dijk and van Kreel, 1978). The development of this concentration gradient has been associated with placental accumulation of the amino acid to levels exceeding the maternal or fetal concentrations. The present study demonstrates that the human placenta can establish a concentration gradient of AIB between the maternal and fetal circulations and that the placental tissue concentrates AIB to levels greater than those of either the maternal or fetal compartments (Table 1).

Perfused human placentae vary in their ability to accumulate AIB (Table 1). Differences between placentae in the degree to which they accumulate AIB have been observed by other investigators as well (Dancis et al. 1968, van Dijk and van Kreel 1978). Factors which may influence amino acid accumulation by the placenta include the intracellular concentration of amino acids, the concentration of transport carrier protein, and the energy supply for the transport system (Miller and Berndt, 1974; Smith and Depper, 1974; Guidotti et al., 1978).

By comparing the tissue AIB concentration at the end of the experiment (Table 1) to the change in total AIB concentration in the fetal compartment (Figure 3), a correlation between the two is apparent. These observations are consistent with the hypothesis of Oxender and Christensen (1959) which predicts for these experiments

---

Figure 3. Total AIB (^{3}H-AIB + ^{14}C-AIB) concentrations in fetal arterial (●) and maternal arterial (○) perfusate samples during in vitro perfusion in six different experiments. The concentration of total AIB in the maternal plasma was made larger than that in fetal plasma to compensate for the initially rapid accumulation of AIB by the tissue.

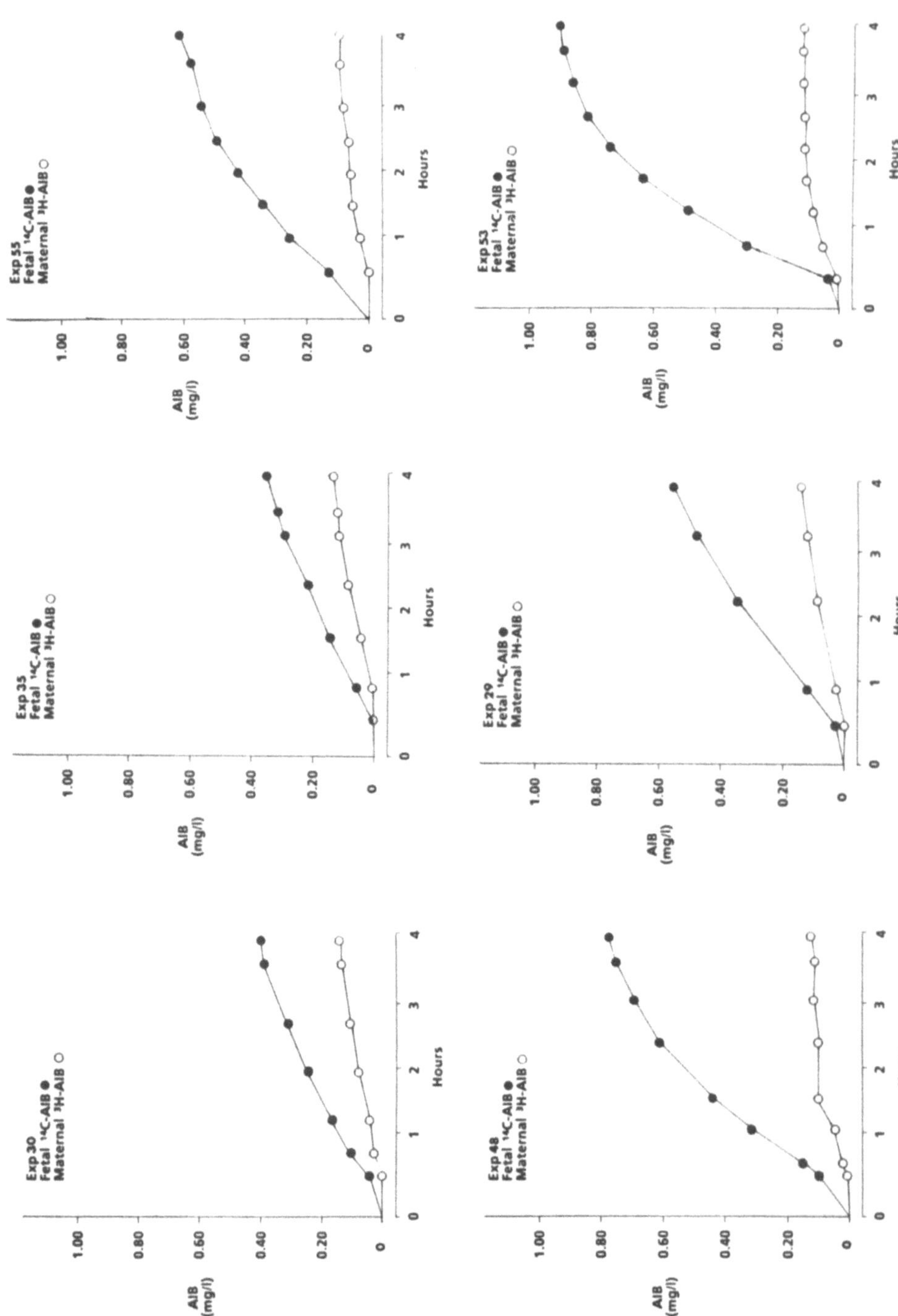
Exp 55
Fetal ¹⁴C-AIB ●
Maternal ³H-AIB ○
Exp 35
Fetal ¹⁴C-AIB ●
Maternal ³H-AIB ○
Exp 30
Fetal ¹⁴C-AIB ●
Maternal ³H-AIB ○
Exp 53
Fetal ¹⁴C-AIB ●
Maternal ³H-AIB ○
Exp 29
Fetal ¹⁴C-AIB ●
Maternal ³H-AIB ○
Exp 48
Fetal ¹⁴C-AIB ●
Maternal ³H-AIB ○
AIB (mg/l)
1.00
0.80
0.60
0.40
0.20
0
Hours
0
1
2
3
4

that the concentration increase in the fetal compartment is determined by the concentration in the placenta. That a perfect correlation between placental and fetal AIB concentrations was not observed may be due to differences in the degree to which the fetal circulation perfused the placental cells concentrating AIB. Unfortunately, in the current study there was no method to quantitatively measure the maternal to fetal perfusion overlap continuously. Nonetheless, the ratio of placental to fetal concentration of AIB was similar in five of six experiments (Table 1).

A number of studies have demonstrated that the movement of amino acids across the placenta is bidirectional (Dancis et al., 1968; Schneider et al., 1979). In particular Dancis et al. (1968) showed that AIB transfer does occur from fetus to mother in the guinea pig but at a rate slower than in the reverse direction. The bidirectional nature of AIB transport across the human placenta is illustrated in Figure 4. The concentration of ^{14}C-AIB transferred into the fetal compartment increases more than the concentration of ^{3}H-AIB transferred into the maternal compartment.

Placental accumulation of amino acid is believed to be dependent upon Na^+ and K^+-activated ATPase which is ouabain sensitive (Miller and Berndt, 1974). While ouabain does reduce placental amino acid accumulation, human placental tissue slices still accumulate AIB 1.4 fold over incubation media containing $1x10^{-5}M$ ouabain (Miller and Berndt, 1974), and ouabain at the same concentration reduces placental transfer of alanine by only 50 per cent in the guinea pig (Kihlström and Kihlström, 1981). In the current study ouabain ($1x10^{-5}M$) reduced AIB accumulation by the perfused human placenta, yet placental tissue still concentrated AIB to a small degree (Table 1). It thus appears that either this concentration of ouabain is insufficent to completely inhibit transport ATPase or possibly a transport ATPase independent mechanism for placental amino acid accumulation exists. Furthermore, the absence of a transplacental AIB concentration gradient reflects equivalent accumulation of AIB from the maternal and fetal circulations in the presence of $1x10^{-5}M$ ouabain (Table 1).

SUMMARY

The placenta plays an active role in the regulation of the amino acid concentration in fetal blood. This regulation is mediated by active accumulation of amino acid by the placenta to levels exceeding the maternal and fetal concentrations. In this study the bidirectional transport of α-aminoisobutyric acid (AIB) wasinvestigated in the dually perfused human placental lobule in vitro. The viability of the placenta during four to six h of perfusion was determined by hemodynamic

Figure 4. Concentrations of ^{14}C-AIB in fetal arterial perfusate (●) and of ^{3}H-AIB in maternal arterial perfusate (o) during six separate perfusions. Initially the maternal perfusate contained only ^{14}C-labeled AIB with unlabeled AIB (total concentration 1.3-1.5 mg/l) and the fetal perfusate contains only ^{3}H-labeled AIB with unlabeled AIB (total AIB was 0.8-1.1 mg/l). Thus the presence of ^{14}C-AIB in the fetal compartment and the presence of ^{3}H-AIB in the maternal compartment reflect bidirectional transfer of AIB by the placenta.

(fetal vasculature integrity), metabolic (oxygen consumption), and morphologic (ultrastructure) evaluations. After four h of perfusion, AIB was accumulated by the placenta to levels 2.8 fold greater than the maternal plasma and 2.3 times greater than the fetal plasma. Thus the concentration of AIB in the fetal circulation was 1.2 times that of the maternal concentration. Ouabain was shown to inhibit placental AIB accumulation and the development of a fetal to maternal concentration gradient. In the presence or absence of ouabain, some movement of AIB occurred from fetal to maternal compartments in addition to the transport from maternal to fetal compartments. The technique of human placental lobule perfusion appears useful for the study of placental transport over an extended period of time (4-6 hours) in vitro.

ACKNOWLEDGMENTS

Appreciation is expressed to Karen Jensen for the preparation of the electron micrographs, to Bradley Cole and Paul Krienberg for their technical assistance in the placental perfusions, and to the staff of the Labor and Delivery floor, especially Barbara Messura, for assistance in obtaining placentae. We acknowledge the loan of some perfusion equipment from SUNY, Buffalo, New York. This work was supported in part by NIH grants: ES 02774, ES 01247, and ES 01248.

REFERENCES

Challier, J.C., Schneider, H., and Dancis, J. (1976) In vitro perfusion of human placenta V. oxygen consumption. *Amer. J. Obstet. Gynecol.* 126,261-265.

Christensen, H.N. and Streicher, J.A. (1948) Association between rapid growth and elevated cell concentrations of amino acids. I. In foetal tissues. *J. Biol. Chem.*.175,95-100.

Dancis, J. Money, W.L., Springer, D., Levitz, M. (1968) Transport of amino acid by placenta. *Amer. J. Obstet. and Gynecol.* 101,820-829.

Dixon, M., (1943) *Manometric Methods*, ed. 2, Cambridge University Press, Cambridge, England.

Enders, R.H., Judd, R.M., Donohue, T.M., and Smith, C.H. (1976) Placental amino acid uptake. III. Transport systems for neutral amino acids. *Amer. J. Physiol.* 230,706-710.

Guidotti, G.G., Borghetti, A.F. and Gazzola, G.C. (1978) The regulation of amino acid tranport in animal cells. *Biochim. Biophys. Acta* 515,329-366.

Hayter, C.J., E.A. Hutchinson, M.J. Karvonen, and Young, M. (1964) Placental transport of a-aminoisobutyric acid in the unanesthetized guinea-pig (Abstract). *J. Physiol.*, London 175,11P-13P.

Hill, P.M.M. and Young, M. (1973) Net placental transfer of free amino acids against varying concentrations. *J. Physiol.* 235,409- 422.

Hill, R.B. and LaVia, M.F (1980) *Principles of Pathobiology*, ed. 3, Oxford University Press, New York.

Karnovsky, M.J. (1965) A formaldehyde-glutaraldhyde fixative of high Osmolarity for use in electron microscopy. *J. Cell Biol.* 27,137A.

Karnovsky, M.J. (1961) Simple methods for "staining with lead" at high pH in electron microscopy. *J. Biophys. Biochem. Cytol.* 11,729-732.

Kihlström, I. and Kihlström, J.E. (1981) An improved technique for perfusion of the guinea pig placenta in situ giving viable conditions demonstrated by placental transport of amino acids (L- and D-alanine). *Biol. Neonate* 39,150-159.

Maulik, D., Contrator, S.F., Lippes, J. and Knight, A. (1981) Extracorporeal perfusion of the whole human placenta-a new model. Placenta Suppl. 3, 353-366.

Miller, R.K. and Berndt, W.O. (1974) Characterization of neutral amino acid accumulation by human term placental slices. *Amer. J. Physiol.* 227,1236-1242.

Miller, R.K., Koszalka, T.R., and Brent, R.L. (1976) The transport of molecules across the placental membranes. In *The Cell Surface in Animal Embryogenesis and Development.* (ed.), G. Poste and G.L. Nicholson, Amsterdam: Elsevier-North Holland Biomedical Press, pp. 145-223.

Oxender, D.J., and Christensen, H.N. (1959) Transcellular concentration as a consequence of intracellular accumulation. *J. Biol. Chem.* 234,2321-2324.

Panigel, M. (1969) Comparative anatomical, physiological, and pharmacological aspects of placenta permeability and haemodynamics in the non-human primate placenta and in the isolated perfused human placenta. In *The Fetal Unit,* International Congress Series, No. 183, (ed.), Pecile A. Finzi, p. 279., Amsterdam: Excerpta Medica Foundation.

Schneider, H., Panigel, M., and Dancis, J. (1972) Transfer across the perfused human placenta of antipyrine, sodium, and leucine. *Amer. J. Obstet. Gynecol.* 114,822-828.

Schneider, H., Mohlen, K.H., and Dancis, J. (1979) Transfer of amino acids across the in vitro perfused human placenta. *Pediat. Res.* 13,236-240.

Schneider, H. and Dancis, J. (1974) Amino acid transport in human placental slices. *Amer. J. Obstet. Gynecol.* 120,1092-1098.

Smith, C.H. and Depper, R. (1974) Placental amino acid uptake. II. Tissue preincubation, fluid distribution, and mechanisms of regulation. *Pediatr. Res.* 8,697-703.

Spurr, A.R., (1969) A low-viscosity epoxy resin embedding medium for electron microscopy. *J. Ultrastruc. Res.* 26,31-43.

van Dijk, J.P. and van Kreel, B.K. (1978) Transport and accumulation of a-aminoisobutyric acid (AIB) in the guinea pig placenta. *Pflügers Archiv.* 377,217-224.

Watson, M.L. (1958) Staining of tissue sections for electron microscopy with heavy metals. *J. Biophys. Biochem. Cytol.* 4,475- 478.

Young, M. and Prenton, M.A. (1969) Maternal and fetal plasma amino acid concentrations during gestation and in retarded fetal growth. *J. Obstet. Gynaecol. Br. Commonw.* 76,333-344.

Young, M. (1981) Placental amino acid transfer and metabolism. Placenta Suppl. 2,177-184.

DISCUSSION

GENBACEV (Zemun): In your distribution studies with ^{14}C-leucine, it appears that the leucine is accumulated by the placenta. What were the levels in the fetal circulation? I would be interested to know how much is transferred and how much is accumulated and incorporated into protein. In our in vitro techniques with tissue slices results appear to be in close agreement with the observations you have made. The percentage of free leucine remaining in our tissue preparation is approximately 15percent, which I believe is similar to your observations after 4 h of perfusion.

WIER (Rochester): In the ^{14}C-leucine studies, we attempted to measure the biosynthetic capability of the placenta during perfusion. The leucine was present in both the fetal and maternal perfusates ($2x10^{-11}$). The incorporation of ^{14}C-leucine into trichloroacetic acid precipitable proteins in the perfused tissue was determined in two experiments. While these results are only preliminary, the use of this amino acid to measure a relative rate of protein synthesis is encouraged because a high percentage (>90percent) of the amino acid was incorporated into placental proteins after four h of perfusion. One problem we have encountered with this protocol is that the placenta accumulates so much amino acid that the concentration gradient between fetal and maternal compartments is between 1.4 and 1.5 within 2 to 3 hours, but decreases thereafter due to continued utilization of ^{14}C-leucine by the placenta.

KELMAN (Richland): Do you clear the maternal and fetal spaces before you begin your recirculation? In one of your figures, it appears that the perfusate has a red color.

WIER (Rochester): The perfusate is a Krebs-Ringer Phosphate Bicarbonate supplemented with glucose and dextran. There is always a small number of red blood cells remaining in the placenta at the start of each experiment. Even when you superficially wash the surface of the placenta with the KRP and do begin the actual perfusion, there is an additional washout of red blood cells from the maternal space. That is why we use a blood filter in our system and do not return the first 20 ml of fetal perfusate to the recirculating system. We have found that this improves our perfusion system perhaps by eliminating damaged red blood cells and vasoreactive substances.

KELMAN (Richland): Have you looked at the composition of your media at the end of your experiments? For example, have you determined the amount of hemoglobin in your perfusion system either on the maternal or the fetal side? Does it look like there is hemoglobin there?

WIER (Rochester): Even though we may have a small amount of red blood cells retained in the maternal perfusate, the perfusate sample after centrifugation is perfectly clear. We have not measured the amount of hemoglobin present.

KELMAN (Richland): Do you believe you could obtain better kinetics if you used a single pass flow on the fetal side and on the maternal side, depending upon which direction you want to examine?

WIER (Rochester): One problem with measuring transport in a recirculating system for both the maternal and fetal circulations is that the placental accumulation of the substrate can interfere with the concentration gradients established since there is a limited amount of substrate available. We are currently not supplementing the perfusates to maintain a constant level of substrate. With a single pass system for the maternal circulation, it is possible to maintain a high level of substrate delivery, and the concentration gradient developed toward the fetal compartment would be maintained without sacrificing that substrate to meet placental demand. Yet the objective developed for this study was to determine the feasibility of prolonged experiments and to document the capability of normal function. We believe that within the first 1.5 to 2 h in this perfusion system you are looking at a stabilization period. Perhaps opening the circuits at 2 h and performing this type of analysis would simulate the conditions you inquired about.

KELMAN (Richland): At 3 hours, in one of your perfusions, you had a reversal of the AIB levels. Do you think this is degeneration of the preparation or it is saturation of a carrier system?

WIER (Rochester): All of the other criteria for monitoring the viability of all six of these preparations are maintained when we observed this decrease. Therefore, if it is a degenerative change, we cannot document that other than by the change that we are looking at in AIB transport. It is possible that we are exceeding the transport maximum of 1×10^{-5} M. We do have some preliminary data where AIB is present in 10^{-8} M to investigate this possibility. As Dr. Cedard discussed earlier, this is a dynamic system with transfer occuring in both directions. These decreases may also be related to the placental demands of the system.

CAREY (Storrs): Do you believe this perfusion system is applicable for the measurement of protein transport?

WIER (Rochester): We have not performed studies in this area; however, Professor Dancis has reported data relating to the transport of proteins and amino acids. We do hope to study the movement of Vitamin B_{12} and transcobalamin II-Vitamin B_{12}. We do know that there are specific binding sites for the transcobalamin II-Vitamin B_{12}. Thus, besides, IgG, transcobalamin II-Vitamin B_{12} may be transferred via receptor mediated endocytotic processes.

BEER (Ann Arbor): We have learned a substantial amount about tissue graft rejection by analyzing lymphocytes which actually can be washed away from an organ. This has been quite helpful in the study of perfused kidneys. Have you or your colleagues examined the profile of lymphocytes that do appear in the perfusate and have you analyzed for the immunoreactivity?

WIER (Rochester): No, we have not examined such issues; however, it does appear that it is feasible to undertake.

ILLSLEY (Harrow): How do you follow the flow-limited clearance of your preparation, e.g., antipyrine, during the course of your studies?

WIER (Rochester): We have not used antipyrine in this system since it would allow for only one evaluation. To measure antipyrine clearance, you must have an open circuit. Otherwise, the buildup of this material could lead to errors in evaluation. We have examined urea in our system. In recent experiments, we have modified our fetal perfusate and now can measure oxygen transport across the placenta. We believe this can be a much better index of perfusion overlap and a measure of flow-limited clearance.

VAN DIJK (Rotterdam): In experiments using the isolated and perfused guinea pig placenta, we have measured the transfer and uptake of AIB (Pflügers Archiv 337:217-224, 1978). In our experiments with tracer labeled amounts of AIB, the fetal levels of AIB exceed the maternal levels within 60 minutes. Thus, during the first 40 to 60 minutes of the perfusion, it appears that a placental compartment is being filled to a concentration of 20 fold higher than the maternal levels. After that point, it is apparent that the AIB is actively transported from mother to fetus. It appears that you are also observing this same phenomenon in the human placenta.

WIER (Rochester): We certainly agree with your observation and as noted in the article, we have compensated for this placental compartment filling by having the maternal levels of AIB begin at 1.4 mg/l and the concentration in the fetal compartment at 1.25 mg/l. Within the first thirty minutes of perfusion, these levels will become approximately 1 mg/l. Thus, there is a large extraction of AIB from both circulations in filling the placental compartment.

Trophoblast Research 1:55-70, 1983

THE EFFECTS OF ANOXIA ON HUMAN PLACENTAL METABOLISM AND FETAL SUBSTRATE PROFILES INVESTIGATED BY AN IN VITRO PLACENTAL PERFUSION TECHNIQUE

Nicholas P. Illsley,[1,3] Paul Penfold,[1] Sara E. Bardsley[1]
Beryl M. Tracey[2], and J.G. Aarnoudse[4]

Division of Perinatal Medicine[1] and Division of Inherited Metabolic Diseases[2], Medical Research Council, Clinical Research Centre, Watford Road, Harrow, HA1 3UJ, Middlesex, U.K.

INTRODUCTION

Placental metabolism has effects beyond the preservation of the materno-fetal exchange and supply functions. As a highly active metabolic unit (Sparks, 1979) the position of the placenta at an early point in the fetal supply line has consequences for the range and types of energy and growth-sustaining substrates utilized by the fetus. Thus, factors which alter placental metabolism may have major effects on the substrate profile available to the fetus.

The extreme form of oxygen deprivation, that is, anoxia, has been used in this study to examine not only the reaction of placental metabolism but also the effects on the types of metabolite released or transferred into the fetal circulation. While the anoxic situation is not one that occurs physiologically, it is helpful in determining the direction and types of changes that should be monitored in the case of less extreme degrees of hypoxia observed clinically.

The in vitro perfusion technique enables us to study the effects of anoxia on carbohydrate metabolism without the intervening effects of fetal or maternal metabolism or hormonal feedback. In a previous report we demonstrated the viability of this preparation, but suggested that anoxia might be deleterious to placental function (Illsley et al., in press). This study assesses the effects of anoxia on placental metabolism, energy production and metabolite profiles.

METHODS

Placentae were obtained from uncomplicated term pregnancies (gestation 38-41 weeks) and utilized immediately after delivery. The methods of cannulation, perfusion and the perfusion system have been described elsewhere (Penfold et al., 1981; Illsley et al., in press). An open maternal circulation was used and the fetal circulation was initiated using an open circuit. The fetal circuit was converted to a closed circuit (containing 150 ml) after the switch was made to the appropriate level of

3. To whom reprints should be addressed

4. Department of Obstetrics, University Hospital, Groningen, The Netherlands.

oxygenation of the fetal medium. In the oxygenated perfusions the maternal circulation was gassed with 95 percent O_2, 5 percent CO_2, and the fetal circulation with a mixture of 95 percent O_2, 5 percent CO_2 and 95 percent N_2, 5 percent CO_2 to achieve a fetal arterial pO_2 of 25-50 mm Hg. In the anoxic perfusions both circulations were gassed with 95 percent N_2, 5 percent CO_2.

The perfusion medium was a Krebs-Ringer phosphate/bicarbonate buffer containing 30 g/l of dextran (molecular weight approximately 70,000) and 0.1 percent bovine serum albumin. Maternal medium contained 4.25 mM (oxygenated) or 4.09 mM (anoxic) glucose. The fetal medium did not contain glucose to enable assessment of the transfer to, and accumulation, of glucose in the fetal circuit. Fetal perfusate pH was maintained between 7.35 and 7.42 by the bicarbonate buffering system. The medium also contained a range of 20 amino acids including glutamine. The amino acid concentrations in the medium were similar to those found in maternal plasma at term (Penfold et al., 1983). Both maternal and fetal circulations initially contained the same range and concentrations of amino acids.

Perfusate pO_2 values were continuously monitored using Clark-type oxygen electrodes (Rank Bros., Bottisham, Cambs) placed in maternal and fetal circuits close to arterial and venous cannulation points. These electrodes had a volume of 4 ml, and the perfusate in the electrodes was continually stirred by magnetic stirrers. Fetal arterial pressure was measured by a pressure transducer (Druck DPI 201 pressure indicator and PDCR 10 transducer) located close to the fetal arterial cannulation point. Fetal arterial pressures ranged between 24 and 50 mm Hg over the series of experiments with the maximum change in any one experiment being 7 mm Hg. Signals from the oxygen electrodes and pressure transducer were fed through an analogue to digital converter and displayed using an Apple II Plus microcomputer. The signals were sampled every 30 seconds and stored for later analysis on a floppy disk system interfaced to the computer.

Fetal and maternal perfusate samples were taken from arterial and venous circulations at the start of fetal recirculation and every 30 minutes thereafter. Samples removed from the fetal circulation were replaced by an equal volume of fetal medium to maintain a constant fetal volume. Samples were centrifuged immediately after removal and frozen for later analysis. At the end of the perfusion, tissue samples from the perfused lobule were frozen in liquid nitrogen for metabolite analysis.

Glucose and lactate were assayed on a Technicon Auto Analyser II using standard glucose oxidase and lactate dehydrogenase methods. After extraction of the frozen tissue into trichloroacetic acid, glycolytic intermediates and ribose-5-phosphate were assayed using the methods described by Lang and Michal (1974), Michal and Beutler (1974), and Racker (1974). Organic acids were analysed in perfusate samples taken at the end of the perfusion. The extraction, derivatisation and chromatographic procedures used were those devised by Chalmers and Watts (1972), and Tracey et al. (in press).

Statistical significance was calculated using one sample or two sample-t-tests.

RESULTS

Glucose metabolism

Maternal and fetal arterial and venous samples taken at 30 min intervals over the course of the perfusions were assayed for glucose. Maternal arterial glucose concentrations were 4.25 ± 0.12 and 4.09 ± 0.11 mM, for the oxygenated and anoxic perfusions respectively. The time course of the maternal venous and fetal arterial glucose concentrations are plotted in Figure 1, and demonstrate the stable nature of placental glucose uptake from the maternal circulation and the equilibration of fetal circuit glucose concentrations with the constant maternal arterial level. Uptake is defined as the rate of removal of glucose from the maternal circulation calculated from the maternal arteriovenous difference, standardized per unit time and tissue weight.

Rates of placental glucose uptake, maternal to fetal transfer and utilization were calculated by the Fick principle. Maternal flow rates of 18.4 ± 0.6 and 20.0 ± 0.6 ml/min, fetal flow rates of 6.1 ± 0.1 and 6.4 ± 0.3 ml/min and lobule weights of 28.6 ± 3.7 and 23.3 ± 3.9 g were used for the oxygenated and anoxic perfusions respectively (Table 1).

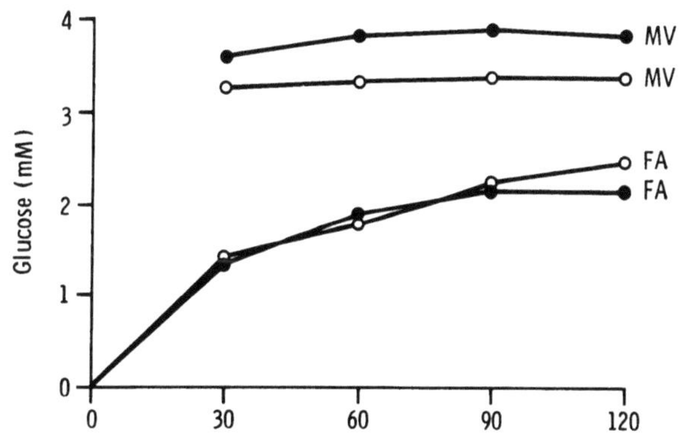

Figure 1. Fetal uptake of glucose from the maternal circulation under oxygenated and anoxic conditions. Changes in the fetal arterial (FA) and maternal venous (MV) concentrations of glucose under oxygenated (●) and anoxic (○) conditions. Values are means of 6 (oxygenated) or 4 (anoxic) perfusions. NB. Open maternal circulation and recirculating fetal circuit.

Table 1. Glucose distribution in oxygenated and anoxic perfusions with time.

Perfusion type	Time*	Uptake µmol/min/kg**	Transfer µmol/min/kg**	Consumption µmol/min/kg**
Oxygenated	30	416±66	118±37	299±56
	60	272±62	30 ±15	242±59
	90	262±52	41 ±21	221±35
	120	282±83	31 ±30	251±56
Anoxic	30	764±81	77 ±15	687±95
	60	670±21	58 ±24	612±48
	90	635±38	34 ±10	601±32
	120	632±23	12 ±14	620±29

Values are means ± SEM of 6 (oxygenated) or 4 (anoxic) perfusions.
All anoxic values for uptake and consumption are greater than values ($P<0.01$).
*Time in min after the start of fetal recirculation
**kg wet weight of tissue

Lactate production

Lactate production over the perfusion period was measured in the same samples as glucose. The rate of lactate production, subdivided into maternal and fetal release, is shown in Table 2. The anoxic perfused tissue displayed a significantly greater production of lactate ($P<0.02$) throughout the perfusion than did the oxygenated tissue.

The increased rate of lactate production observed in the anoxic perfusion was reflected in the differences in maternal and fetal circuit lactate concentrations (Figure 2).

Oxygen consumption

Maternal and fetal arterial and venous pO_2 values were obtained every 30 seconds from the in-line oxygen electrodes. In the oxygenated perfusions, the average arterial pO_2 ranged between 565 and 590 mm Hg, while the fetal arterial pO_2 varied between 36 and 49 mm Hg. Anoxic perfusates were free of oxygen during placental transit.

The oxygen consumption and transfer were calculated using the maternal and fetal flow rates and lobule weights (Table 3). Rates of oxygen transfer and consumption were stable throughout the perfusion period.

Table 2. Lactate production in oxygenated and anoxic perfusions.

Perfusion type	Time*	Maternal µmol/min/kg**	Fetal µmol/min/kg**	Total µmol/min/kg**
Oxygenated	30	272±29	69.0±12	341±35
	60	292±61	50.0±13	342±71
	90	242±30	33.0±4	275±30
	120	304±21	31.0±3	335±21
Anoxic	30	488±44	120.0±17	608±58
	60	585±68	35.0±13	620±57
	90	567±53	27.0±5	594±51
	120	575±46	37.0±15	612±60

Values are means ± SEM of 6 (oxygenated) or 4 (anoxic) perfusions. All anoxic values for maternal and total are greater than oxygenated values ($P<0.02$).
*Time in min after the start of fetal recirculation
**kg wet weight of tissue

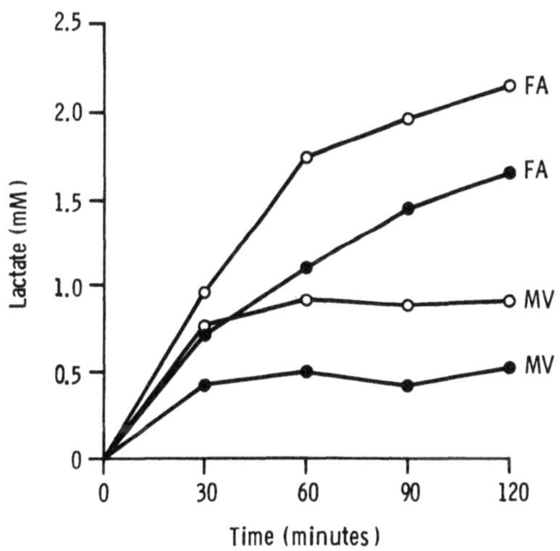

Figure 2. Lactate concentrations in maternal and venous circulations in oxygenated and anoxic conditions. Changes in the fetal arterial (FA) and maternal venous (MV) concentrations of lactate under oxygenated (●) and anoxic (○) conditions. Values are means of 6 (oxygenated) or 4 (anoxic) perfusions. Maternal venous lactate; anoxic > oxygenated ($P<0.01$). Fetal arterial lactate; anoxic > oxygenated at 60, 90 and 120 min ($P<0.01$). NB. Fetal perfusate was recirculated, maternal circulation was open.

Table 3. Oxygen transfer and consumption in oxygenated perfusions

Time	Oxygen consumption	Oxygen transfer
30	215±32	21±5
60	203±34	15±6
90	202±23	14±8
120	206±22	15±8

Values are means ± SEM of 6 perfusions expressed in terms of μmol O_2/min kg wet weight of tissue. Time is the period (in min) after the start of fetal recirculation.

Glucose balance

The glucose, lactate and oxygen consumption values reported above were used to quantify the distribution of glucose uptake through the major pathways of glucose metabolism (Figure 3). Lactate production, oxygen consumption (assuming glucose oxidation as the only oxygen consuming process) and glucose transfer accounted for 84 percent of the glucose taken up during oxygenated perfusions. The remaining 16 percent must also include the glucose demands of glycogen synthesis, the pentose phosphate pathway and pyruvate production.

In the anoxic perfusions, however, lactate production and glucose transfer accounted for only 54 percent of the glucose uptake. Assuming that the 16 percent of glucose uptake unaccounted for in the oxygenated perfusions (and ascribed to other pathways) could be applied to the anoxic perfusion, the shortfall in anoxic glucose balance still amounted to some 30 percent of the glucose uptake.

Glucose metabolites

Tissue samples from oxygenated and anoxic perfused placentae were extracted with trichloroacetic acid and assayed for a series of glycolytic intermediates to discover whether the glucose uptake which was unaccounted for in the anoxic perfusions remained in the tissue as hexose, pentose or triose phosphate derivatives. The results (Table 4) showed that there were no differences in tissue content between the two perfusion types for glucose-6-phosphate, fructose-6-phosphate, glucose-1-phosphate, phosphoenolpyruvate and pyruvate. Concentrations of two metabolites were reduced in the anoxic samples; dihydroxyacetone phosphate was decreased by 26 percent and fructose-1, 6-diphosphate by 42 percent compared to the samples from

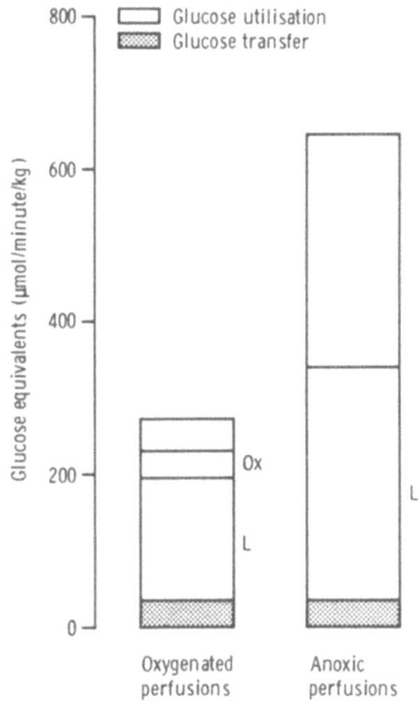

Figure 3. Distribution of glucose uptake in oxygenated and anoxic perfusions. Division of total glucose uptake in oxygenated and anoxic perfusions and subdivision of glucose utilization. L, lactate; OX, aerobic glycolysis. Values were averaged over the time course of 6 (oxygenated) or 4 (anoxic) perfusions. Lactate glucose - equivalents = lactate production/2. Oxygen glucose - equivalents = oxygen consumption/6.

oxygenated tissue. Assays were also conducted to measure the tissue content of ribose-5-phosphate, an indicator of the flux through the pentose phosphate pathway, but no differences were found between oxygenated and anoxic samples.

Placental production of organic acids

Fetal perfusate of samples for organic acid analysis were taken at the end of the perfusion. Gas-liquid chromatography produced chromatograms similar to those seen in Figure 4. Chromatogram peak areas were normalized, using an internal standard added prior to extraction (undecanedioic acid). Preliminary identification of the peaks was made by comparison of retention times and retention time indices with those determined previously for a range of organic acids.

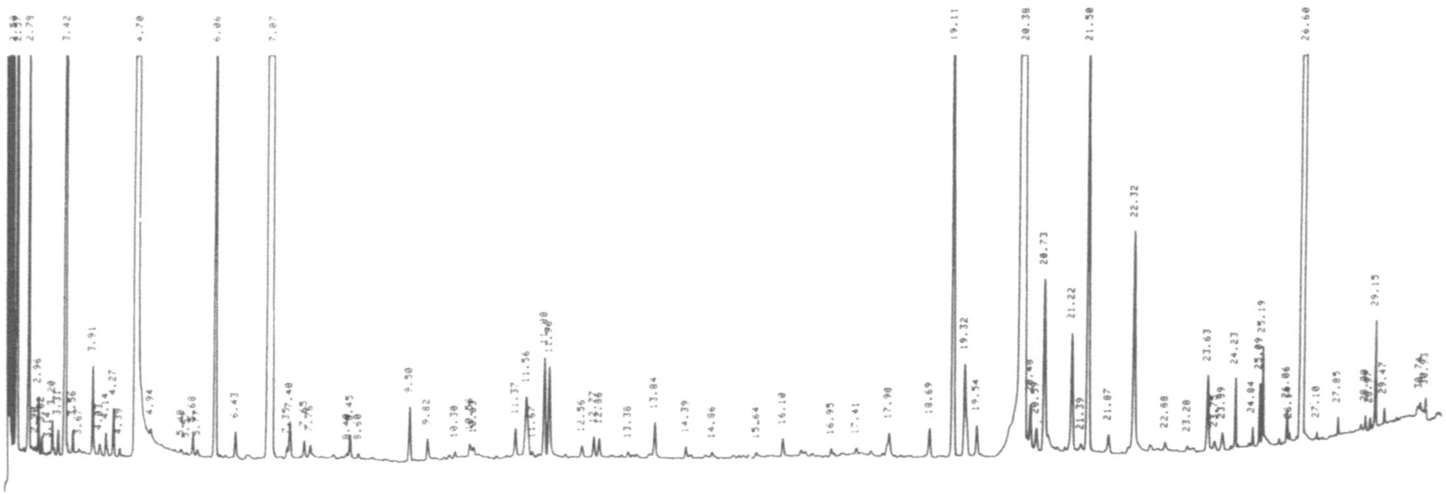

Figure 4. Chromatogram of a sample taken from an anoxic perfusate. Column retention times increase from left to right

Table 4. Perfused tissue metabolites

Metabolite	Oxygenated nmol/min/kg*	Anoxic nmol/min/kg*
Glucose-1-phosphate	4.8±0.8	6.7±0.9
Glucose-6-phosphate	14.4±0.9	13.4±0.6
Fructose-6-phosphate	11.9±1.8	9.8±0.6
Fructose-1,6-diphosphate	119.0±8**	69.0±13
Dihydroxyacetonephosphate	15.0±1**	11.0±1
Phosphoenolpyruvate	18.0±5	18.0±3
Pyruvate	29.0±8	10.0±1
Ribose-5-phosphate	1122.0±98	1184.0±67

Values are means ± SEM of 5 (oxygenated) or 4 (anoxic) samples.
*kg wet weight of tissue
**Oxygenated values > anoxic values ($P<0.1$)

On the basis of these preliminary identifications a comparison was made of organic acids found in the fetal perfusate after aerobic and anaerobic perfusion. A more rigorous analysis must await solution of the problems of detection caused by the very low concentrations of circulating organic acids. Nevertheless, these data provide a guide to the changes in the nature of organic acid metabolites being released by the placenta into the fetal circulation.

A 15 ml sample of perfusate plus 1 ml of the undecanedioic acid (containing 1 mg of the standard) was extracted and derivatized for gas-liquid chromatography. The 2 µl sample which was used produced a peak area for the undecanedioate of 1000 units representing 5 mg of the standard. Although the areas for other peaks cannot be related to the quantities present using these values, the areas do bear a similar relationship to the amount present in the sample. This means that the quantities present in the sample were, in several cases, in the low nanogram range, at the limits of detectability using this method. This also means that there were very small quantities in the fetal perfusate, in the low microgram range.

The organic acids of interest here which have been identified are shown in Table 5. The anoxic perfusions contained less of the tricarboxylic acid cycle acids, citrate, cis-aconitate and malate, but increased levels of succinate and 2-oxoglutarate. Both 3-hydroxybutyrate and acetoacetate were substantially increased in the anoxic perfusion. Uric acid, an indicator of hypoxia (Saugstad, 1975) showed an increase from undetectable levels in the oxygenated perfusions to significant levels in the anoxic perfusates.

Table 5. Organic acid components in oxygenated and anoxic fetal perfusates.

Metabolite	Peak area (ox)	Peak area (anox)	An/Ox (%)
2-Phosphoglyceric	0.9	1.7	188
Lactic	514.4	558.9	109
Pyruvic	4.2	7.3	171
Cis-aconitic	1.3	1.1	78
Citric	6.3	5.3	83
2-Oxoglutaric	0.9	2.5	279
Succinic	4.3	7.0	162
Fumaric	3.0	2.9	98
Malic	10.7	9.0	84
3-Hydroxybutyric	1.1	2.2	202
Acetoacetic	0.2	0.5	258
Linoleic	1.0	1.1	118
Oleic	n.d.*	0.2	-
Stearic	0.4	n.d.	-
Gluconic	0.3	0.5	189
Glucuronic	10.7	12.3	114
Uric	n.d.	3.2	-
Undecanedioic	1000**	1000	

Values are the mean peak areas (in arbitrary units) of 6 (oxygenated) or 4 (anoxic) samples calculated after subraction of an initial perfusate blank.
*n.d.- not detectable; **1000 units of peak area represents 5 nanograms of undecanedioic acid.

DISCUSSION

One of the most striking aspects of placental carbohydrate metabolism is the magnitude of placental glucose utilization. The glucose utilization rate for oxygenated tissue of 238 µmol/min/kg is 5-10 fold higher than the glucose turnver observed in the fetal lamb (Warnes et al., 1977) with 42 µmol/min/kg or the 27-44 µmol/min/kg estimated for the human neonate (Sparks, 1979). Placental utilization rates are closer to the value of 295 µmol/min/kg found for the brain tissue in the fetal lamb or that found for the brain tissue of adult animals (Makowski et al., 1972).

Under normal conditions fetal brain tissue uses glucose as an energy source almost exclusively (Hay, 1979), thereby providing a major drain on the glucose supplied to the fetus. The increase in placental glucose utilization to 611 µmol/min/kg in anoxic conditions, although an extreme case, demonstrates the response of the placenta to oxygen deprivation. Increases in placental utilization of glucose during a period of oxygen deprivation could therefore reduce the availability of glucose for fetal metabolism, especially for dependent tissues such as the brain. This has been reported clinically by Lumley and Wood (1967) when, by halving the arterial pO_2 of women in labor, they produced a rise in maternal blood glucose, but a fall in fetal blood glucose. The fetal brain may be able to use other substrates such as oleic acid or 3-hydroxybutyrate (Bossi et al., 1982) which we demonstrated were increased in anoxic fetal perfusates. While this may be important in a hypoglycemic situation, under hypoxic conditions, placental removal of glucose would only tend to exacerbate the oxygen deprivation.

A corollary of the increased placental glucose consumption in anoxic conditions is the alteration in lactate production by the placenta. The rate of lactate production was nearly doubled in anoxic conditions compared to the production in oxygenated tissue. The majority of lactate, over 85 percent in oxygenated perfusions and over 90 percent in anoxic perfusions, was removed via the maternal circulation, similar to the lactate production observed by Schneider et al. (1981) although different in magnitude. Despite maternal flow rates equivalent to or greater than those observed in vivo (McFadyen, 1979) and the presence of an increasing gradient between fetal and maternal arterial circulations, lactate accumulated in the fetal circulation to levels observed in normal umbilical arterial blood (Lin et al., 1980). Under normoxic conditions, the removal of fetal lactate by placental transfer and fetal metabolism is able to maintain lactate concentrations at a safe level. In anoxic (or hypoxic) conditions, our results suggest that much greater concentrations of lactate would enter the fetal circulation due to increased placental production and to the diminished ability of the fetus to oxidize lactate. Furthermore, the existence of high placental lactate concentrations could hinder the feto-maternal transfer of lactate and lead to the accumulation of toxic concentrations in fetal blood and tissues. Such a situation has been observed in the guinea pig during hypoxia (Moll and Kastendieck, 1978) where the authors found that placental transfer slowed lactate accumulation to only a minor extent. Lactate accumulation was primarily determined by the rate of lactate production. Myers (1978) noted in experimental monkeys that beyond a certain level of oxygen deficiency, serum glucose and lactate concentrations were of much more importance than the degree of oxygen deprivation in determining pathologic outcome. Once the tricarboxylic acid cycle was impaired, carbohydrate status became more important than oxygen status. Our results, in agreement with Myers, tend to suggest that lactate (and the fall in pH) are the potentially damaging agents rather than oxygen deficiency itself. The fall in fetal pH after glucose infusions in labor (Sabata et al., 1967; Shelley, 1973) may be reflections of this effect.

The rates of oxygen consumption observed in the oxygenated perfusions (202 µmol/min/kg) are lower than those reported. Schneider et al. (1981) reported an oxygen consumption of 430 µmol/min/kg. Our results suggest, however, that there is no rigid requirement for oxidative metabolism. The level of oxygen consumption is not important, provided that a sufficient supply of glucose exists to maintain the placental energy supply through anaerobic glycolysis. Our reasoning is based on two observations. At the lower levels of oxygen consumption shown here, the system was able to maintain a normal ultrastructure as determined by electron microscopy, throughout the perfusion period (Fox, Illsley and Penfold, unpublished data). The placenta also demonstrated a functional viability at this level of oxygen consumption through the ability to transfer and concentrate a range of amino acids in the fetal circulation. The placental transfer and fetal accumulation of amino acids, an energy requiring process, was maintained over the length of oxygenated and anoxic perfusions to the same degree (Penfold et al., 1983). Thus, placental structure and function was maintained without oxygen in the presence of physiological concentrations of glucose. This confirms the suggestion by Longo et al., (1973) that anaerobic glycolysis was capable of supporting amino acid accumulation in placental tissue.

As an addition to the previous observation, we would also suggest that the yield of energy obtained by complete placental oxidation of glucose is probably overestimated. If it is assumed that the increased utilization of glucose seen in the anoxic perfusions was able to compensate for lost oxygen consumption, (as the maintained amino acid transfer would suggest) then the energy produced by anaerobic consumption of the extra glucose should be equivalent to that generated by the oxygen consumption. This equivalence produces an efficiency for aerobic glycolysis of only 58 percent. This result is supported by evidence that the efficiency of oxidative phosphorylation in placental mitochondria is lower than that shown for adult animal or human mitochondria (Illsley et al., 1983; Olivera and Meigs, 1975). It is also possible that the decreased efficiency of mitochondrial respiration might apply to fetal as well as placental tissues (Pollack, 1975; Aprille and Asimakis, 1980) thus devaluing, in part, the role of oxygen in fetal energy generation.

The measurements of intermediate glycolytic metabolites showed that the glucose uptake which is unaccounted for in the anoxic perfusions is not present in the tissue as hexose or triose phosphates. The tissue content of ribose-5-phosphate, a component of the pentose phosphate pathway and a precursor of purine and pyrimidine nucleotide synthesis, is not different in oxygenated and anoxic tissue. This is in contrast to aerobic tumor tissue, which can exhibit a large accumulation of several hexose, pentose and triose phosphates (Eigenbrodt and Glossman, 1980).

In the absence of insulin control, increased uptake of glucose was most probably stimulated by intracellular processes such as the increased activity of the regulatory enzymes hexokinase and phosphofructokinase (Newsholme and Start, 1975). However, despite the increased uptake of glucose in anoxia, glucose was not detectable in oxygenated or anoxic tissue extracts (data not shown). In combination with the data on glycolytic intermediates, this indicates that placental glycolysis is capable of concerted adaptation to a higher pathway flux, as evidenced by the increased lactate output, without the need for protein synthesis, although this may occur as a longer term consequence as suggested by Diamant and Kissilevitz (1981). The removal of a major part of lactate output through the maternal circulation and the maintenance of a normal physiological pH through the bicarbonate buffering system permitted an accelerated glycotic flux in the anoxic perfusion (Rovetto et al., 1975).

The concentration of organic acids in the fetal perfusate at the end of the perfusion, with the exceptions of lactate and glycerol, was in the range of 20-200 ng/ml. Determination of organic acids at these low levels is difficult using current methods of extraction, and capillary gas chromatography and further optimization of the procedures is required. Nevertheless, it is possible to speculate on the patterns suggested here. The increases in succinate and 2-oxoglutarate and decreases in other tricarboxylic acid cycle acids are similar to the patterns observed in rat heart when it is made anoxic (Freminet, 1981), and probably represent the independent operation of sections of the cycle which participate in other pathways. The increase in ketone bodies and the altered profile of fatty acids is indicative of increased lipolysis and/or fatty acid oxidation by placental tissue. Whether the precursors of these ketone bodies are stored in the placenta or whether they are in transit across is impossible to tell. It is interesting to note, however, that the fatty acid oxidation which produces these fragments is activated comparatively rapidly and in the presence of a large transplacental glucose flux. This raises the question of the initial activation of a process which is normally accepted as being hormonally stimulated. The increase in uric acid in the anoxic fetal perfusate is a recognized marker for anoxic or hypoxic metabolism (Saugstad, 1975), although the true levels of uric acid production may be masked by the requirement for oxygen in urate synthesis. In general these data, including the changes in a number of peaks which have not yet been identified, suggest potentially important changes in the fetal substrate profile during anoxia.

SUMMARY

Placental glucose utilization rates in the in vitro perfusion were high compared to whole body rates of glucose consumption and were similar to the rate of utilization by brain tissue. During anoxia, placental utilization increased more than two-fold.

Nearly 70 percent of placental glucose was metabolized to lactate under oxygenated conditions. In anoxic conditions lactate output was almost doubled, although it accounted for only 50 percent of the anoxic glucose consumption. The majority of lactate was removed from the placenta by the maternal circulation, but the quantities which passed into the fetal circulation accumulated to produce in vivo umbilical arterial levels.

Placental oxygen consumption was not necessary to maintain placental structure and the major placental function. A sufficient supply of glucose, removal of lactate, and maintenance of normal pH permitted an acceleration of glycolysis under anoxic conditions without damage to the placenta. Placental aerobic glycolysis operated at only 60 percent of its theoretical efficiency under oxygenated conditions.

The change from oxygenated to anoxic conditions altered the output of organic acid metabolites released into the fetal circulation during perfusion and confirmed the shift in tissue metabolism to the anaerobic mode.

REFERENCES

Aprille, J.R. and Asimakis, G.K. (1980) Postnatal development of rat liver mitochondria: State 3 respiration, adenine nucleotide translocase activity and the net accumulation of adenine nucleotides. *Arch. Biochem. Biophy.* 201, 654-577.

Bossi, E., Zuppinger, K., Siegrist, H.P., Wiesmann, U. and Herschkowitz, N. (1982) Age-dependent utilization of 3- hydroxybutyrate and oleic acid as glucose substitutes by neonatal mouse brain cultures. *Ped. Res.* 16, 579-582.

Chalmers, R.A. and Watts, R.W.E. (1972) The quantitative extraction and gas-liquid chromatographic determination of organic acids in urine. *Analyst* 97, 958-967.

Diamant, Y.Z. and Kissilevitz, R. (1981) The placenta in intrauterine fetal deprivation. *Acta Obstet. Gynecol. Scand.* 50, 141-147.

Eigenbrodt, E. and Glossman, H. (1980) Glycolysis - one of the keys to cancer? *Trends Pharm. Sci.* 1, 240-245.

Freminet, A. (1981) Carbohydrate and amino acid metabolism during acute hypoxia in rats: Blood and heart metabolites. *Comp. Biochem. Physiol.* 70B, 427-433.

Hay, W.H. (1979) Fetal glucose metabolism. *Sem. Perinatol.* 3, 157-176.

Illsley, N.P., Aarnoudse, J.G., Penfold, P., Bordsley, S.E., Coade, S.B., Stacey, T.E., and Hytten, F.E. Mechanical and metabolic viability of an in vitro placental perfusion system under oxygenated and anoxic conditions. *Placenta* (in press).

Illsley, N.P., Coade, S.B. and Harkness, R.A. (1983) The maturation of oxidative phosphorylation in human mitochondria and its relation to increased adenine nucleotide concentration. *Biochem. Soc. Transac.* 11, 294.

Lang, G. and Michal, G. (1974) D-glucose-6-phosphate and D- fructose-6-phosphate. In *Methods of Enzymatic Analysis* (ed.), Bergmeyer, H.U., pp. 1238-2342. New York: Academic Press.

Lin, C-C., Moawad, A.H., Rosenow, P. and River, P. (1980) Acid-base characteristics of fetuses with intrauterine growth retardation during labor and delivery. *Amer. J. Obstetr. Gynecol.* 137, 553-559.

Longo, L.D., Yuen, P. and Gusseck, D.J. (1973) Anaerobic glycogen dependent transport of amino acids by the placenta. *Nature* 243, 409-411.

Lumley, J.M. and Wood, C. (1967) Influence of hypoxia on glucose transport across the placenta. *Nature* 216, 403-404.

McFayden, I.R. (1979) Maternal blood flow to the uterus. In *Placental Transfer.* (ed.), Chamberlain, G.V.P. and Wilkinson, A.W., pp. 31-44. Tunbridge Wells: Pitman Publishing.

Makowski, E.L., Schneider, J.M., Tsoulos, N.G., Colwill, J.R., Battaglia, F.C. and Meschia, G. (1972) Cerebral blood flow, oxygen consumption and glucose utilization of fetal lambs in utero. *Amer. J. Obstet. Gynecol.* 114, 292-303.

Michal, G. and Beutler, H-O. (1974) D-fructose-1,6-diphosphate, dihydroxyacetone phosphate and D-glyceraldehyde-3-phosphate. In: *Methods of Enzymatic Analysis.* (ed.), Bergmeyer, H.U., pp. 1314-1319. New York: Academic Press.

Moll, W. and Kastendieck, E. (1978) Accumulation and disappearance of lactate in a fetus with a hemochorial placenta. The role of placental transfer and fetal metabolism. *J. Perinatal Med.* 6, 246-254.

Myers, R.E. (1978) Lactic acid accumulation as cause of brain edema and cerebral necrosis resulting from oxygen deprivation. In *Advances in Perinatal Neurology.* (ed.), Korobkin, R. and Guilleminault, C., pp. 85-114. New York: S.P. Medical and Scientific Books.

Newsholme, E.A. and Start, C. (1975) *Regulation in Metabolism.* pp. 3449, London: Wiley-Interscience.

Olivera, A.A. and Meigs, R.A. (1975) Mitochondria from human term placenta. I. Isolation and assay conditions for oxidative phosphorylation. *Biochem. Biophys. Acta* 376, 426-435.

Penfold, P., Drury, L., Simmonds, R.J. and Hytten, F.E. (1981) Studies of a single placental cotyledon in vitro: I. The preparation and its viability. *Placenta Suppl.* 2,149-154.

Penfold, P., Illsley, N.P., Purkiss, P. and Jennings, P. (1983) Human placental amino acid transfer and metabolism in oxygenated and anoxic conditions. *Trophoblast Res.* (this volume).

Pollack, J.K. (1975) The maturation of the inner membrane of foetal rat liver mitochondria. *Biochem. J.* 150, 477-488.

Racker, E. (1974) D-ribose-5-phosphate. In *Methods of Enzymatic Analysis.* (ed.), Bergmeyer, H.U., pp. 1342-1343. New York: Academic Press.

Rovetto, M.J., Lamberton, W.F. and Neely, J.R. (1975) Mechanisms of glycolytic inhibition in ischemic rat hearts. *Circul. Res.* 37,742-751.

Sabata, V., Znamenacek, K., Pribylova, H. and Melichar, V. (1967) The effect of glucose infusion administered to the mother during delivery on metabolism of premature newborns. In *Intrauterine Dangers to the fetus.* (ed.) Horsky G. and Stembera, H., pp. 435- 439. Amsterdam: Excerpta Medica.

Saugstad, O.D. (1975) Hypoxanthine as a measurement of hypoxia. *Pediat. Res.* 9,158-161.

Schneider, H., Challier, J-C. and Dancis, J. (1981) Transfer and metabolism of glucose and lactate in the human placenta studied by a perfusion system in vitro. *Placenta Suppl.* 2, 129-138.

Shelley, H.J. (1973) The use of chronically catheterized foetal lambs for the study of foetal metabolism. In *Foetal and Neonatal Physiol.* (ed.) Comline, K.S., Cross, K.W., Dawes, G.S. and Nathanielsz, P.W., pp. 360-397. Cambridge: Cambridge University Press.

Sparks, J.W. (1979) Augmentation of the glucose supply in the fetus and newborn. *Sem. Perinatol.* 3, 141-155.

Tracey, B.M., Stacey, T.E. and Chalmers, R.A. Urinary and plasma organic acids in dizygotic twin siblings with 3- hydroxy-3-methylglutaric aciduria, studied by gas chromatography and mass spectrometry using fused silica capillary columns. *J. Inherit. Metab. Dis.* (in press).

Warnes, D.M., Seamark, R.F. and Ballard, F.J. (1977) Metabolism of glucose, fructose and lactate in vivo in chronically cannulated foetuses and in suckling lambs. *Biochem. J.* 162, 617- 626.

DISCUSSION

PANIGEL (Paris): Have you measured the volumes that you are perfusing on both the fetal and maternal sides? How long is the perfusion stable?

ILLSLEY (Harrow): Our perfusion is stable over the entire two hour period. We have currently modified our techniques using antipyrine clearance. We load the maternal resevoir with cold antipyrine in high concentration and then perfuse it in an open circuit. The fetal circuit is also open. We use a UV monitor at 280 to measure the antipyrine. Therefore, we can determine the clearance of antipyrine directly.

PANIGEL (Paris): You are to be congratulated for this comparison between hypoxic and hyperoxygenated experiments. Where is the missing glucose? Do you suspect that it mainly goes to lactate? How many perfusions did you do? I see six and four are in your presentation.

ILLSLEY (Harrow): When we have performed other experiments without amino acids, we have used nine and ten perfusions. The same sort of effects are seen in all of our studies. The figures for glucose utilization and lactate production are slightly different and lower. But the pattern is exactly the same. Some of these changes may be due to the slightly smaller fetal volume that we are using at this time.

DANCIS (New York): What are the oxygen consumption data for your placental studies? I would suggest that you are probably dealing with hypoxia vs. anoxia rather than hyperoxia vs. anoxia. I am curious why you did not use radioactive glucose to follow these metabolic studies.

ILLSLEY (Harrow): We were not expecting to find the results we did find. The next experiments should involve these radiolabelled studies. We hope to use blood to simulate more closely the physiologic situation. However, using blood has innumerable other problems unfortunately.

Trophoblast Research 1:71-80, 1983

CLEARANCE OF α-AMINOISOBUTYRIC ACID DURING IN SITU PERFUSION OF THE GUINEA PIG PLACENTA

Bruce J. Kelman and Melvin R. Sikov

Biology and Chemistry Department
Pacific Northwest Laboratory
Richland, Washington 99352

INTRODUCTION

Studies of the transport of amino acids across the placenta in a variety of species have provided little evidence of differences in amino acid transport among species with hemochorial placentae. A non-metabolized neutral amino acid (α-aminoisobutyric acid - AIB) has been used as a model compound in several studies of amino acid transport. Several studies exist which show that AIB transport from mother to fetus has characteristics often found in active transport systems, and it is now widely believed that AIB is actively transported across the hemochorial placenta. For example, tissue slices from both the human and guinea pig placenta are capable of concentrating AIB against a gradient, and this concentration follows saturation kinetics (Dancis et al., 1968; Miller and Berndt, 1974). Further, specific amino acid transport systems present in several types of isolated cells and tissues (the A, L., and ASC systems) are also present in the placenta. The A system has been shown to mediate AIB transport in the human placenta (Enders et al., 1976).

Transport of AIB has been studied in the guinea pig placenta both in vivo and in vitro (Dancis et al., 1968; van Dijk and van Kreel, 1978). It is clear that AIB transport in the placenta is responsible for accumulation of AIB in the fetus (Dancis et al., 1968). When AIB transport from mother to fetus was studied in the intact animal (by in situ perfusion of the fetal circulation alone) and in the isolated placenta artificially perfused from both sides, AIB was actively accumulated in placental cells and moved from maternal to fetal side of the placenta against a concentration gradient (van Dijk and van Kreel, 1978). AIB transport showed saturation kinetics from both the maternal and fetal sides at 5 mmol/l concentrations. Calculated kinetic parameters or AIB transport ranged from 0.20 to 0.40 mmol/min for Vmax and 285-500 mmoles/l for Km. Accumulation of AIB appeared to take place predominantly from the maternal side of the placenta; followed by release into the maternal and fetal circulations in equal amounts. This view may have to be modified, since a recent publication by Eaton and Yudilevich (1981) presents a convincing argument that amino acid efflux from placental tissue is asymmetric, and preferably directed towards the fetal side of the placenta. Although this study did not use AIB, it included other neutral amino acids expected to be transported by the A system.

Most existing data strongly support the concept that transport of AIB from mother to fetus involves an active component, although the magnitude of this active component relative to passive components in the guinea pig placenta under physiological conditions is not apparent from the literature. As a step towards clarifying the relative roles of active and passive movements of amino acids across the guinea pig placenta, concurrent measurements of transplacental movements of a substance which crosses the placenta directly by simple diffusion and of a substance which is actively transported were obtained.

METHODS

Outbred Hartley guinea pigs were bred during the estrus occuring immediately after farrowing so that gestational age was known within 24 hours. The animals used in this study had been pregnant for 60 (± 1) days.

The perfusion technique and mathematical analyses used in these experiments have been extensively described (Kelman, 1977; Kelman and Walter, 1977b; Kelman and Walter, 1980). A schematic diagram of the perfusion system is shown in Figure 1. The pregnant dam, anesthetized with a combination of sodium pentabarbital injected intraperitoneally and InnovarVet (Pittman-Moore; fentanyl citrate and droperidol) injected intramuscularly, was tied in a supine position to a plastic rack. The rack was placed in a bath of mammalian Ringers solution (37°C) which covered the lower legs and part of the posterior abdomen. One uterine horn was exteriorized through an incision in the lateral abdominal wall and one fetus exposed through an incision in the uterine wall and amniotic sac. The uterus, placenta, and fetus were all immersed in the Ringers solution and an umbilical artery cannulated with flexible polyethylene tubing (0.023 inch id, 0.038 inch od). The remaining umbilical artery was tied. The cannula was attached to Tygon tubing which passed through a peristaltic pump and then to a reservoir. The umbilical vein was then cannulated and the venous cannula

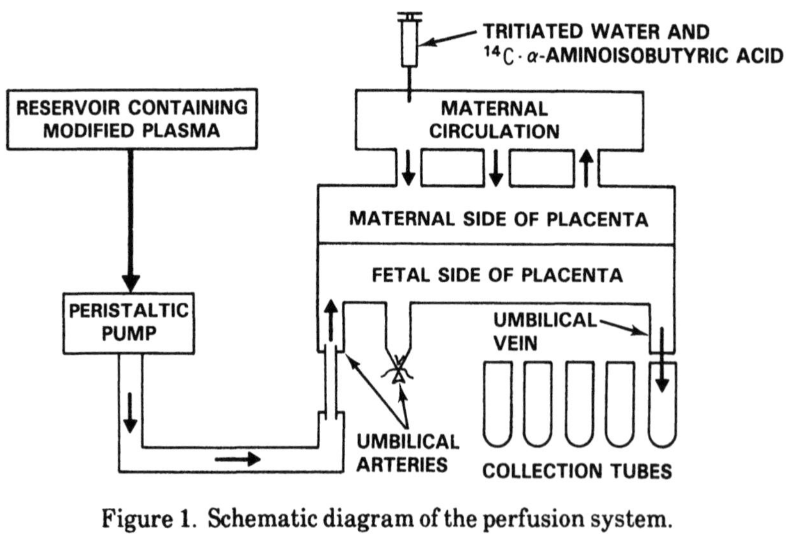

Figure 1. Schematic diagram of the perfusion system.

was then elevated to a height sufficient to maintain venous pressure at approximately normal levels (110 mm above the center of the placenta) as described previously (Kelman, 1977). After cannulation of the umbilical vein, perfusion fluid was pumped through the placenta and collected as a series of discrete samples. When the patency of the system had been established, 10 μCi of tritiated water and 40 μCi of ^{14}C-AIB (specific activity 35 mCi/mg) were injected into the maternal jugular vein. The dose was allowed to mix in the maternal circulatory system for approximately 4 min. before sampling was begun. (Previous use of this system has shown that this period of time allows uniform mixing of the dose with the maternal blood volume). Maternal blood samples were drawn at 1-10 min. intervals from a cannulated carotid artery and immediately centrifuged and aliquots of plasma were obtained. Maternal plasma samples and perfusate were analyzed by standard liquid scintillation techniques including quench correction.

Perfusion pressure, maternal electrocardiogram, blood pressure, and heart rate were monitored continuously. Umbilical flow rates were adjusted throughout the perfusion in an effort to keep them constant to allow for easier mathematical handling of the data. Umbilical flow rates used in these experiments overlapped the physiological range of umbilical flow rates for the guinea pig at this gestational age (as previously discussed by Kelman, 1977). At the completion of each experiment, placentae were collected and analyzed for AIB content by standard liquid scintillation techniques.

The perfusion fluid consisted of sterile, filtered plasma from adult guinea pigs with the pH adjusted to 7.35. Preparation of this solution was identical to that previously described (Kelman and Walter, 1977b).

Calculations and statistical analyses

The clearance of tritiated water from maternal to fetal circulation (T_{MF}) was calculated as has been previously described (Kelman and Walter, 1977b). The clearance of ^{14}C-AIB from maternal to fetal circulation (AIB_{MF}) was calculated in an analogous manner. Clearances were calculated according to the following formula:

$$\text{Clearance} = \frac{P}{M} \times R$$

where clearance is equivalent to the volume of maternal plasma that would contain an amount of radiolabel equal to that entering the perfusate per min (ml/min), P is the ^{3}H or ^{14}C concentration (μCi/ml) measured in the perfusing solution, and M is the average maternal tritium or ^{14}C concentration (μCi/ml) as determined from either a series of linear approximations, or a graph of tritium or ^{14}C concentration in maternal plasma vs. time. In no case did the use of linear as opposed to curvilinear approximations change the calculated clearance by more than 7 percent. R is the flow rate of the perfusate (ml/min) as determined by the volume of perfusion solution collected per minute and is equivalent to the umbilical flow rate.

Data were evaluated by regression analysis using a linear model in a manner analogous to studies with other materials previously reported (Kelman and Walter,

1980). Curvilinear models appeared to fit the data better than a linear model in some cases, but inclusion of additional polynominal coefficients could not be justified statistically.

RESULTS

Data were obtained from studies in nine placentae in seven dams. AIB_{MF} ranged from 0.23 to 0.55 ml/min (Table 1). Regression and correlation coefficients, umbilical flow rates, the probability of a non-zero regression coefficient,and the AIB_{MF} at tritiated $water_{MF}$ (T_{MF}) = 0 (i.e. intercept of the linear regression) are shown in Table 2. All regression coefficients were significantly less than 1.0 ($P < 0.01$). In all perfusions, umbilical flow rates were kept approximately constant so that changes in maternal blood flow to the placenta could be detected more readily than if the umbilical flow rates were varied over a wide range.

Figures 2 and 3 show typical data obtained in these experiments. In Figure 2 there was a mechanical interference in the position of the arterial cannula between approximately 20 and 30 min after administration of AIB due to a vigorously contracting uterus. In this experiment, the preparation appeared to begin degenerating about 85 min after the injection of AIB. In Figure 3 a change in T_{MF} occurred between approximately 28 and 34 min. after administration of AIB which was independent of a change in umbilical flow rate .

Upon completion of perfusions, all functional placentae were collected and analyzed for ^{14}C content (Table 3). All placentae tended to accumulate more AIB with increasing time (correlation coefficient = 0.64 for a linear model, $P < 0.06$), although this relationship was significant only when perfused placentae alone were considered

Table 1
Clearance of ^{14}C-AIB from mother to fetus (AIB_{MF})*

Dam/Placenta	AIB_{MF}(mean ± SE) ml/min
1/1	0.44 ± 0.25
2/1	0.55 ± 0.09
2/2	0.23 ± 0.04
3/1	0.52 ± 0.15
4/1	0.32 ± 0.07

* at T_{MF} = 0.20 or greater

Table 2
Relationship between the clearance of ^{14}C-labeled α-aminoisobutyric acid from dam to fetus (AIB_{MF}) and the clearance of tritiated water from dam to fetus (T_{MF})

Dam/ Placenta	Regression Coefficient (b)*	$AIB_{MF} \pm SE$** ml/min (a)*	Correlation Coefficient (r)	P	Number of Samples	Umbilical Flow Rate (mean ± SD) ml/min
1/1	0.237	0.254 ± 0.041	0.89	<0.001	46	1.43 ± 0.22
2/1	0.720	-0.004 ± 0.015	0.93	<0.001	10	1.86 ± 0.12
2/2	0.166	0.151 ± 0.023	0.62	<0.05	10	1.63 ± 0.14
3/1	0.272	0.169 ± 0.021	0.73	<0.001	60	1.91 ± 0.09
4/1	0.204	0.064 ± 0.008	0.73	<0.001	66	1.76 ± 0.12
5/1	0.639	0.020 ± 0.006	0.95	<0.001	18	1.64 ± 0.11
6/1 ($T_{MF} > 0.2$)	0.150	0.051 ± 0.007	0.86	<0.001	40	2.13 ± 0.17
6/1 ($T_{MF} < 0.2$)	0.202	0.019 ± 0.005	0.96	<0.001	14	1.81 ± 0.13

* $AIB_{MF} = a + b\,T_{MF}$
** at $T_{MF} = 0$

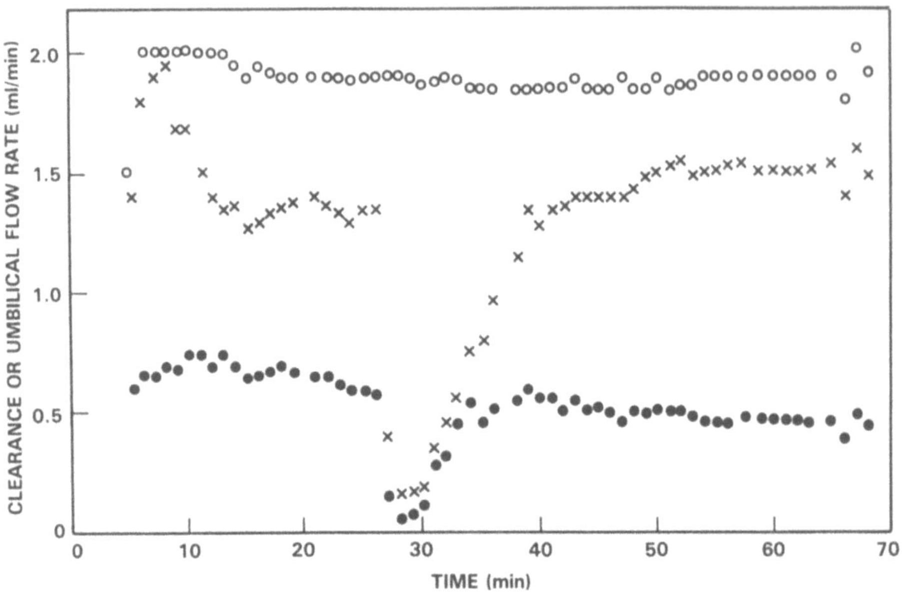

Figure 2. Dam #4. Clearance of labeled α-aminoisobutyric acid (AIB_{MF}, ●) and tritiated water (T_{MF}, ×) from dam to fetus, and umbilical flow rate (○).

(correlation coefficient = 0.95 for a linear model, $P < 0.025$). All placentae accumulated significantly higher concentrations of AIB than were present in maternal plasma.

DISCUSSION

Data obtained in these experiments agree well with data reported in the literature. In experiments analogous to ours, van Dijk and van Kreel reported clearance of AIB from maternal to fetal circulation of the placenta to ranges from 0.3 to 0.8 ml/min and placental concentration factors ranging from 8 at 240 min to 25 at 180 min. Analogous clearances in our experiments ranged from 0.23 ± 0.04 ml/min to 0.55 ± 0.09 ml/min and concentration factors calculated in an analogous manner ranged from 3 at 55 min to approximately 50 at 180.

Previous experience has shown that tritium clearance is a linear function of umbilical flow rate in experiments in which maternal blood flow to the placenta does not vary greatly (Kelman, 1977; Kelman and Walter, 1977b; Kelman and Walter, 1980). At the umbilical flow rates and perfusion ratios expected in these experiments, calculations by Moll and Kostendieck (1977) have shown that a linear model is a reasonable approximation. Since umbilical flow rates were maintained at nearly constant rates in these experiments, changes in ^3H clearance could only be due to changes in maternal blood flow to the placenta.

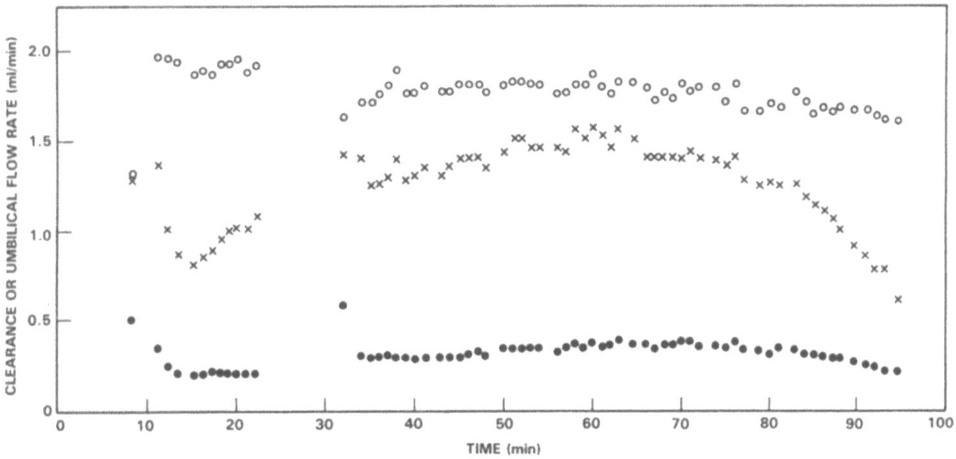

Figure 3. Dam #6. Clearance of Labeled α-Aminoisobutyric Acid (AIB_{MF}, ●) and Tritiated Water (T_{MF}, ×) from Dam to Fetus, and Umbilical Flow Rate (○). Note the change in T_{MF} unaccompanied by a change in umbilical flow rate between 26 and 34 minutes, which represents a large change in maternal blood flow to this placenta.

Table 3

^{14}C-AIB Content of perfused guinea-pig placentae

Dam/ Placenta	Treatment	^{14}C-AIB Placental (nCi/gm)	^{14}C-AIB Maternal Plasma (nCi/gm)	Time Post Injection Minutes
2/1	Nonperfused	179.4	8.4	180
2/2	Perfused	197.7	8.4	180
3/1	Perfused	55.4	13.9	69.5
3/2	Nonperfused	99.1	13.9	69.5
3/3	Nonperfused	142.6	13.9	69.5
4/1	Perfused	39.1	20.3	97.3
7/1	Nonperfused	153.9	16.9	54.6
7/2	Perfused	25.8	16.9	54.6

Table 4
Estimated AIB clearances at normal and zero placental flow rates in the perfused guinea pig placenta

Dam/ Placenta	AIB_{MF} at $T_{MF}=0$ml/min (ml/min)	AIB_{MF} at $T_{MF}=1.8$ml/min (ml/min)	Relative Contribution of AIB_{MF} at $T_{MF}=0$(%)
1/1	0.25	0.68	37%
2/2	0.16	0.45	36%
3/1	0.17	0.66	26%
4/1	0.06	0.43	14%
6/1	0.08	0.38	16%

Several inferences can be drawn from the correlations observed between T_{MF} and AIB_{MF}. The correlation between T_{MF} and AIB_{MF} over the range measured in our experiments suggests (but does not prove) that the two materials move across the placenta in a similar manner. The sensitivity of AIB_{MF} to changes in flow on the maternal side of the placenta at very low concentrations of AIB in the maternal plasma (Table 3; Figure 2) is most consistent with the presence of a large diffusional component of AIB clearance. However, this does not imply that no indications of active AIB transport were found. Since water diffuses relatively freely across the placenta, one would expect that T_{MF} should approach zero only when the blood flow on at least one side of the placenta is zero (ignoring the minute contribution which the volume of the compartment representing the vasculature within the placenta would contribute). The correlation coefficients in Table 2 indicate that a linear model is a reasonable description of the relationship between AIB_{MF} and T_{MF}. In these experiments, flow on the fetal side of the placenta was always greater than zero since a flow greater than zero is required in order to obtain perfusate samples for analysis. However, one can obtain an estimation of the value of AIB_{MF} at $T_{MF} = 0$ by calculating the intercept of the regression of AIB_{MF} on T_{MF}. This AIB clearance then represents a maximal non-diffusional component (i.e. most likely a transport mechanism) since diffusional forces should be minimal when there is no flow on at least one side of the placenta.

Table 4 lists experiments in which AIB_{MF} at $T_{MF} = 0$ were significantly different from zero ($P < 0.01$). Using historical data (Kelman and Sikov, 1981), T_{MF} at a flow rate of 2 ml/min is approximately 1.8 ml/min, with normal maternal blood flow to the placenta. Using a T_{MF} of 1.8, the regression equations from experiments in Table 2 can be used to calculate an expected AIB_{MF} at a T_{MF} of 1.8 as shown in Table 4. Inspection of Table 4 will show that the AIB_{MF} at $T_{MF} = 0$ is approximately 15-35% of the AIB_{MF} expected at flow rates within the lower limit of a physiological range. Thus, it appears that under physiological conditions in the intact animal a substantial portion of AIB_{MF} is due to passive means. Assuming that AIB is a model compound for neutral amino acids, it, therefore, appears that one need not invoke active transport mechanisms to account for a large supply of amino acids to the fetus.

SUMMARY

Transport of a number of amino acids across the placenta appears to involve an active component. Extensive investigation of the transport of α-aminoisobutyric acid (AIB; a nonmetabolized amino acid) has shown that AIB is actively transported from mother to fetus across the hemochorial placenta of the guinea pig. Nevertheless, the relative magnitude of the contribution of active and passive movements in the placenta under physiological conditions in the intact animal is not apparent from the literature. As a step towards clarifying the relative roles of active and passive movements of amino acids across the placenta, it was considered useful to obtain concurrent measurements of transplacental movements of a substance which crosses the placenta rapidly by simple diffusion (water) and of a substance which is actively transported across the placenta (AIB). In our study, placentae from guinea pigs between 59 and 61 days of gestation were perfused in situ through cannulated umbilical vessels with the maternal circulation left intact. Tritiated water and ^{14}C-AIB were injected into a maternal jugular vein and maternal blood samples were obtained at 1 to 10 minute intervals; perfusate samples were collected sequentially after one pass through the placenta. Clearance of ^{14}C-AIB from mother to fetus (AIB_{MF}) and AIB concentrations in placental tissue, maternal plasma, and perfusate were consistent in magnitude with data obtained by other investigators who have clearly shown an active transport of AIB in the placenta. On the other hand, in this study AIB_{MF} ranged from approximately 50% to 96% of the clearance of ^{3}H-labeled water from mother to fetus (T_{MF}) and changes in AIB_{MF} correlated closely with changes in T_{MF} in all perfusions. Thus, it appears that AIB_{MF} closely paralleled T_{MF} and our data suggest that a relatively large component of AIB_{MF} is of passive origin in the in situ placenta. It is hypothesized that under physiological conditions the existence of active transport mechanisms in the intact animal does not need to be invoked in supplying large quantities of amino acids to the fetus.

ACKNOWLEDGMENTS

This research was supported by the U.S. Department of Energy under Contract Number DE-AC06-76RLO-1830 and NIH under Grant Number 2R01 GM20661.

REFERENCES

Dancis, J., Money, W.L., Springer, D., and Levitz, M. (1968) Transport of amino acids by placenta. *Amer. J. Obst. Gynec.* 101, 820-829.

Eaton, B.M. and Yudilevich, D.L. (1981) Uptake and asymmetric efflux of amino acids at maternal and fetal sides of placenta. *Amer. J. Physiol.* 241, C106-C112.

Enders, R.H., Judd, R.M., Donohue, T.M. and Smith, C.H. (1976) Placental amino acid uptake. III. Transport systems for neutral amino acids. *Amer. J. Physiol.* 230, 706-710.

Kelman, B.J. (1977) Inorganic mercury movements across the perfused guinea pig placenta in late gestation. *Tox. Appl. Pharm.* 41, 659-665.

Kelman, B.J. and Walter, B.K. (1977b) Passage of cadmium across the perfused guinea pig placenta. *Proc. Soc. Exper. Biol. Med.* 156, 68-71.
Kelman, B.J. and Walter, B.K. (1980) Transplacental movements of inorganic lead from mother to fetus. *Proc. Soc. Exper. Biol. Med.* 163, 278-282.
Kelman, B.J. and Sikov, M.R. (1981) Plutonium movements across the haemochorial placenta of the guinea pig. *Placenta* Suppl. 3, 319-326.
Miller, R.K. and Berndt, W.O. (1974) Characterization of neutral amino acid accumulation by human term placental slices. *Amer. J. Physiol.* 227, 1236-1242.
Moll, W. and Kastendieck, E. (1977) Transfer of N_2O, CO, and HTO in the artificially perfused guinea pig placenta. *Resp. Physiol.* 29, 283-302.
van Dijk, J.P. and van Kreel, B.K. (1978) Transport and accumulation of α-aminoisobutyric acid (AIB) in the guinea pig placenta. *Pflügers Arch.* 377, 217-224.2

Trophoblast Research 1:81-100, 1983

FACTORS AFFECTING THE UPTAKE OF α-AMINO ACIDS BY HUMAN PLACENTAL VILLUS: ACETYLCHOLINE, PHOSPHOLIPID METHYLATION, Ca^{++} AND CYTOSKELETAL ORGANIZATION

B. V. Rama Sastry, Stanley L. Barnwell and Robert D. Moore

Department of Pharmacology
Vanderbilt University School of Medicine
Nashville, Tennessee 37232, U.S.A.

INTRODUCTION

Efficient transport of amino acids by the placenta is necessary for growth of the fetus. Information on the regulatory mechanisms of amino acid transport in human placenta is relatively limited. Several investigators have studied the uptake of amino acids by isolated placental villi or slices from human placenta using mainly α-aminoisobutyric acid (AIB) (Miller and Berndt, 1974; Smith and Depper, 1974; Schneider and Dancis, 1974; Gusseck et al., 1975; Rowell and Sastry, 1978, 1981; Welsch et al., 1981a; Barnwell and Sastry, 1982). These studies have provided variables which influence the uptake of AIB by placenta. They have also provided information on optimum temperature (37°C) and optimum pH (7.4 to 7.8) for AIB uptake and oxidative energy sources for the uptake of AIB (Longo et al., 1973; Miller and Berndt, 1974). According to Christensen's (1973) nomenclature, AIB is transported primarily by the A system. It can also fit the ASC and L systems, and, therefore, it has equal or greater access to transport systems than many of the natural neutral amino acids.

During the past decade, considerable progress has been made toward delineation of the cholinergic system in human placenta and its role in the regulation of amino acid transport in placenta (Sastry and Sadavongvivad, 1979; Fant and Harbison, 1981). ACh has been positively identified in human placenta by gas chromatography and mass spectrometry (Sastry et al., 1976; Welsch and Wenger, 1980). The kinetic properties of human placental choline acetyltransferase (ChA) are similar to those of mammalian brain ChA (Sastry and Henderson, 1972, 1976). There is some evidence that there are cholinergic receptors of the muscarinic type, possibly different from those in nervous tissue, in human placenta (Sastry and Sadavongvivad, 1979). High concentrations of nicotine (10^{-4}M) and atropine (5 x 10^{-4}M) inhibited ACh release and AIB uptake by isolated placental villus. Nicotinic receptor antagonists like d-tubocurarine and mecamylamine did not exert any effect on ACh release or AIB uptake (Sastry et al., 1977; Olubadewo and Sastry, 1978; Rowell and Sastry, 1978). Selective inhibitors of ChA depressed AIB uptake by the placental villus (Rowell and Sastry, 1981; Welsch et al., 1981a; Leventer et al., 1982). However, the relationships between ChA inhibition, changes in ACh levels, ACh release, and depression of AIB uptake have not been established. Extracellular Ca^{++} is critical for the release of ACh from the placental villus. It is not known if AIB uptake by placental villus is depressed in the absence of extracellular Ca^{++}.

Preincubation of human placental tissue for several hours has been noted to increase accumulation of AIB (Smith et al., 1973), possibly due to an increase in transport sites synthesized during the incubation period (Smith and Depper, 1974; Gusseck et al., 1975). Therefore, this system may afford a method of manipulating the synthesis of membrane associated carrier proteins, their translocation, and their insertion into the lipid bilayer of the plasma membrane. The lipid bilayer is mainly composed of phospholipids which provide a fluid matrix for proteins and their movement (Singer and Nicolson, 1972). Membrane phospholipids are mainly composed of phosphatidylethanolamine (PE) and phosphatidylcholine (PC). They are asymmetrically distributed in the membrane, PE facing the interior and PC facing the exterior of the cell. In several cell membranes, there are two methyltransferases which methylate PE to PC in a step-wise fashion when S-adenosyl-L-methionine (SAM) is present (Hirata and Axelrod, 1980; Axelrod and Hirata, 1981). PE N-methyltransferase (Methyltransferase I), located in the interior bilayer of the membrane, converts PE to phosphatidyl-N-methylethanolamine (PME). PME N-

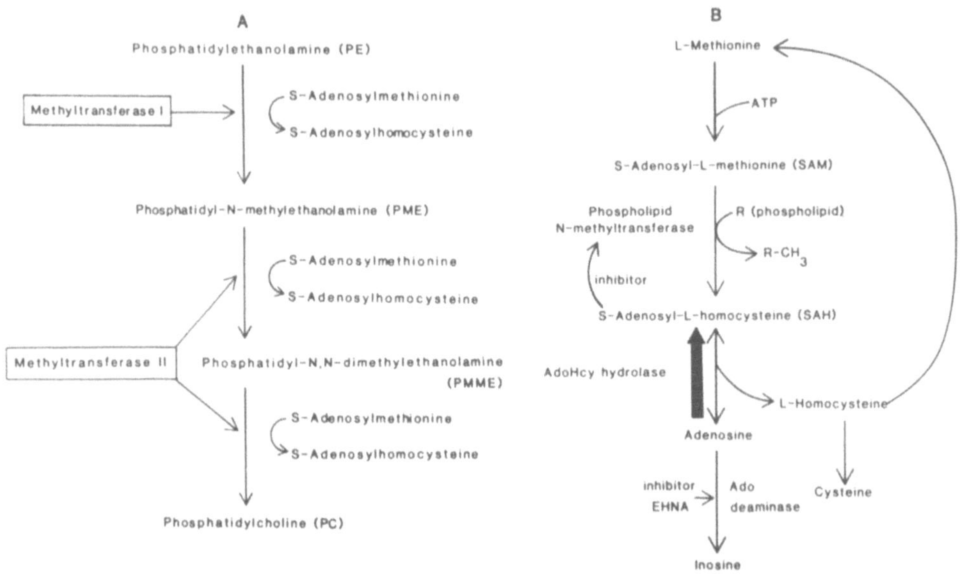

Figure 1. Metabolic pathways: A. Stepwise methylation of membrane phosphatidylethanolalmine (PE) to form phosphatidylcholine (PC). B. Formation of S-adenosyl-L-methionine (SAM) and S-adenosyl-L-homocysteine (SAH).

methyltransferase (Methyltransferase-II) converts PME into phosphatidyl-N, N-dimethylethanolamine (PMME) and PC (Figure 1A). Transient accumulation of PME during transmethylation within the membrane, due to the difference in the affinities of SAM to the two methyltransferases, has been found to increase membrane fluidity (Hirata and Axelrod, 1978; Sastry et al., 1981a; Jaiswal et al., 1982). Changes in phospholipid methylation and membrane fluidity have been known to influence Ca^{++} fluxes and Ca^{++}-ATPase activity (Strittmatter et al., 1979). Biosynthesis of PC via the methylation pathway occurs in plasma (Barnwell and Sastry, 1981a) and microsomal (Welsch et al., 1981b) membranes of human placenta. Further, the plasma membrane of human placental villus has been shown to contain both phospholipid methyltransferases (Barnwell and Sastry, 1981a,b). There is also evidence for the presence of Ca^{++}-ATPase in human term placenta (Miller and Berndt, 1973). All of these observations suggest that inhibition of phospholipid methylation may interfere with Ca^{++} entry and exit from the trophoblast cell, ACh release and AIB uptake.

Calcium ions are required for the formation of microtubular assembly and secretory processes. If the microtubular organization is necessary for amino acid uptake, its disruption should depress AIB uptake.

The effects of several factors, linked to one another in cellular function, on the uptake of amino acids by the placental villus were studied in the experiments described in this communication. These effects include the inhibition of (a) ACh synthesis and release, (b) phospholipid methylation, and (c) formation of microtubular assembly on amino acid uptake. In view of the central role of Ca^{++} in ACh secretion, AIB uptake by the placental villus in a Ca^{++}-free medium was also examined as part of this investigation. In all cases, AIB uptake was depressed, indicating that these cellular processes are internally linked for optimum uptake of amino acids by the human placental villus.

METHODS

Radiolabeled compounds

All radiolabeled amino acids were obtained from Amersham (Amersham, England). These included 2-amino (1-^{14}C) isobutyric acid (61 mCi/mmol), L-(U-^{14}C)lysine monohydrochloride (340 mCi/mmol), L-(U-^{14}C)isoleucine (342 mCi/mmol), [6,6'(n)-^{3}H]sucrose (9.7 Ci/mmol).

(^{14}C)ACoA (about 54.4 µCi/mmole, chemical purity 97.5 percent) was obtained from New England Nuclear Corp. (Boston, MA) in 2.5 ml of aqueous solution at pH 4.0. This was diluted to 7.5 ml with phosphate buffer to obtain the stock solution (Sastry and Henderson, 1972).

S-Adenosyl-L-(methyl-^{3}H)methionine (SAM) (64 Ci/nmol) was purchased from New England Nuclear Corp. (Boston, MA). All other reagents were of analytical grade.

Choline acetyltransferase inhibitors

2-Benzoylethyltrimethylammonium (BETA) and α-napthtoylethyltrimethylammonium (α-NETA) were synthesized in our laboratory (Chaturvedi et al., 1978; Janson et al., 1982).

Chemicals used for the formation of S-adenosyl-L-homocysteine (SAH), an inhibitor of enzymatic methylations

Erythro-9-(2-hydroxy-3-nonyl)adenine (EHNA) was supplied by Burroughs Wellcome Co. (Research Triangle Park, NC). L-Homocysteine thiolactone (L-HCT) and adenosine were obtained from Sigma Chemical Co. (St. Louis, MO). SAH was formed in the placental cells along the pathways shown in Figure 1B when the tissue was incubated with adenosine, L-HCT and EHNA.

Preparation of human placental villi

Full term human placentae were collected after either vaginal or Cesarean section deliveries at Vanderbilt University Hospital and transported immediately to the laboratory. They were kept at 4°C for less than 1 h before use. The amniochorion was dissected along the border of each placenta. Erythrocytes are known to accumulate AIB, and unperfused placenta displayed characteristics different from those of blood free placenta (Gustke and Kowalewski, 1970). Therefore, each placenta was perfused to remove fetal blood. The two umbilical arteries were cannulated with suitable polyethylene tubes, and the placenta was flushed with ice-cold 0.9 percent saline containing 0.5 U/ml beef lung heparin (Upjohn, Kalamazoo, MI) until the effluent from the umbilical vein was clear of blood. About 3-4 liters of perfusate was usually required for each placenta. The chorionic and basal plates were removed, and the villous tissue was diced into small fragments (0.1 - 0.3 g) and placed in a beaker of cold, oxygenated Krebs Ringer bicarbonate (KRB) medium containing NaCl, 118.50 mM; KCl, 4.87 mM; $CaCl_2$, 2.54 mM; $MgSO_4$, 1.19 mM; KH_2PO_4, 1.19 mM; $NaHCO_3$, 24.88 mM; dextrose, 11.11 mM and maintained at pH 7.4. The tissue was again washed with ice-cold KRB solution, transferred to a 500 ml flask containing KRB medium and preincubated at 37°C for 90 min. while the medium was continuously aerated with 95 percent O_2/5 percent CO_2. At the end of the preincubation period, the tissue was washed with 250 ml of cold KRB and transferred to the incubation chambers as described below.

Incubation chambers were 50 ml glass syringe barrels (50 cc hypodermic luer syringes, Eisele, Nashville, TN) arranged inverted in a 37°C water bath. The gas mixture (95 percent O_2/5 percent CO_2) was introduced from the tip of the syringe needle into the chamber. The rim of each chamber was coated with a thin line of silicon gel to retard bubbling. There were both control and experimental chambers. Each chamber was filled with 45 ml of KRB. Up to 2 ml of KRB containing dissolved drug were added to each experimental chamber. Two ml of KRB without the drug were added to each control chamber. Sufficient preincubated placental tissue was transferred to each chamber to bring the volume to 50 ml. The tissue was allowed to equilibrate for 5 min before 200 µl of a stock solution (2.5×10^{-2}M) of a labeled amino acid and the corresponding carrier were added to each chamber. The final concentration of the amino acid in each chamber was $10^{-4}M$. The radioactivity in the medium was about 46,640 dpm/ml.

Uptake of the nonmetabolizable amino acid, α-aminoisobutyric acid (AIB)

Details of AIB uptake by isolated placental villus have been described in several papers published from our laboratory (Rowell and Sastry, 1978, 1981; Barnwell and Sastry, 1982). The present studies use minor modifications of these procedures.

The radioactivity of ^{14}C-AIB in the tissue was measured by homogenizing the desiccated tissue with a Brinkmann Polytron. A 0.5 ml aliquot of the homogenate was placed in a glass scintillation vial with 2 ml of "NCS" solubilizer (Amersham Searle Co., Arlington Heights, IL) and dissolved overnight at 50°C. Chemiluminescence was decreased by acidifying the sample with 34 µl of glacial acetic acid per ml of NCS used, waiting until chemiluminescence decayed before counting, and counting samples in the dark. Decolorization was performed by adding 0.5 ml of 30-35 percent H_2O_2. Ten ml of liquid scintillation cocktail were added, and samples were counted in a Beckman CPM-100 Liquid Scintillation System. Quenching by the samples was determined by adding an internal carbon-14 standard of known specific activity and measuring the counting efficiency.

The distribution of AIB was expressed as the intracellular concentration of amino acid in the villous tissue (I) divided by its extracellular concentration (O), to give an I/O ratio. The extracellular space was determined using radiolabeled sucrose as described by Rowell and Sastry (1981). The intracellular space was calculated as described by Smith et al. (1973). The I/O ratio is a measure of the concentrating ability of the active transport carrier in the villous membrane.

Uptake of the metabolizable amino acids--aspartic acid, isoleucine and lysine

For those amino acids which are metabolized, the uptake as a function of time was also expressed as an I/O ratio calculated by the same method used for AIB. However, this expression was complicated by virtue of the entrance of these amino acids into cellular metabolic pathways. Therefore, the distribution of the amino acids between the trichloroacetic acid (TCA) soluble (TCA supernatant) and precipitable (TCA pellet) portions of the placental tissue in the presence or absence of inhibitors was studied. In this procedure, the dessicated tissue was homogenized in 10 ml of ice-cold 20 percent TCA for 1 min using a Brinkman Polytron. A 0.5 ml aliquot of the homogenate was added to a scintillation vial. Another aliquot was centrifuged at 15,000 x g for 30 min in a Sorvall RC-5B refrigerated centrifuge. Samples from the pellet and supernatant were placed in scintillation vials for counting. The samples from the homogenate and pellet were dissolved in 2 ml NCS overnight at 50°C. Samples were handled as described for the determination of AIB in the homogenate.

Determination of ACh

The tissue ACh and ACh released from placental tissue into the incubation medium were extracted and identified by pyrolysis gas chromatography as described by Sastry et al (1976) and Olubadewo and Sastry (1978).

Assay for choline acetyltransferase (ChA) and carnitine acetyltransferase (CaA)

The activity of ChA or CaA was determined by a modification of methods described by Schrier and Shuster (1967), and Sastry and Henderson (1972) in which the labeled acetyl group was enzymatically transferred from 1-^{14}C-acetyl-CoA to choline or carnitine.

Phospholipid methylation

The details of techniques used for separation of membrane phospholipids by thin layer chromatography, their identification, and the assay for phospholipid methyltransferases have been described in earlier papers from our laboratory (Sastry et al., 1981a,b).

Phospholipid N-methyltransferases were assayed by ^{3}H-methyl groups transferred from ^{3}H-SAM to the endogenous phosphatidylethanolamine in the membrane. The total methylation was measured by the incorporation of ^{3}H-methyl groups into phospholipids at 202.24 μM SAM. Methyltransferase I was assayed by the amount of phosphatidyl-N-(^{3}H-methyl)ethanolamine formed at 2.24 μM SAM. Methyltransferase II was assayed by the amount of phosphatidyl-(^{3}H)choline formed.

Protein determinations

Protein content in the homogenates was established according to the method of Lowry et al. (1951).

Statistics

Results are expressed as means and standard errors wherever possible. The significance of the difference between the mean values was calculated by Student's t test. A result was considered significant if its p value was < 0.05.

RESULTS

Effects of 2-benzoylethyltrimethylammonium (BETA) on placental AIB uptake, ChA activity, ACh levels and release of ACh

BETA was found to be a stable, potent and very slowly reversible inhibitor of ChA (Rowell and Sastry, 1978). It had an I_{50} of about 3 μM for inhibiting ChA in vitro, and it caused complete inhibition of partially purified placental ChA at 100 μM. In order to evaluate the effect of ChA inhibition on active amino acid uptake in placental villus, the influence of BETA on I/O ratios for AIB uptake was studied. BETA decreased I/O ratios for AIB uptake by placental villus in a concentration dependent fashion (Figure 2A). A concentration of 0.5 mM BETA caused a maximum decrease in the I/O ratio (72 percent of control). No further decrease in I/O ratio was observed when the concentration of BETA was increased to 1.0 mM. These data support previous observations reported by Rowell and Sastry (1981).

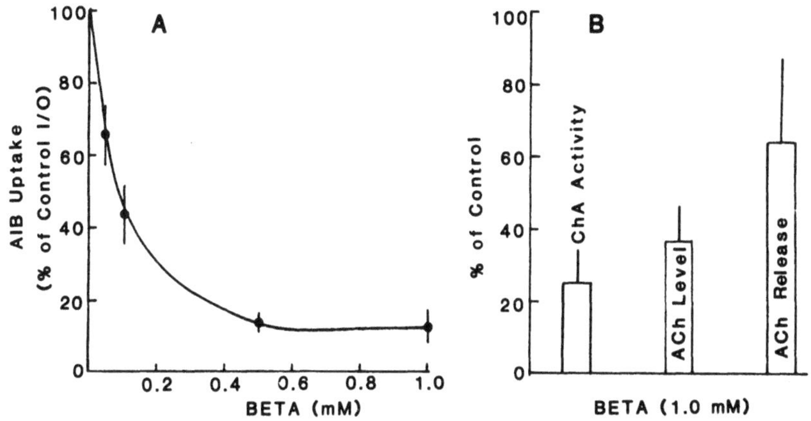

Figure 2. Inhibition of AIB uptake, ChA activity, ACh level and the rate of ACh release by BETA in isolated placental villus. Each point is a mean ± standard error from 4 to 6 values. Villi from the same placenta were used in the control and experimental conditions. A) Concentration-response curve for the inhibition of AIB uptake by BETA. The ordinate represents the percent of control I/O ratio (I: inside concentration; O: outside concentration). The control I/O ratio was 6.24 ± 0.52. All other I/O ratios were expressed as a percentage of this value. The preincubation period was 90 min. At the end of the preincubation period, the tissue was washed and transferred to the incubation chamber. Incubation continued for 2 h in the presence of 0.1 mM AIB with or without BETA. At the end of 2 h, the uptake of AIB was measured by observing changes in the concentration of amino acid in the medium. BETA was present in both the preincubation and incubation medium. B) ChA activity, the rate of ACh release from the trophoblast, and ACh levels were measured from villi of different placentae. The ACh level and ACh release are summarized from Olubadewo (1976).

When AIB uptake was maximally depressed by 1.0 mM BETA, ChA activity in the tissue was decreased by only 66-75%, indicating that all of the enzyme in situ was not accessible to BETA (Figure 2B). The ACh content in the villus was reduced by 52-63%, so 37- 48 percent was still present in the tissue. The original rate of release of ACh was depressed by only 14-36%.

The above observations indicate that BETA was more potent for inhibiting AIB uptake than ChA in situ. Reduction in tissue ACh levels and the rate of ACh release do not completely explain the depression of AIB uptake. Mechanisms other than ChA inhibition may be involved in decreasing placental AIB uptake by BETA.

Depression of AIB uptake and inhibition of ChA by α-naphthoylethyltrimethylammonium (α-NETA)

The α-NETA is a potent inhibitor of ChA (Janson et al., 1982; Moore and Sastry, 1982). It has an I_{50} of 9 μM on partially purified ChA (Figure 3A), and its inhibition is not reversible by dialysis. It did not significantly inhibit highly purified carnitine acetyltransferase (CaA) from pigeon breast muscle. It completely inhibited ChA in vitro and also completely inhibited the active uptake of AIB at 10^{-3} M. The I/O ratio was not significantly lower than one (Figure 3B). The IC_{50} for depression of the I/O ratio of AIB uptake was about 10^{-4}M. However, the tissue concentration of α-NETA estimated by ChA assay was about 8 x 10^{-5}M. Still, α-NETA was about 90 times more potent for inhibiting the purified enzyme than the in situenzyme. ACh levels and ACh release in the presence of α-NETA have yet to be investigated.

Inhibition of the uptake of ^{14}C-labeled neutral, acidic and basic amino acids by BETA, and distribution of radioactivity in TCA pellet and supernatant fractions

BETA, at a concentration of about 60 μM, decreased the I/O ratio of AIB by about 50 percent after 2 h of incubation. The same dose of BETA decreased the I/O ratios of isoleucine, lysine, and aspartic acid by 52, 61, and 72 percent respectively, indicating that BETA is seemingly more effective in depressing the uptake of neutral amino acids than basic and acidic amino acids.

In order to determine to what extent the amino acids entered cellular metabolic pathways, the distribution of ^{14}-C-amino acids between the TCA soluble and insoluble fractions was determined (Figure 4). With AIB, most of the administered radioactivity (99-106%) was recovered in the TCA-supernant fraction. Although BETA (0.1 mM) decreased the I/O ratio for AIB uptake by 50%, it did not alter the distribution of AIB. With lysine, isoleucine and aspartic acid, 46, 43 and 66 percent respectively of the total radioactivity taken up was in the TCA-supernatant fraction. Thirty-eight, 56, and 21 percent respectively was in the TCA-pellet fraction. With lysine and isoleucine, the total radioactivity taken up by the tissue could be accounted for by the radioactivity in these two fractions. With aspartic acid, about 9-11 percent of the total radioactivity was not recovered, possibly because of a decarboxylation step in its metabolism. The presence of BETA lowered the amount of radioactivity incorporated into the TCA-pellet fraction and increased the radioactivity in the TCA-supernatant fraction. These effects of BETA were significant when the tissue was incubated with lysine or isoleucine. These observations indicate that BETA inhibited protein synthesis in placenta.

Role of Ca^{++} in the uptake of AIB by placental villus

In view of the importance of Ca^{++} for the release of ACh (Olubadewo and Sastry, 1978) and the role of ACh in AIB uptake (Rowell and Sastry, 1978, 1981), the uptake of AIB in Ca^{++}-free medium and in the presence of 2.54 mM Ca^{++} (control) was studied (Figure 5A). The Ca^{++}-free medium contained Na^+, K^+, and Mg^{++}. It also contained disodium EDTA or EGTA (2.05 mM). In the Ca^{++}free medium AIB uptake was depressed. The I/O ratio was about 10 percent of the control after 1 h of incubation, and there was no further decrease after 2 h. The I/O ratio for AIB uptake was restored to its normal value within one h by adding 2.5 or 7.5 mM Ca^{++} to the incubation medium.

The rate of ACh release was inhibited by about 96-98 percent when the tissue was incubated for 2 h in a Ca^{++}-free medium (Figure 5B).

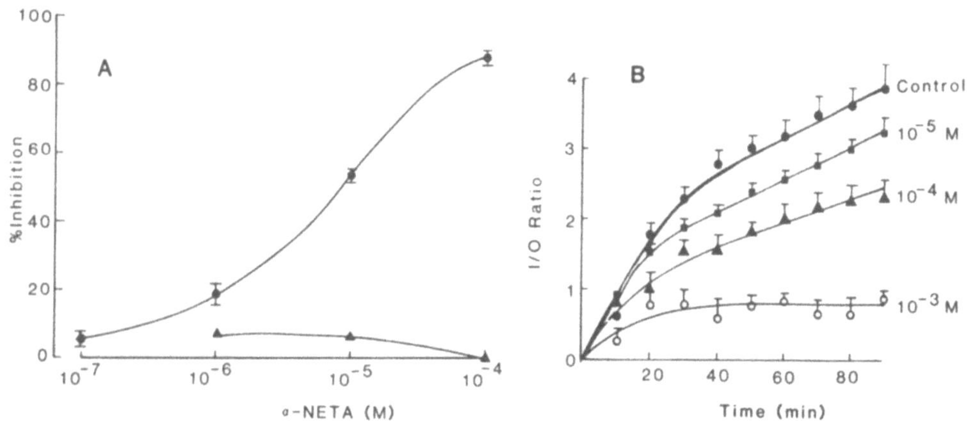

Figure 3. A) Inhibition of partially purified placental ChA by α-NETA (upper curve) and highly purified pigeon breast carnitine acetyltransferase (lower curve). B) I/O Ratios for the uptake of AIB as a function of time. The conditions for this experiment are similar to those described for BETA in the legend for Figure 2.

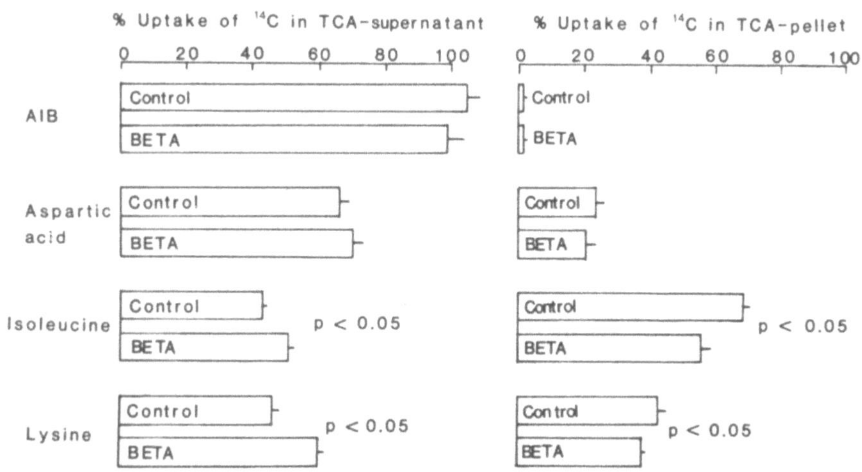

Figure 4. Distribution of the ^{14}C-activity of the amino acids AIB, aspartic acid, isoleucine, and lysine into the tricholoracetic acid (TCA) pellet and TCA-supernatant when the placental villus was incubated with BETA (0.1 mM) for 2 h. All values are expressed as percent of total uptake of the radioactivity into the tissue.

Preincubation in the absence of amino acid increases the uptake of amino acids and protein synthesis. Incubation of placental villus in a Ca^{++}-free medium did not increase the ACh level, but incubation of the tissue in the presence of Ca^{++} increased the ACh level by about 250 percent in 2 h (Figure 5C). It is not known if incubation of placental villus in normal Ca^{++} induces the synthesis of ChA.

Depression of AIB uptake by inhibition of phospholipid methylation

As discussed in the introduction, phospholipid methylation regulates Ca^{++} fluxes in some tissues. Ca^{++} is required both for increasing ACh levels and ACh release in placenta. Therefore, the effect of the inhibition of phospholipid methylation by S-adenosyl-L-homocysteine (SAH) on AIB uptake by placental villus was studied. SAH does not enter the cells efficiently. Therefore, the intracellular level of SAH was increased by incubating the tissue with L-homocysteine thiolactone (L-HCT, 100 µM), adenosine (100 µM), and erythro-9-(2-hydroxy-3-nonyl) adenine (EHNA, 10 µM), an inhibitor of adenosine deaminase, for 2 h (Pike et al., 1978) (Figure 1B). AIB uptake by the placental villus was enhanced by about 25-30 percent when the tissue was incubated with adenosine alone for 1 h (Figure 6A1) or 2 h (Figure 6A2). Neither L-HCT nor EHNA had a significant effect on AIB uptake. When the tissue was incubated with a mixture of adenosine, L-HCT, and EHNA, the I/O ratio for AIB uptake was depressed by 40 percent after 2 h (Figure 6A2).

After 2 h of incubation, the tissue extracts were analyzed for SAH by HPLC (Figure 6, B1-B5). Standard SAH has a retention time of 20 minutes. When the tissue was incubated alone (Figure 6B1, control) or in the presence of L-HCT (Figure 6B3), EHNA (Figure 6B4) or adenosine (Figure 6B5) alone, the presence of SAH could not be detected in HPLC chromatograms. When the tissue was incubated with a mixture of adenosine, L-HCT and EHNA, a large peak in the HPLC chromatogram was observed (Figure 6B2). These observations indicate that SAH was formed in the tissue when adenosine, L-HCT and EHNA were present in the incubation medium and phospholipid methylation was inhibited.

The tissue was also analyzed after two hs of incubation for phospholipid methyltransferases. PME formation was inhibited by 60 percent at a 1 µM SAM concentration. Methyltransferase I was inhibited by about 60%. PC formation was inhibited by about 40 percent at a 51 µM SAM concentration. Methyltransferase II was inhibited by about 40%. The rate limiting enzyme in stepwise phospholipid methylation is Methyltransferase I (Sastry et al., 1981a,b). This enzyme is considered to regulate membrane fluidity and Ca^{++} fluxes. This enzyme was inhibited to a greater extent in the present experimental conditions.

Influence of colchicine on the uptake of AIB by isolated placental villus

Microtubules are known to regulate certain types of cellular movement and secretory processes (Wilson and Meza, 1973). Colchicine disrupts microtubules. The effect of colchicine on AIB uptake was studied in order to evaluate the role of microtubules in amino acid uptake by placental villus. Colchicine (2.4×10^{-4}M) inhibited about 30 ± 3 percent of AIB uptake. This indicates that the microtubular system may be necessary for "amplification" of the uptake of AIB by the placental villus.

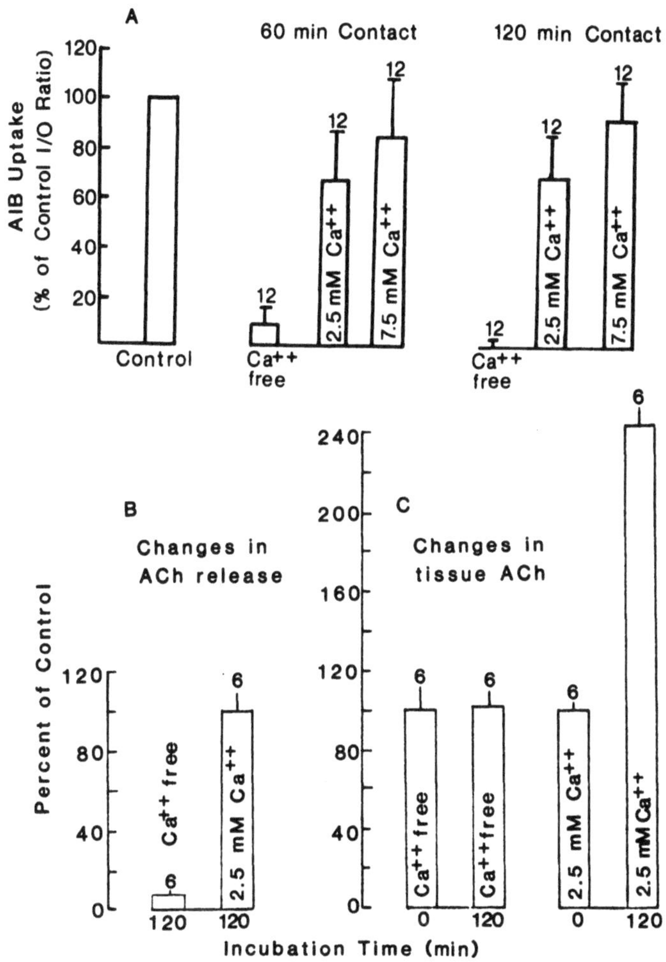

Figure 5. Effects of Ca^{++} on A) AIB uptake, B) changes in ACh release, and C) changes in tissue ACh. The control I/O ratio for AIB uptake for placentae in panel A was 10.2 ± 0.6 at 60 min and 15.2 ± 0.7 at 120 min. Villi from the same group of placentae were used for control and experimental groups. All experimental values are expressed as percentage of control values determined with villi from the same placenta. Bars are means, and the vertical lines are standard errors from the number of observations indicated over the bars.

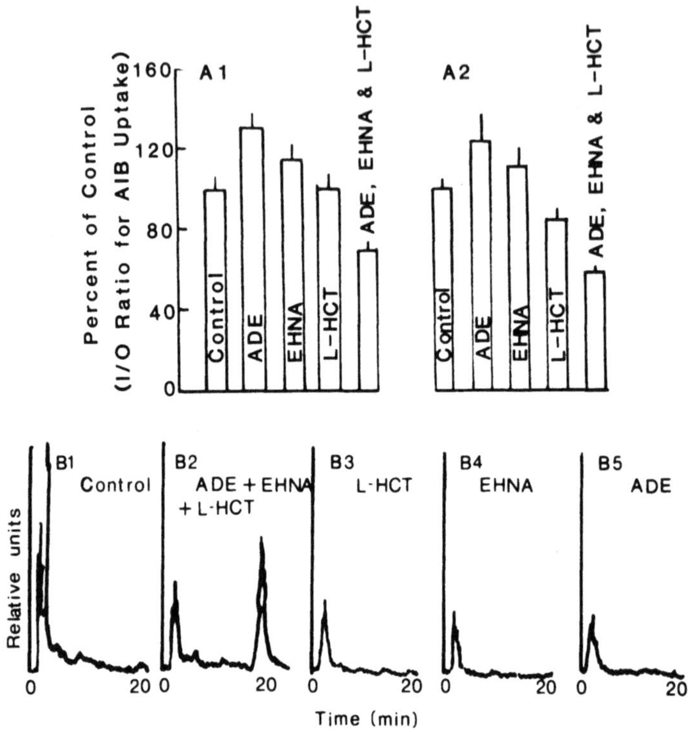

Figure 6. Depression of AIB uptake by the isolated placental villus when it was incubated for 1 h (A1) or 2 h (A2) with adenosine (ADE), erythro-9-(2-hydroxy-3-nonyl)adenine (EHNA), and L-homocysteine thiolactone (L-HCT) individually or together. The control I/O ratio for placentae in panels A1 and A2 were 4.5 ± 0.1 at 1 h and 7.1 ± 0.2 at 2 h. Villi for control and drug-treated groups were obtained from the same group of placentae. Each bar is a mean ± standard error from 5 values. In the presence of all three, a peak demonstrating the presence of S-adenosylhomocysteine (SAH) in extracts of the placental villus tissue appeared on an HPLC chromatogram with a retention time of 20 min (B2). The peak at 20 minutes was not detectable when the issue was incubated with buffer (B1), or buffer containing L-HCT (B3), EHNA (B4) or ADE (B5) individually.

DISCUSSION

Several factors influence the uptake of amino acids into placental villus. Of these, requirements for oxidative energy sources and optimum conditions for AIB uptake are well established. Several other factors necessary for optimum uptake of AIB by placental villus--ACh, membrane phospholipid methylation, extracellular Ca^{++} ions, and microtubules--are not well understood. These constituents seem to regulate AIB, and they seem to be related to one another. Extracellular Ca^{++} may occupy a central position in their interrelationships.

Entry of extracellular Ca^{++} is necessary for spontaneous or drug (e.g., nicotine) induced release of ACh from placental villus (Sastry et al., 1977; Olubadewo and Sastry, 1978). According to the present investigations, AIB uptake is depressed in the absence of extracellular Ca^{++}. Although there is no direct evidence that phospholipid methylation affects Ca^{++} fluxes in human placental villus, phospholipid methylation increased Ca^{++} efflux and Ca^{++}-ATPase activity in erythrocytes (Strittmatter et al., 1979). The maximum increase in ATPase activity was achieved at a low concentration of SAM when PME accumulated in the membrane. In the present investigation, inhibition of phospholipid methylation depressed AIB uptake by the placental villus, and the formation of PME was inhibited to a greater degree than the formation of PC.

Microtubules are arbitrarily divided into two classes, labile and stable. Microtubules found in the axons and dendrites of the nervous system, the mitotic apparatus of dividing cells, and the cytoplasm of animal as well as plant cells fall into the labile category (Wilson and Meza, 1973). It is generally believed that labile microtubules are in a state of dynamic equilibrium. Colchicine produces disruption of microtubules and thereby interferes with mitosis, certain types of cellular movement and secretory processes. It does not disrupt intact microtubules by directly binding to the tubule. Rather, it binds to monomer tubulin in soluble pools, thereby destroying the sensitive equilibrium that exists between monomer and polymer (Wilson et al., 1974). If the dynamic microtubular assembly is present in the cytoplasm of the syncytiotrophoblast and is necessary for the secretion of ACh and the uptake of AIB by the trophoblast, colchicine should interfere with these processes. In the present investigation, AIB uptake was depressed by colchicine, indicating that the formation of a microtubular assembly may be necessary for the efficient uptake of AIB. There is additional indirect evidence that intact cellular organization is necessary for efficient uptake of AIB. According to Olubadewo (1976), subcellular fractionation of homogenates of human placental villus results in the localization of ACh in the cytosol, and calcium pump activity is localized in the microsomes. Attempts to discover if uptake activity could be localized in one of the subcellular fractions were not successful. None of the subcellular fractions exhibited efficient AIB uptake activity. Active uptake was observed only with minced placenta, which contained intact placental cells. These observations indicate that there are no intracellular sequestering sites for AIB, and the intact plasma membrane is required for AIB uptake. Mechanisms for ACh release, calcium pump activity, and amino acid uptake are linked only in intact cells.

ACh storage vesicles, which are comparable to synaptic vesicles, were not isolated from placental villus by subcellular fractionation of its homogenates. There is no anatomical equivalent of the synaptosome, from which ACh vesicles could be liberated, in the syncytiotrophoblast. However, there is some indirect evidence that ACh is present in a bound form in placenta. Cold storage (4°C) of placenta for 72 h did not significantly alter placental ACh levels (Sastry et al., 1976). On the other hand, freezing-thawing treatments led to total destruction of placental ACh. Stone (1955) has reported similar observations on ACh in the brain. These findings indicate some form of tissue storage for placental ACh which has not yet been investigated.

Olubadewo (1976) prepared a highspeed supernatant fraction of human placental homogenate and subjected it to equilibrium dialysis. The concentration of ACh (nmol/ml) remaining inside the dialysis bags exceeded the concentration outside of the bag by about 37%. This indicates some ACh binding to cytoplasmic proteins or other macromolecules. These observations indicate that there are at least two forms of ACh in syncytiotrophoblast, free and bound ACh. The present study indicates that there are two fractions of ACh in placenta, one releasable and one stored. These two fractions can be influenced independently of one another. According to the present studies, preincubation of the placental villus increases both the rate of ACh release and the level of ACh in the tissue as a function of time. The ChA inhibitor BETA depressed ACh levels to a greater degree than its rate of release. Similar observations were reported by Welsch et al. (1981a) and Leventer et al. (1982). When placental tissue was incubated in a Ca^{++}-free medium, ACh levels were not altered, whereas the rate of ACh release was completely eliminated.

A question arises whether the rate of ACh release or the ACh level is more significant for the regulation of AIB uptake by placental villus tissue. In consideration of the effects of ACh in the nervous system, it is reasonable to expect that the rate of ACh release is more physiologically relevant and is linked to amino acid transport systems in the placenta. In a Ca^{++}-free medium, both the rate of ACh release and AIB uptake were depressed. ACh levels were unchanged. In preincubation experiments, both releasable and stored pools of ACh in the villus were increased, and the rate of AIB uptake cannot be completely explained by ChA inhibition and the corresponding decrease in tissue ACh levels, especially at high concentrations of BETA. BETA in a concentration of 520 μM caused full blockade of muscarinic receptors (EC50, 260 μM) in innervated structures (Rowell et al., 1978). According to Fant and Harbison (1981), trophoblast membrane vesicles contain muscarinic receptors which are similar to those in innervated structures in certain aspects. Cholinergic receptors involved in the regulation of ACh release from placenta were also blocked by high concentrations of nicotine (Olubadewo and Sastry, 1978). At 240 μM, it caused full blockade of nicotinic receptors (EC50, 120 μM) in the innervated structures. Although BETA did not inhibit acetylcoenzyme A formation by ATP-citrate lyase, it inhibited 99 percent of acetate thiokinase in brain at 100 μM (Sastry, Janson and Chaturvedi, unpublished observations). It is possible, therefore, that BETA may reduce the pool of acetylcoenzyme A available for ACh synthesis in placenta. Therefore, part of the effect of BETA on AIB uptake may be due to blockade of cholinergic receptors and synthesis of acetylcoenzyme A in syncytiotrophoblast. The relationships between ChA inhibition and the depression of AIB uptake by α-NETA are still under investigation. However, the available data suggest that ACh synthesis and release are linked to amino acid uptake systems in the placental villus. Detailed conclusions can be made only after more information becomes available on (a) different ACh pools in placental villus, (b) links between the releasable pool and the stored pool, (c) the nature of the placental cholinergic receptors and (d) the selectivity of BETA and α-NETA for inhibiting ChA.

Increasing the intracellular levels of SAH inhibited phospholipid methylation and AIB uptake by the placental villus. This observation suggests that inhibition of AIB uptake by placental villus was partly due to the inhibition of phospholipid methylation in the plasma membrane. The extent of the part played by inhibition of phospholipid methylation cannot be assessed from the available data, because SAH inhibits all SAM mediated methylations (Pugh et al., 1978; Diliberto et al., 1979; Eiden et al., 1979; Sastry et al., 1982). Methylation of COOH, -SH and >NH groups in proteins can alter surface charges and affect the structure and function of membranes. Protein carboxymethylation has been shown to be involved in neurosecretory processes. There are no studies which indicate that inhibition of protein carboxymethylation may decrease ACh release from placental villus, thus contributing to the inhibition of AIB uptake. Preincubation of the placental villus in the absence of amino acids does increase the synthesis of carrier proteins (Smith and Depper, 1974; Gusseck et al., 1975). The present experiments were conducted in the presence of AIB. Therefore, inhibition of nuclear protein methylation by SAH may not play a significant role in the inhibition of AIB uptake by placenta.

SUMMARY

Placental insufficiency for the transport of amino acids may contribute to intrauterine fetal growth retardation. Therefore, effects of several factors on the uptake of amino acids by isolated placental villus using mainly the nonmetabolizable α-aminoisobutyric acid (AIB) were studied. In a limited number of experiments, aspartic acid, isoleucine and lysine were used. The following results were obtained: (1) 2-Benzoylethyltrimethylammonium (BETA), an inhibitor of choline acetyltransferase (ChA) inhibited AIB uptake and lowered ChA and acetylcholine (ACh) levels and decreased ACh release. (2) BETA inhibited incorporation of metabolizable amino acids into proteins, possibly by lowering ACh levels. (3) α-Naphthoylethyltrimethylammonium (α-NETA) inhibited ChA and AIB uptake by placental villus. There was a positive relationship between the inhibition of ChA and the depression of AIB uptake by the villous tissue. The inhibition of placental ChA by α-NETA was not reversed by washing the tissue or by dialyzing the homogenates. (4) Placental villus contains two phospholipid N-methyltransferases (PMT I and II). In the presence of S-adenosyl-L-methionine, PMT I converted phosphatidylethanolamine into phosphatidyl-N-methylethanolamine (PME), and PMT II converted PME into phosphatidylcholine. Inhibiting PMTs in plasma membrane by increasing the intracellular levels of S-adenosyl-L-homocysteine (SAH) in the placental villus inhibited AIB uptake. (5) Ca^{++} is required for both release of ACh and AIB uptake. (6) Inhibition of the microtubular assembly by colchicine depressed AIB uptake. (7) Whole placental trophoblast cells are necessary for efficient active uptake of AIB. These observations indicate that (1) ACh synthesis, its release, and its activation of the cholinergic receptor; (2) membrane phospholipid methylation, Ca^{++} transport, and amino acid transport systems; and (3) an organized cytoskeletal system are linked to one another for effective transport of AIB across human placental trophoblast.

ACKNOWLEDGMENTS

This investigation was partially supported by a grant from the Council for Tobacco Research, U.S.A., Inc. and by United States Public Health Service Research Grants ES-03172, HD-10607 and RR-05424. Two of the authors (S.L.B. and R.D.M.) were supported by a predoctoral traineeship from the National Institutes of Health Grant GM0058 from the National Institutes of General Medical Sciences.

REFERENCES

Axelrod, J. and Hirata, F. (1981) Phospholipid methylation and receptor mediated transmission of biological signals through membranes. In *Drug Receptors and Their Effectors* (ed.), Birdsall, N.J.M., pp. 51-58, London and Basingstoke: MacMillan Publishers LTD.

Barnwell, S.L. and Sastry, B.V.R. (1981a) The role of enzymatic phospholipid methylation on amino acid uptake in human placental villus. *Fed. Proc.* 40, 667.

Barnwell, S.L. and Sastry, B.V.R. (1981b) Depression of the active uptake of α-amnioisobutyric acid by the isolated placental villus during inhibition of phospholipid methylation. *Proc. Eighth Internat. Cong. Pharm., Japanese Pharmacological Society and Science Council of Japan,* Abstracts, p. 814.

Barnwell, S.L. and Sastry, B.V.R. (1982) Influences of nicotine and tobacco gases on the uptake of neutral amino acids by isolated placental villus. *J. Environ. Pathol. Oncol.* 5, 549-563.

Chaturvedi, A.K., Rowell, P.P. and Sastry, B.V.R. (1978) Relationships between chemical structure and inhibition of human placental choline acetyltransferase by keto-analogs of acetylcholine. *J. Pharm. Sci.* 67, 657-660.

Christensen, H.N. (1973) On the development of amino acid transport systems. *Fed. Proc.* 32, 19-28.

Diliberto, E.J., Jr., O'Dea, R.F. and Viveros, O.H. (1979) The role of protein carboxy-methylase in secretory and chemotactic eukarotic cells. In *Transmethylation* (ed.), Usdin, E., Borchardt, R.T. and Creveling, C.R., pp. 529-538, New York: Elsevier/North Holland.

Eiden, L.E., Borchardt, R.T. and Rutledge, C.O. (1979) Protein carboxymethylation in neurosecretory processes. In *Transmethylation* (ed.), Usdin, E., Borchardt, R.T. and Creveling, C.R., pp. 539-546, New York: Elsevier/North Holland.

Fant, M.E. and Harbison R.D. (1981) Syncytiotrophoblast membrane vesicles: A model for examining the human placental cholinergic system. *Teratology* 24, 187-199.

Gusseck, D.J., Yuen, P. and Longo, D. (1975) Amino acid transport in placental slices. Mechanisms of increased accumulation by prolonged incubation. *Biochim. Biophys. Acta* 401, 278-284.

Gustke, H. and Kowalewski, S. (1970) Effect of perfusion on biochemical composition of the human placenta. *Biol. Neonate* 30, 116-122.

Hirata, F. and Axelrod, J. (1978) Enzymatic methylation of phosphatidylethanol-amine increases erthrocyte membrane fluidity, *Nature* (London) 275, 219-220.

Hirata, F. and Axelrod, J. (1980) Phospholipid methylation and biological signal transmission. *Science* 209, 1082-1090.

Jaiswal, R.K., Sastry, B.V.R. and Landon, E.J. (1982) Changes in microsmal membrane microviscosity and phospholipid methyltransferases during rat liver regeneration. *Pharm. (Basel)* 24, 355-365.

Janson, V.E., Jaiswal, N. and Sastry, B.V.R. (1982) Depression of human sperm motility by α-naphthoylethyltrimethylammonium and its tertiary analog, novel inhibitors of choline acetyltransferase. *The Pharmacologist* 24, 238.

Leventer, S.M., Rowell, P.P. and Clark, M.J. (1982) The effect of choline acetyltransferase inhibition on acetylcholine synthesis and release in term human placenta. J. *Pharma. Exp. Therap.* 32, 301-305.

Longo, L.D., Yuen, P. and Gusseck, D.J. (1973) Anaerobic, glycogen-dependent transport of amino acids by the placenta. *Nature* 243, 531-533.

Lowry, O.H., Rosebrough, N.J., Farr, A.L. and Randall, R.J. (1951) Protein measurement with the Folin phenol reagent. *Biol. Chem.* 193, 265-275.

Miller, R.K. and Berndt, W.O. (1973) Evidence for a Mg^{++} dependent, Na^{++} K^{+} activated ATPase and Ca^{++}-ATPase in human term placenta. *Proc. Soc. Exp. Biol. Med.* 143, 118-122.

Miller, R.K. and Berndt, W.O. (1974) Characterization of neutral amino acid accumulation by human term placental slices. *Amer. Physiol.* 277, 1236-1242.

Moore, R.D. and Sastry, B.V.R. (1982) Depression of the uptake of α-aminoisobutyric acid in human placental villus by novel inhibitors of choline acetyltransferase, *The Pharmacologist* 24, 101.

Olubadewo, J. (1976) Human placental cholinergic system: Occurrence, distribution, variation with gestational age and release of acetylcholine. Ph.D. Thesis, Vanderbilt University, Nashville, Tennessee, University Microfilms, Ann Arbor, Michigan, No. 76-22359.

Olubadewo, J.O. and Sastry, B.V.R. (1978) Human placental cholinergic system: Stimulation-secretion coupling for release of acetylcholine from isolated placental villus, *J. Pharm. Exp. Therap.* 204, 433-455.

Pike, M.C., Kredich, N.M. and Snyderman, R. (1978) Requirements of S-adenosyl-L-methionine mediated methylation for human monocyte chemotaxis. *Proc. Nat. Acad. Sci. U.S.A.* 75, 3928-3932.

Pugh, C.S.G., Borchardt, R.T. and Stone, H.O. (1978) Sinefungin, a potent inhibitor of Virion mRNA (guanine) methyltransferase, mRNA (nucleoside-2')-methyltransferase, and viral multiplication. *J. Biol. Chem.* 253, 4075-4077.

Rowell, P.P., Chaturvedi, A., and Sastry, B.V.R. (1978) (2-Benzoylethyl)-trimethylammonium chloride: A new, selective and stable inhibitor of human placental choline acetyltransferase. *J. Pharm. Exp. Therap.* 205, 624-634.

Rowell, P.P. and Sastry, B.V.R. (1978) The influence of cholinergic blockade on the uptake of α-aminoisobutyric acid by isolated human placental villi. *Tox. Appl. Pharm.* 45, 79-93.

Rowell, P.P. and Sastry, B.V.R. (1981) Human placental cholinergic system: Depression of the uptake of α-aminoisobutyric acid in isolated human placental villi by choline acetyltransferase inhibitors. *J. Pharm. Exp. Therap.* 216, 232-238.

Sastry, B.V.R. and Henderson, G.I. (1972) Kinetic mechanisms of human placental choline acetyltransferase. *Biochem. Pharm.* 21, 787-802.

Sastry, B.V.R. and Henderson, G.I. (1976) Mechanisms of acetylcholine synthesis and its regulation by products and inhibitors. In *Drugs and Central Synaptic Transmission* (ed.), Bradley, P.B. and Dhawan, B.N., pp. 89-98, Baltimore: University Park Press.

Sastry, B.V.R. and Sadavongvivad, C. (1979) Cholinergic systems in non-nervous tissues. *Pharm. Rev.* 30, 65-132.

Sastry, B.V.R., Olubadewo, J.O. and Boehm, F.H. (1977) Effects of nicotine and cocaine on the release of acetylcholine from isolated human placental villi. *Arch. Inter. Pharm. Therap.* 229, 23-36.

Sastry, B.V.R., Owens, L.K. and Janson, V.E. (1982) Enhancement of the responsiveness of the rat diaphragm by L-methionine and phospholipid methylation and their relationships to aging. *J. Pharm. Exp. Therap.* 221, 629- 636.

Sastry, B.V.R., Olubadewo, J., Harbison, R.D. and Schmidt, D.E. (1976) Human placental cholinergic system: Occurrence distribution and variation with gestational age of acetylcholine in human placenta. *Biochem. Pharmacol.* 25, 425-431.

Sastry, B.V.R., Statham, C.N., Meeks, R.G. and Axelrod, J. (1981a) Changes in phospholipid methyltransferases and membrane microviscosity during induction of rat liver microsomal cytochrome P-450 by phenobarbital and 3-methylcholanthrene. *Pharm. (Basel)* 23, 211-232.

Sastry, B.V.R., Statham, C.N., Axelrod, J. and Hirata, F. (1981b) Evidence for two methyltransferases involved in the conversion of phosphatidylethanolamine to phosphatidylcholine in the rat liver. *Arch. Biochem. Biophys.* 21, 762-774.

Schneider, H. and Dancis, J. (1974) Amino acid transport in human placental slices. *Amer. J. Obstet. Gynecol.* 120, 1092-1097

Schrier, B.K. and Shuster, L. (1967) A simplified radiochemical assay for choline acetyltransferase. *J. Neurochem.* 14, 977-985.

Singer, S.J. and Nicolson, G.L. (1972) The fluid mosaic model of the structure of cell membranes: Cell membranes are viewed as two dimensional solutions of oriented globular proteins and lipids. *Science* 175, 720-731.

Smith, C.H, Adcock, E.W., Teasdale, F., Meschia, G. and Battaglia, F.C. (1973) Placental amino acid uptake: tissue preparation, kinetics and preincubation effect. *Amer. J. Physiol.* 224, 558-564.

Smith, C.H. and Depper, R. (1974) Placental amino acid uptake. II. Tissue preincubation, fluid distribution and mechanisms of regulation. *Pediat. Res.* 8, 697-703.

Stone, W.E. (1955) Acetylcholine in the brain. I. "Free," "bound" and total acetylcholine. *Arch. Biochem. Biophys.* 59, 181-192.

Strittmatter, W.J., Hirata, F. and Axelrod, J. (1979) Increased Ca^{++}-ATPase activity associated with methylation of phospholipids in human erthrocytes. *Biochem. Biophys. Res. Comm.* 88, 147-153.

Welsch, F. and Wenger, W.C. (1980) Acetylcholine in human placenta. Identification by pyrolysis gas chromatography/mass spectrometry and tissue levels following different modes of delivery. *Naunyn-Schmiedeberg's Arch. Pharm.* 311, 113-118.

Welsch, F., Wenger, W.C. and Stedman, D.B. (1981a) Acetylcholine in human term placenta: Tissue levels in intact fragments after inhibition in vitro of choline acetyltransferase and relationship to (^{14}C)α-aminoisobutyric acid uptake. *Placenta (Supple. 3)* 339-351.

Welsch, F., Wenger, W.C. and Stedman, D.B. (1981b) Choline metabolism in placenta: evidence for the biosynthesis of phosphatidylcholine in microsomes via the methylation pathway. *Placenta* 2, 211-221.

Wilson, L. and Meza, I. (1973) The mechanism of action of cholchicine: Colchicine binding properties of sea urchin sperm tail doublet tubulin. *J. Cell. Biol.* 58, 709-719.

Wilson, L., Bamburg, J.R., Mizel, S.B., Grisham, L.M. and Creswell, K.M. (1974) Interaction of drugs with microtubule proteins. *Fed. Proc.* 33, 158-166.

DISCUSSION

PANIGEL (Paris): As a cytologist, I am interested in your reported effect of colchicine on microtubular assembly, which leads to depression in the AIB uptake and in the uptake of amino acids in general. Do you have any electron microscopic evidence corresponding to the effects of colchicine and the measurements you have shown in this report? Is this effect on microtubular assembly an assumption or observation? This is important because the cytoskeleton of the syncytiotrophoblast has a very particular appearance as shown by Ockleford and associates (*Biology of the Trophoblast*, Chapter 3, 1983). Do you have these parallel biochemical and electron microscopic studies?

SASTRY (Nashville): Colchicine has been studied in several other tissues. At the present time, it is an assumption we are making. We have to perform the histological and electron microscopic studies.

MILLER (Rochester): In your presentation, you indicated that calcium plays an integral role in the uptake of AIB by human placental slices. We have previously noted (*Amer. J. Physiol.*, 1974) that this transport process is also quite dependent upon magnesium. Have you determined whether magnesium is important in the control of acetylcholine in the placenta?

SASTRY (Nashville): Magnesium does have a marked effect on acetylcholine release in the nerve. In the human placenta, it is not as effective on releasing acetylcholine. I have not investigated this in detail, but it should certainly be explored further.

VAN KREEL (Rotterdam): Do you know the isoelectric point of AIB? When we have measured the uptake of ions, the cell potential is of importance. If you altered the extracellular calcium concentration, you may also alter the cell potentials. You can expect an effect on uptake of any charged molecules, so I suggest that it is important to determine how specific the calcium effect is on AIB uptake. Calcium may have an effect on uptake of other ions as well.

SASTRY (Nashville): We were thinking that calcium has an effect on acetylcholine release which in turn opens up the gates or pores on the membrane. Then again, calcium may have a direct effect on amino acid transport.

Trophoblast Research 1:101-120, 1983

DEPRESSION OF AMINO ACID UPTAKE IN HUMAN PLACENTAL VILLUS BY COCAINE, MORPHINE AND NICOTINE

Stanley L. Barnwell and B.V. Rama Sastry[1]

Department of Pharmacology, Vanderbilt University School of Medicine
Nashville, Tennessee 37232 U.S.A.

INTRODUCTION

There are several drugs which are known to cause intrauterine growth retardation in experimental animals and man (Tuchmann-Duplessis, 1975). This retarded growth may predispose neonates to perinatal morbidity and mortality. Morphine is known to be associated with retarded intrauterine growth, the extent of which is apparently related to the amount of exposure (Stone et al., 1971). Nicotine and smoking are also implicated in intrauterine fetal growth retardation (Tuchmann-Duplessis, 1975; Hasselmeyer et al., 1979). Prior studies in our laboratory have demonstrated dose-related inhibition of the uptake of the amino acid, α-aminoisobutyric acid (AIB), by components of tobacco smoke (Barnwell and Sastry, 1982). Intrauterine fetal growth retardation among cocaine addicts has not been well documented. However, its use as an euphoric drug has recently become more popular, and greater numbers of pregnant females may be exposing their offspring to the drug (Ellinwood and Kilbey, 1975). Amino acids for fetal protein synthesis and metabolic energy have to be transported from maternal blood to the fetal circulation through the placenta. There is, however, little information on the effects of the above drugs on amino acid transport in human placenta.

Amino acid transport in the placenta and its regulation has been the subject of numerous studies. The transport has been shown to be stereospecific (Page et al., 1957) and capable of generating higher concentrations of amino acids in the fetal blood compared to the maternal blood (Dancis et al., 1968). There is a net unidirectional flow of AIB from maternal blood to the fetus as inferred from in vivo studies using pregnant guinea pigs and radiolabeled AIB (Hayter et al., 1964). The uptake of AIB, a nonmetabolizable amino acid, by human placental slices, has been shown to be dependent on sodium and potassium ions in the medium, and dependent on both aerobic and anaerobic mechanisms (Miller and Berndt, 1974). In the placenta, there are at least three amino acid transport systems (Enders et al., 1976) corresponding to the systems described by Christensen (1975). That regulation occurs for amino acid transport is partly suggested by the preincubation effect: an increase in the uptake of AIB after preincubating the placental villus tissue for up to 24 h in the absence of amino acids (Smith et al., 1973). This preincubation effect has been shown to be limited to one of the transport systems, the "A" system (Enders et al., 1976). Other tissues which exhibit a similar preincubation effect for the uptake of AIB by the "A" system include chick embryo hearts (Gazzola et al., 1972) and estrogen-primed uterus of the rat (Riggs and Pan, 1972).

1. To whom reprints should be addressed.

The role of the cholinergic system in regulating placental amino acid transport in human placenta was proposed several years ago (Harbison et al., 1975) and has been developed along several lines. Human placental tissue contains high concentrations of acetylcholine (ACh) (Sastry et al., 1976) and releases this ACh into the maternal circulation (Olubadewo and Sastry, 1978). Regulation of amino acid transport is just one of the many roles in which the placental cholinergic system is involved (Sastry and Sadavongvivad, 1979). Cholinergic blockade by ACh (2 mM and atropine (500 μM) inhibited accumulation of AIB by human placental villus tissue 34 percent and 61 percent respectively (Rowell and Sastry, 1978). 2-Benzoylethyltrimethylammonium (BETA) has been shown to be a selective inhibitor of choline acetyltransferase (ChA) (Rowell et al., 1978). This agent has recently been shown to inhibit AIB uptake by placental villus (ED_{50}, 62 μM) (Rowell and Sastry, 1981) and to lower placental ACh levels (Welsch et al., 1981; Leventer et al., 1982; Sastry et al., 1983). Involvement of cholinergic function in the transport of substances other than amino acids has recently been described (Welsch, 1980). In that study, the clearance of ^3H-antipyrine from an in vitro maternal circulation was reduced by ACh (70 μM ACh produced a 24 percent depression) and physostigmine (10 μM physostigmine produced a 12 percent depression).

To further elucidate the role of the cholinergic system in the placenta, we have studied the effects of cocaine, morphine and nicotine on amino acid transport. Cocaine (28 μM) inhibited the spontaneous release of ACh from placental villus tissue by 34 percent (Sastry et al., 1977). Morphine, in a concentration as low as 0.1 μM, decreased ACh release from cholinergic nerve endings in guinea pig ileum and interfered with the muscle stimulation by the nerve (Paton, 1957; Schaumann, 1957). Nicotine (58 μM) increased spontaneous ACh release (34 percent) from placental tissue (Olubadewo and Sastry, 1978). In higher concentrations, nicotine (2.5 mM) produced cholinergic blockade and depressed AIB uptake by placental tissue (Rowell and Sastry, 1978). The release of ACh from placental villi was absolutely dependent on extracellular Ca^{++} (Olubadewo and Sastry, 1978).

The amino acids for the present study include AIB, aspartic acid, isoleucine, and lysine. AIB transport appears to be mediated mainly by the "A" system as described by Christensen (1975), while isoleucine transport is mediated by the "L" system (Enders et al., 1976). The transport of lysine occurs by at least two systems in Escherichia coli, and at least one is specific for lysine (Rosen, 1971). In cell cultures, this sytem has been termed the "LYS+" system (Borghetti et al., 1980). In certain bacteria, the uptake of aspartic acid occurs by two systems, one of which is shared by neutral amino acids (Ring et al., 1977).

METHODS AND MATERIALS

Chemicals

Krebs-Ringer Bicarbonate (KRB) solution was prepared with the following composition: NaCl, 118.50 mM; KCl, 4.87 mM; $CaCl_2$, 2.54 mM; $MgSO_4$, 1.19 mM; KH_2PO_4, 1.19 mM; $NaHCO_3$, 24.88 mM; dextrose, 11.11 mM. All amino acids used were from a commercial source: α-aminoisobutyric acid (United States Biochemical Corporation, Cleveland, OH), L-isoleucine (ICN, Cleveland, OH), L-aspartic acid

(Aldrich, Milwaukee, WI), L-lysine monohydrochloride (Calbiochem, La Jolla, CA). Morphine sulfate and cocaine hydrochloride were obtained from Mallinckrodt (St. Louis, MO). Nicotine was obtained from Eastman (Rochester, NY). ACS aqueous counting scintillant (Amersham, England) was used for liquid scintillation counting.

Radiolabeled amino acids

All radiolabeled amino acids were obtained from Amersham (Amersham, England). These included 2-amino(1-^{14}C)isobutyric acid (61 mCi/mmol), L-(U-^{14}C)lysine monohydrochloride (340 mCi/mmol), L-(U-^{14}C)aspartic acid (227 mCi/mmol, L-(U-^{14}C)isoleucine (342 mCi/mmol), (6,6'(n)-^{3}H)sucrose (9.7 Ci/ mmol).

Preparation of human placental villi

Full term human placentae were obtained immediately after either vaginal or Cesarean section deliveries at Vanderbilt University Hospital. They were kept at 4°C for not more than one h before isolated villus tissues were incubated as described below. The amniotic membrane was trimmed along the border of each placenta. Each placenta was perfused to remove fetal blood, since erythrocytes are known to take up AIB, and unperfused placentae display characteristics different from those of blood-free placentae (Gustke and Kowalewski, 1970). Perfusion was accomplished by cannulating the two umbilical arteries with polyethylene tubing of the appropriate size and flushing the placenta with ice cold 0.9 percent saline containing 0.5 U/ml beef lung heparin (Upjohn, Kalamazoo, MI) until the effluent from the umbilical vein was clear of blood. About 3-4 liters of perfusate were usually required. Several blood-free cotyledons from the placentae were used as the source of the villus tissue. The chorionic and basal plates were removed, and the remaining portion, the villus region, was diced into small fragments of 0.1 to 0.3 g and placed in a beaker of cold, oxygenated KRB. The tissue was again washed with ice -cold saline and transferred to a 500 ml flask containing KRB solutions for preincubation. Preincubation was continued at 37°C for 90 min while the medium was continuously aerated with 95 percent O_2 -5 percent CO_2. At the end of the preincubation period, the tissue was washed with 250 ml of cold KRB and transferred to the incubation chambers as described below.

While the villus tissue was preincubating, the incubation chambers in which uptake was measured were prepared. These chambers were 50 ml glass syringe barrels (50 cc hypodermic luer syringe, Eisele, Nashville, TN) arranged to be inverted in a heated water bath maintained at 37°C such that the gas mixture (95 percent O_2/5 percent CO_2) could be introduced from the tip of the syringe needle into the chamber. The rim of each chamber was coated with a silicon gel to retard bubbling. These chambers were divided into two groups, control and experimental. Each chamber was filled with 45 ml of KRB. Up to 2 ml of KRB containing dissolved drug was added to each experimental chamber. To each control chamber, 2 ml of KRB without drug was added. Sufficiently preincubated placental tissue was transferred to each chamber to bring the volume to 50 ml. The tissue was allowed to equilibrate for 5 min before 200 µl of a stock solution (25 mM) of labeled amino acid and the corresponding carrier was added to each chamber. The final concentration of the amino acid in each chamber was 0.1 mM. The radioactivity in the medium was about 2.12 Ci/l.

Measurement of the uptake of the nonmetabolizable amino acid, AIB

After the amino acid was added, a sample of the medium was taken from the chamber. The time of this first sampling was denoted as "time 0." At time 0, and again at various intervals thereafter (up to 120 minutes), 0.5 ml of the medium was removed and placed in a scintillation vial for counting. After the last sample was obtained, all of the placental tissue was removed from each chamber and blotted dry. The wet weight and dry weight after dessication for 10 h at 85°C were determined. The extracellular space for each placenta was determined using ^3H-sucrose, and the intracellular fluid was calculated according to Smith et al. (1973).

Quantitating the uptake of amino acids by the placental tissue as a function of time was accomplished by determining the decrease in the concentration of the amino acid in the medium as the amino acid left the medium and entered the tissue. From these measurements, a distribution of amino acid between the tissue and medium was derived. The distribution was expressed as the ratio (I/O) of the intracellular concentration of amino acid inside the tissue (I) divided by its extracellular concentration (O). The I/O ratio is a measure of the concentrating ability of the active transport pump in the villus membrane.

The validity of amino acid uptake by depletion in the bath was also verified by actually measuring the amino acid in the tissue. When AIB uptake calculated by the above method was compared with the uptake from direct measurements of ^{14}C-AIB in placental tissue, there were no significant quantitative differences in uptake. The method used for direct measurement of ^{14}C-AIB in the villus tissue was that described by Smith et al. (1973).Further details of these procedures are described in previous papers from our laboratories (Rowell and Sastry, 1978 and 1981).

The radioactivity of ^{14}C-AIB in the tissue was measured by homogenizing the dessicated tissue with a Brinkmann Polytron. A 0.5 ml aliquot of the homogenate was placed in a glass scintillation vial with 2 ml NCS and dissolved overnight at 50°C. Chemiluminescence was decreased by acidifying the sample with 34 µl of glacial acetic acid per ml of NCS used, waiting until chemiluminescence decayed before counting, and counting samples in the dark. Decolorization of the samples was performed by adding 0.5 ml of 30-35 percent H_2O_2. Ten ml of liquid scintillation cocktail was added, and samples were counted in a Beckman CPM-100 Liquid Scintillation System. Quenching by the samples was determined by adding an internal ^{14}C standard of known specific activity and measuring the counting efficiency.

Tests for viability of isolated villus tissue preparations

The viability of isolated placental villus preparations was demonstrated by several biochemical, physiological and pharmacological criteria: (a) the AIB uptake was measured under the influence of dinitrophenol and a nitrogen atmosphere, both of which depressed active uptake of AIB (Harbison et al., 1975); (b) the active uptake of AIB was depressed when the villus tissue was suspended in a KRB medium at 3°C, and this effect could be reversed by increasing the temperature of the KRB medium to 37°C (Rowell and Sastry, 1978); (c) determination of lactate dehydrogenase (LDH) concentrations in villus tissue and the KRB medium in which villus tissue was incubated for 90 min indicated that no significant amount of LDH leaked out of the cells, and the preparation contained 99 percent viable cells (Rowell and Sastry, 1981); (d) The presence of extracellular Ca^{++} is critical both for spontaneous and electrically evoked release of ACh from the nerve and the placenta. No significant amounts of spontaneous, electrically evoked (by field stimulation) or chemically evoked (e.g., 17-63 mM K^+, 58 μM nicotine) release of ACh was observed when the placental villus was incubated in Ca^{++}-free KRB. When normal concentrations of Ca^{++} (2.54 mM) were restored to the medium, ACh was released under the above three conditions (Olubadewo and Sastry, 1978; Sastry et al., 1983).

Measurement of the uptake of the metabolizable amino acids, aspartic acid, isoleucine, and lysine

For those amino acids which are metabolized, the uptake as a function of time was also expressed as an I/O ratio calculated by the same method as was used for AIB. However, this expression is complicated by virtue of the entrance of these amino acids into cellular metabolic pathways. We, therefore, also studied the distribution of the amino acids between the trichloroacetic acid (TCA) soluble and precipitable portions of the placental tissue in the presence and absence of drugs. In this procedure, the dessicated tissue was homogenized in 10 ml of ice cold 20 percent TCA for 1 min using a Brinkmann Polytron. A 0.5 ml aliquot of the homogenate was added to a scintillation vial. Another aliquot was centrifuged at 1,500 x g for 30 min in a Sorval RC5B refrigerated centrifuge. The pellet was washed in 20 percent TCA, homogenized and recentrifuged. Samples from the pellet and supernatants were placed in scintillation vials for counting. The samples from the homogenate and pellet were dissolved in 2 ml NCS overnight at 50°C. Samples were handled as described above for determining ^{14}C-α-aminoisobutyric acid in the homogenate.

Measurement of the initial linear velocity for active uptake of AIB by placental villus, and K_m and V_{max} for the active process

The rate of AIB uptake was determined and plotted as a function of time for 2 h. The time at which the I/O ratio was 1.0 was marked on this plot. At this time point (T) the rate of entry of AIB into the tissue by diffusion and the rate of efflux of AIB were considered to be minimal. The net uptake of AIB was mainly due to active uptake. The initial linear velocity (V) for active uptake was measured by the slope of the line at T. In individual experiments, T appeared between 15 and 20 mins on the time scale.

Statistical analysis

In all figures, means ± standard errors are presented. Straight lines were established with linear regression analysis by the method of least squares using a DEC-10 computer. Since K_m and V_{max} are considered to be constants and seemed to be specific for each placenta, they were expressed for individual placentae. Differences between means were tested using Student's t test, and they were considered significant when $p < 0.05$.

RESULTS

Uptake of amino acids in the presence and absence of cocaine, morphine and nicotine

To determine the concentrations of the drugs effective to inhibit the uptake of amino acids, dose response relationships on the uptake of AIB were studied. Nicotine (Figure 1), morphine and cocaine (Figure 2) all produced dose related depressions in the I/O ratios achieved after 2 h of incubation. At low concentrations of the drugs, there was a large depression in the I/O ratio. At the highest concentrations used, all three drugs completely inhibited uptake. Cocaine had an ED_{50} for inhibiting uptake of AIB of about 3.5 mM. The ED_{50} for morphine was between 2 and 3 mM. Nicotine was the least potent inhibitor of AIB uptake with an ED_{50} of about 20 mM.

For other amino acids aspartic acid, isoleucine and lysine the concentrations of cocaine and morphine used were close to their ED_{50}s for inhibition of AIB uptake. For nicotine, the ED_{50} for inhibiting AIB uptake (20 mM) was high, but lower concentrations produced significant depression. Therefore, a 5 mM concentration of nicotine was selected. With the exception of cocaine at 13 mM, no concentrations of the drugs reduced the I/O ratio below unity. The effects of AIB uptake were reversed when the tissue was washed with KRB after treatment with nicotine (84 percent), morphine (>90 percent) and cocaine (>90 percent).

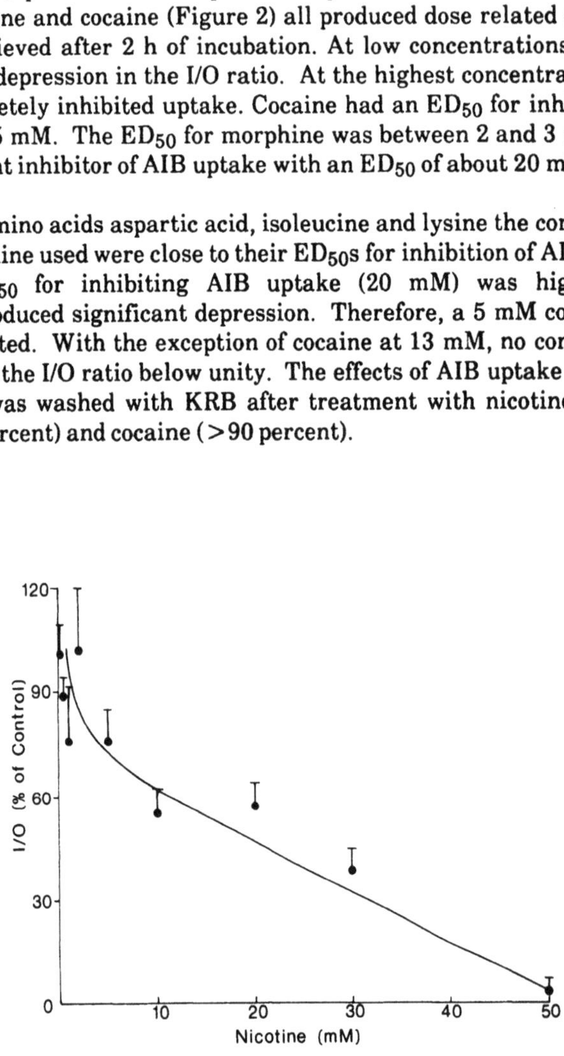

Figure 1. Dose response curve for the uptake of α-aminoisobutyric acid in the presence of nicotine. Ordinate represents the percent of control I/O ratio (I: intracellular concentration; O: extracellular concentration) for the uptake of α-aminoisobutyric acid (uptake when no drug is present). No nicotine was present in the baths during preincubation. Exposure time = 2 h. Points are means ± SE from a minimum of 10 values. The control I/O ratio was 6.8 ± 0.5. The I/O ratio at the highest doses of nicotine was not significantly different from 1.0.

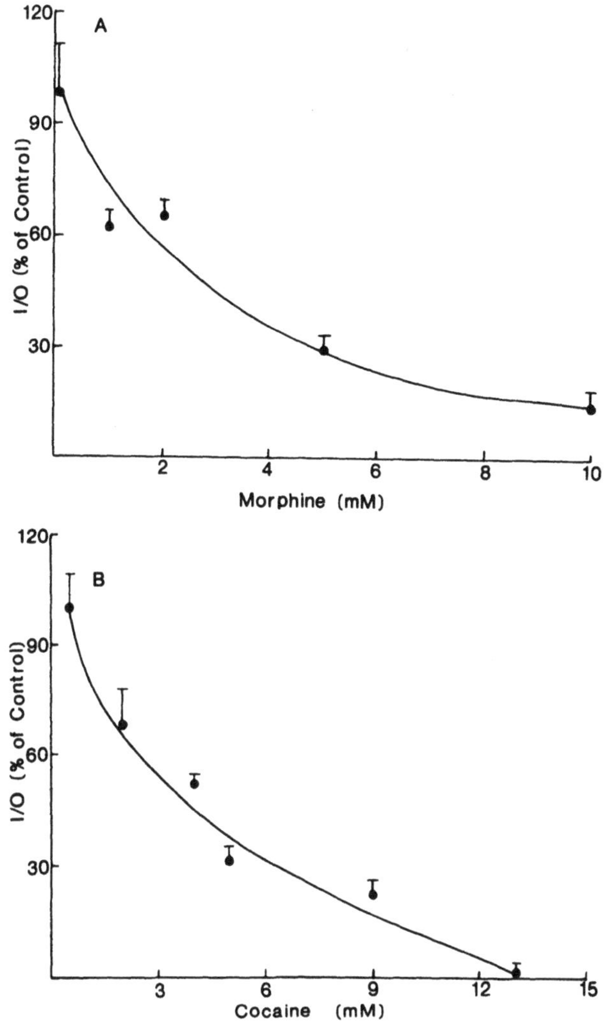

Figure 2. Dose response curves for the uptake of α-aminoisobutyric acid in the presence of morphine (A) and cocaine (B). No drug was present in the preincubation medium. The ordinate represents the percent of control I/O ratio (I: intracellular concentration; O: extracellular concentration) for the uptake of α-aminoisobutyric acid (uptake when no drug is present). The abscissa represents the increasing concentration of drugs. Exposure time = 2 h. Points are means ± SE from 12 experiments. The control I/O ratio in A was 7.7 ± 0.7. In B it was 5.4 ± 0.8. the I/O ratios with 10 mM morphine and 9 mM cocaine were significantly higher than unity.

Effects of nicotine, morphine and cocaine on the uptake of AIB, aspartic acid, isoleucine and lysine as a function of time

Time courses for the uptake of AIB, isoleucine (Figure 3), aspartic acid, and lysine (Figure 4) in the absence of drugs were determined. Two different phases in the uptake curves were observed. During the first phase (0-20 min) the uptake of amino acids was both passive and active. At about 20 min, the I/O ratio was more than unity. The uptake was mainly active during the second phase (20-120 min.). During this phase, the amino acids were taken up by the placental villus against a concentration gradient.

The I/O ratios varied from amino acid to amino acid and from placenta to placenta for each amino acid. Therefore, the placental villi from the same group of placentae were used to measure the uptake of each amino acid in the presence and absence of the drugs. All three drugs inhibited the uptake of all four amino acids as a function of time (Figures 3, 4). In general, morphine and cocaine were more effective than nicotine in inhibiting uptake of all four amino acids. After two h of incubation, all three agents depressed the I/O ratios for all four amino acids (Figures 5,6). These observations indicate that these agents interfered with the active uptake of these amino acids.

Effects of nicotine, morphine and cocaine on the incorporation of amino acids into the trichloroacetic acid-precipitable fraction of placental villi

Of the amino acids studied, only AIB is not metabolized. Aspartic acid, isoleucine and lysine are available to the cell for protein synthesis and catabolism. Calculating uptake as an I/O ratio is complicated for those amino acids which enter cell metabolism. If all of the amino acid which entered the cell was immediately incorporated into the tissue protein, active uptake, defined as transport against a concentration gradient, might not function. Rather, the transport could be explained by simple diffusion or facilitated transport. To determine to what extent the amino acids enter cellular metabolic pathways, the distribution of amino acids between the TCA-soluble and the TCA-insoluble fractions were studied (Table 1). AIB, the nonmetabolizable amino acid, remained in the TCA-soluble fraction. The total radioactivity of AIB recovered was 99-106 percent. 66 percent of the total radioactivity of the aspartic acid, 43 percent of the isoleucine, and 46 percent of the lysine was present in the TCA-soluble fractions. The total recoveries of the radioactivities of the three metabolizable amino acids were higher than 89 percent.

Morphine significantly altered ($p < 0.05$) the distribution of isoleucine between the TCA-soluble and insoluble fractions. It decreased incorporation of the radioactivity into the insoluble fraction (supernatant). Morphine also changed the distribution of aspartic acid between the TCA fractions. Again, there was a relative increase in the proportion of radioactivity in the supernatant and a decrease in the pellet. The proportion of lysine in the supernatant increased significantly ($p < 0.05$) in the presence of each of the drugs. However, there was no concomitant significant decrease in the proportion of lysine in the pellet.

Apparent K_m and V_{max} for the active uptake of AIB by placental villus

The type of inhibition of the active uptake affected by cocaine, morphine, and nicotine was studied by measuring uptake in the presence of a single concentration of the drug and several AIB concentrations. Lineweaver-Burke plots were constructed for the uptake of various concentrations of AIB in the presence and absence of drug (Figure 7). All three drugs changed both slopes and intercepts. The lines did not

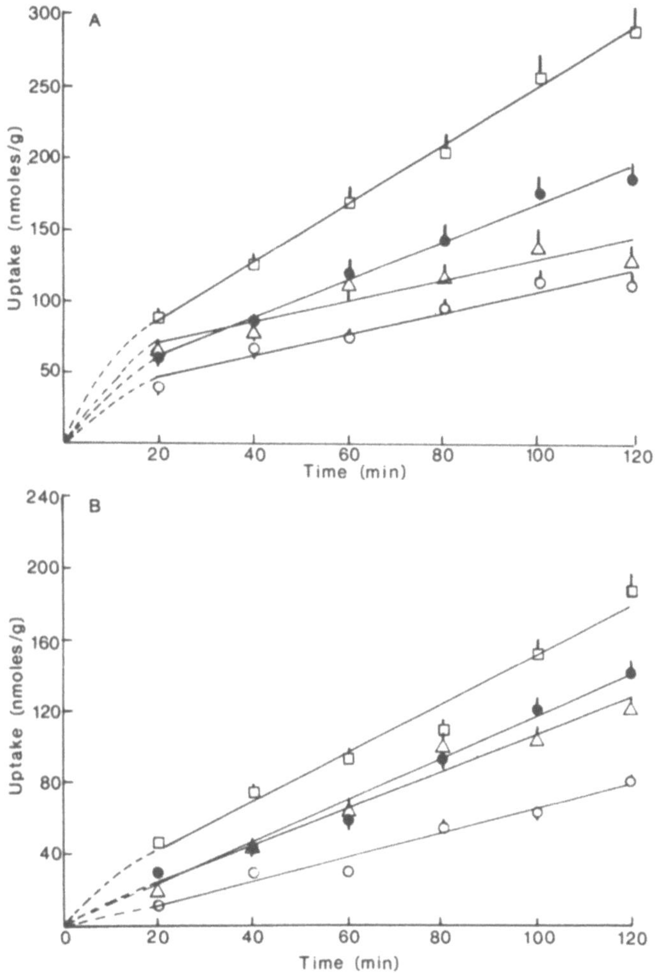

Figure 3. Uptake of neutral amino acids by human placental villus as a function of time in the presence of nicotine (5 mM, ● — ●), morphine (2mM, Δ — Δ), and cocaine (3.5 mM, ○ — ○) and in the absence of any drug (□ — □). Uptake was expressed in nmol/g wet tissue. Villus tissue from the same group of placentae was used in the presence and absence of drugs. Each value is a mean from a minimum of 6 experiments. A = α-Aminoisobytyric acid (0.1 mM). B = Isoleucine (0.1 mM).

intersect on the abscissa or ordinate (Figure 7, Table 2). These results indicate that the nature of inhibition is neither simple competitive nor noncompetitive. The inhibition by these drugs may not be due to their competition with AIB for the transport sites on the carrier.

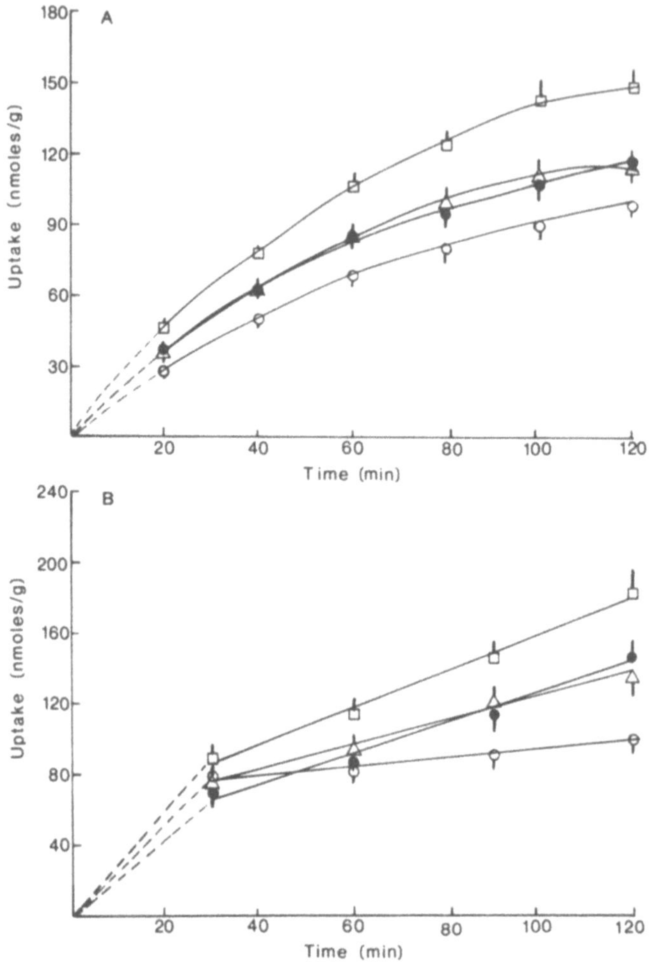

Figure 4. Uptake of acidic and basic amino acids by human placental villi as a function of time in the presence of nicotine (5 mM, ●—●), morphine (2mm, Δ—Δ), and cocaine (3.5 mM, ○—○) and in the absence of drugs (□—□). Villi from the same group of placentae were used in the presence and absence of drugs. Each value is a mean from a minimum of 6 experiments. A = Aspartic acid (0.1 mM). B = Lysine (0.1 mM).

Slopes V_{max} and K_m for AIB uptake in the presence and absence of each drug suggest that the inhibition cannot be classified as simple competitive, noncompetitive or uncompetitive. In each case, the results from one placenta is presented as representative of several placentae.

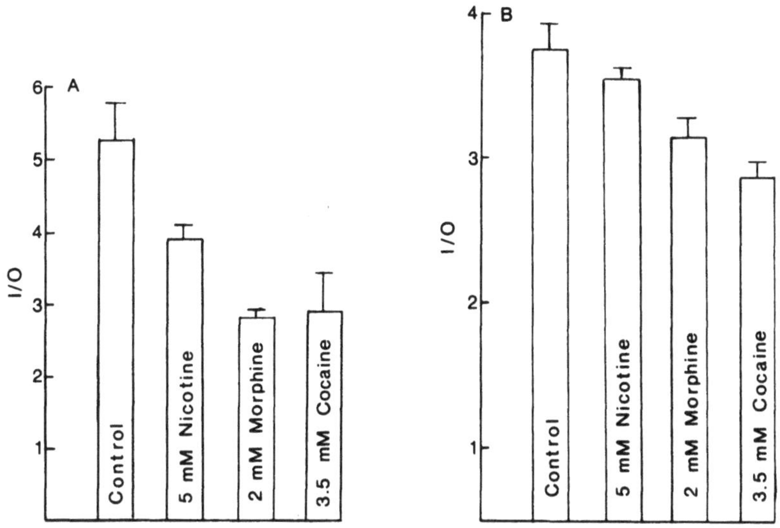

Figure 5. Inhibition of the active uptake of neutral amino acids in the isolated human placental villi by nicotine (5 mM), morphine (2 mM), and cocaine (3.5 mM). The ratio of the concentrations of the amino acid inside (I) and outside (O) was considered as the indicator of the active uptake. Villi from the same group of placentae were used in the control and drug-treated experiments. Each bar is a mean from a minimum of 6 values. The vertical lines represent SE. A = α-Aminoisobutyric acid (0.1 mM). B = Isoleucine (0.1 mM).

There are large variations between placentae as indicated by rather large differences for the K_m and V_{max} values obtained with tissue from different placentae. Because of these differences, the same placenta served as the source of villus tissue for both the control and drug exposed studies. In all placentae, cocaine, morphine and nicotine decreased the maximal velocity of uptake and increased the apparent affinity of the transport sytem for the substrate (Table 2).

DISCUSSION

Amino acids serve as substrates for the synthesis of proteins and for formation of metabolic energy for the developing fetus (Dancis and Shafran, 1958; Gresham et al., 1972). Other reports have demonstrated the uptake of various amino acids by isolated human placenta (Schneider et al., 1979; Schneider and Dancis, 1974; Enders et al., 1976). In this report, we have shown the inhibition of amino acid transport by several drugs of abuse at high concentrations and implicated the cholinergic system in the regulation of placental amino acid transport.

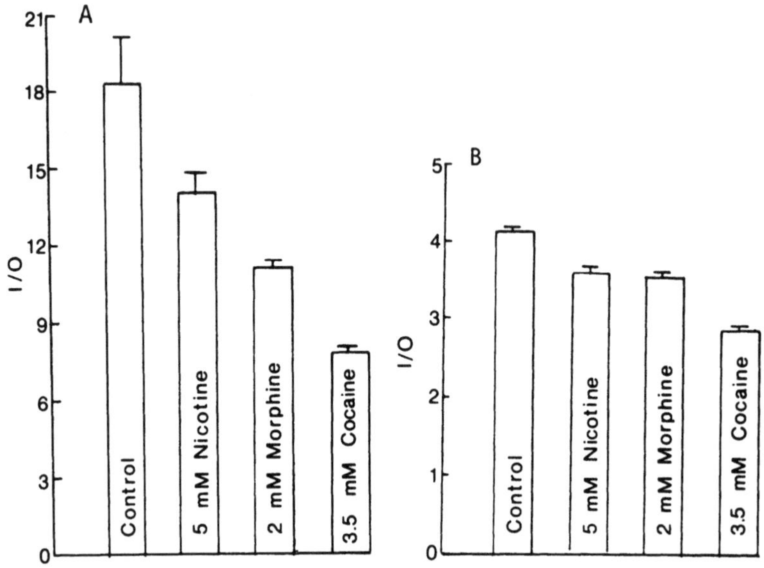

Figure 6. Inhibition of the active uptake of acidic and basic amino acids by nicotine (5 mM), morphine (2 mM), and cocaine (3.5 mM). The ratio of the concentrations of the amino acid inside (I) and outside (O) was considered as the indicator of the active uptake. Villi from the same group of placentae were used in the control and drug-treated experiments. Each bar is a mean from a minimum of 6 values. Vertical lines represent SE. A = Aspartic acid (0.1 mM). B = Lysine (0.1 mM).

Figure 7. Typical double reciprocal plots for the uptake of α-aminoisobutyric acid (AIB) in the presence and absence of drugs. Concentration is expressed as µmol/l; velocity as rate of uptake in µmol/g/min. The straight lines were established with linear regression analysis by the method of least squares using a DEC-10 computer. In neither case did these lines cross on the abscissa or the ordinate. A. In the presence of 5 mM nicotine, the slope of the line increased from 2.2 x 10^4 to 2.8 x 10^4 g-min/l. Both K_m and V_{max} decreased in the presence of nicotine. (Control: V_{max} = 12 x 10^{-9} mol/g/min, K_m = 0.26 x 10^{-3} mol/l; 5 mM; Nicotine: V_{max} = 8.4 x 10^{-9} mol/g/min, K_m = 0.23 x 10^{-3} mol/l). B. In the presence of 2 mM morphine, the slope of the line increased from 7.6 x 10^4 to 11 x 10^4 g/min/l. Both K_m and V_{max} decreased in the presence of morphine (Control: V_{max} = 80 x 10^{-9} mol/min/g, K_m = 6.1 x 10^{-3} mol/l; 2 mM; Morphine: V_{max} = 4.5 x 10^{-9} mol/min/g, K_m = 0.49 x 10^{-3} mol/l). C. In the presence of 3.5 mM cocaine, the slope of the line increased from 4.1 x 10^4 to 7.9 x 10^4 g-min/l. Both K_m and V_{max} decreased in the presence of cocaine (Control: V_{max} = 128 x 10^{-9} mol/g/min, Km = 0.53 x 10^{-3} mol/l; 3.5 mM; Cocaine: V_{max} = 53 x 10^{-9} mol/g/min, K_m = 0.42 x 10^{-3} mol/l).

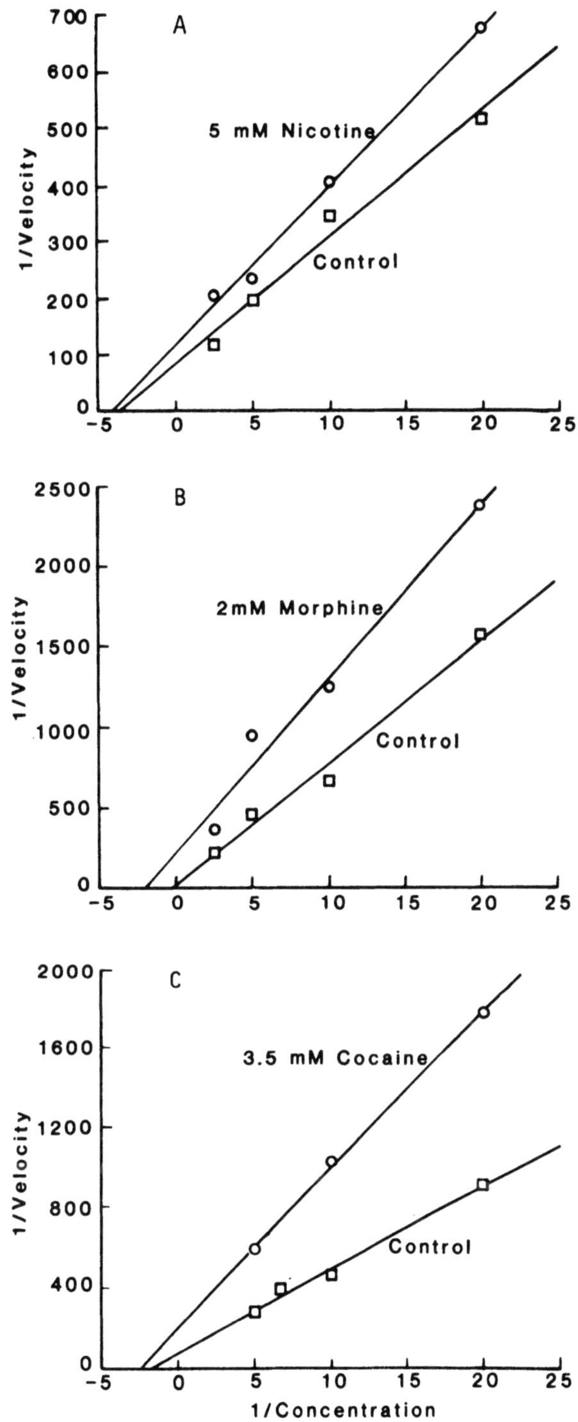
A
5 mM Nicotine
Control
1/Velocity
700
600
500
400
300
200
100
0
-5
0
5
10
15
20
25
B
2mM Morphine
Control
1/Velocity
2500
2000
1500
1000
500
0
C
3.5 mM Cocaine
Control
1/Velocity
2000
1600
1200
800
400
1/Concentration

Table 1. Distribution of the radioactivity of ^{14}C-amino acids between TCA-soluble and TCA-insoluble fractions of placental homogenates[a]

Treatment	TCA fraction	Amino acid (% of uptake) M ± SE			
		AIB	Isoleucine	Lysine	Aspartic Acid
Control[b]	Soluble	105 ± 3	43 ± 1	46 ± 1	66 ± 3
	Insoluble	1 ± 0.1	69 ± 2	43 ± 9	24 ± 2
Nicotine (5 mM)	Soluble	100 ± 2	46 ± 2	51 ± 2[c]	69 ± 2
	Insoluble	1 ± 0.1	62 ± 1	52 ± 2[e]	22 ± 2
Morphine (2 mM)	Soluble	101 ± 1	57 ± 2[c]	51 ± 1[c]	76 ± 2[c]
	Insoluble	1 ± 0.1	54 ± 2[c]	41 ± 4	16 ± 2[c]
Cocaine (3.5 mM)	Soluble	99 ± 1	54 ± 2[c]	58 ± 3[c]	64 ± 2
	Insoluble	1 ± 0.1	63 ± 4	42 ± 3	25 ± 2

[a]Each value is a mean ± SE from 5 experiments. Concentrations of amino acids: 0.1mM.

[b]Control I/O ratios: AIB, 7.8 ± 0.4; Isoleucine, 2 ± 0.2; lysine, 3 ± 0.2; aspartic acid, 19.5 ± 1.0.

[c]Significant from the corresponding control at $p < 0.05$.

The uptake of each amino acid studied was inhibited by the drugs - cocaine, morphine, and nicotine, at mM concentrations. The degree of inhibition varied with the amino acid studied. AIB uptake was the most sensitive to the effects of the drugs. Aspartic acid, which is taken up to the greatest extent, was least sensitive to the effects of the drugs. The uptake of isoleucine and lysine was inhibited to degrees intermediate between the inhibition of AIB and aspartic acid. Differential degrees of inhibition are not unexpected considering the different transport systems involved in the uptake of these amino acids (Enders et al., 1976; Miller and Berndt, 1974). The "A" system, which transports AIB, appears to be most sensitive to the effects of the drugs. It is possible that this transport system is more susceptible to regulatory influences than the "L" system which also functions in the placenta. Enders et al. (1976) have shown that uptake by the "A" system is specifically increased after preincubation of the tissue, the "L" and "ASC" transport systems do not exhibit this increase. The preincubation effect on AIB uptake was seen not only with term placenta but was also observed with placenta of an early gestation period (18-22 weeks) (Miller et al., 1976). This increase results from an increased V_{max} and a decreased Km (Smith et al., 1973). The "A" system may be more finely tuned and more accessible to interference by specific drugs. Of the drugs tested, morphine was most effective for inhibiting the uptake of AIB (ED_{50}, 2 mM), followed closely by cocaine (ED_{50}, 3.5 mM). Nicotine had an ED_{50} of 20 mM. The nature of inhibition of AIB uptake is neither simple competitive nor noncompetitive. These drugs decrease the maximal velocity of uptake and increase the apparent affinity of the transport system for the substrate. These findings suggest a more complex interaction between the drugs and the transport process.

Table 2. Influence of nicotine, morphine, and cocaine on K_m and V_{max} for uptake of AIB in placental villus

Placenta Number	Drug and Concentration (mM)	Rate of Uptake(nmol /g/min)[a]	K_m/V_{max} (g-min/l)	V_{max} (nmol/ min/g)	K_m (nmol/l)
1	Nicotine (0)	2.3	3.9×10^4	71	2.8
	Nicotine (2.5)	2.3	3.8×10^4	46	1.7
2	Nicotine (0)	1.9	4.1×10^4	17	0.69
	Nicotine (2.5)	2.7	3.0×10^4	19	0.56
3	Nicotine (0)	2.3	4.0×10^4	182	7.3
	Nicotine (5)	1.8	4.9×10^4	70	3.4
4	Nicotine (0)	2.9	2.2×10^4	12	0.26
	Nicotine (5)	2.5	2.8×10^4	8	0.23
5	Nicotine (0)	2.4	3.3×10^4	12	0.40
	Nicotine (7.5)	1.2	7.8×10^4	14	0.17
6	Nicotine (0)	2.0	3.4×10^4	3.9	0.14
	Nicotine (7.5)	1.1	4.3×10^4	2.4	0.10
7	Nicotine (0)	1.6	5.8×10^4	6.4	0.37
	Nicotine (7.5)	1.2	5.0×10^4	2.6	0.13
8	Nicotine (0)	1.2	8.0×10^4	13	1.0
	Nicotine (10)	0.6	2.4×10^4	1.1	0.02
9	Morphine (0)	4.2	2.3×10^4	25	0.59
	Morphine (4)	0.57	13.8×10^4	3.4	0.47
10	Morphine (0)	1.5	7.6×10^4	80	6.1
	Morphine (2)	0.8	11.0×10^4	4.6	0.49
11	Morphine (0)	4.2	2.5×10^4	260	6.5
	Morphine (2)	1.9	1.7×10^4	12	0.21
12	Cocaine (0)	2.5	4.1×10^4	138	5.7
	Cocaine (3)	1.2	7.5×10^4	39	2.9
13	Cocaine (0)	2.2	4.1×10^4	128	0.53
	Cocaine (3.5)	1.0	7.9×10^4	53	0.42
14	Cocaine (0)	2.0	5.4×10^4	18	0.98
	Cocaine (3.5)	0.73	4.9×10^4	0.75	0.036

[a]AIB concentration, 10^{-4}M.

[b]The V_{max} for AIB uptake for 14 control placentae was 69 ± 8 nmol/min/g. Treatment with nicotine, morphine and cocaine lowered it to 20 ± 9 (n=8), 7 ± 4 (n=3) and 31 ± 16 (n=3) respectively.

[c]The K_m for AIB uptake for 14 control placentae was 2.4 ± 0.7 nmol/l. This was lowered to 0.79 ± 0.42 (n=8), 0.39 ± 0.09 (n=3) and 1.1 ± 0.9 (n=3) by treatments with nicotine, morphine and cocaine, respectively.

Morphine and nicotine altered the metabolism of the amino acids to a small yet significant extent. These alterations manifested as an increase in amino acid content in the TCA-soluble fraction and a concomitant decrease in the amino acid in the insoluble fractions. These small alterations probably do not account for the decreased uptake in the presence of the drugs. AIB, which is not metabolized, demonstrates an uptake in control conditions and inhibition of uptake in the presence of the drugs. The mechanism by which the drugs exert inhibition on amino acid transport is not well understood.

Cocaine may act as a Ca^{++} antagonist in smooth muscle (Hurwitz et al., 1962). Depletion of Ca^{++} ions results in loss of active uptake of AIB by the villus tissue (Sastry et al., 1983). The selective Ca^{++} chelator, EGTA, was present in both control and Ca^{++} free incubation chambers to exclude its role in directly inhibiting AIB uptake. The effect of morphine may be mediated through the recently described opioid receptor in placental tissue (Valette et al., 1980; Ahmad et al., 1981). Endogenous opioid-like peptides in the placenta have been described by several investigators (Nakai et al., 1978; Odagiri et al., 1979; Sastry et al., 1980, 1981). Objections to some of these reports have been raised since the finding that fragments of immunoglobulin G may interfere with the radioimmunoassay for opioid-like peptides (Julliard et al., 1980). However, reports by Sastry et al. (1980, 1981), which include evidence of biological activity of the placental extracts from which the peptides were measured, are consistent with their having opioid-like activity. Nicotine also produces a depression in the uptake of amino acid. In low concentrations, nicotine can act as a cholinergic agonist, but at the high concentrations used, it acts as an antagonist at cholineregic receptors both directly and indirectly by producing a large outflow of ACh (Rowell and Sastry, 1978).

A common link between each of these drugs is an action involving the cholinergic system. The placenta has a highly developed cholinergic system, including enzymes for the synthesis and degradation of ACh and high levels of ACh, which is released from the villus tissue (Sastry et al., 1976; Olubadewo and Sastry, 1978; Sastry and Sadavongvivad, 1979). Cocaine decreases the release of ACh from placental villi (Sastry et al., 1977). This action may arise from blockade of Ca^{++} influx into the syncytiotrophoblast (Sastry et al., 1977). Ca^{++} is necessary for the release of ACh and normal uptake of AIB (Sastry et al., 1983). Replenishing tissue depleted of calcium returned uptake activity to control levels, ruling out irreversible tissue damage from the absence of Ca^{++}. Similarly, high concentrations of nicotine decrease ACh release from placenta (Olubadewo and Sastry, 1978) and depress AIB uptake. Morphine is known to decrease ACh release from neuronal tissue, possibly by interfering with Ca^{++} influx (Paton, 1957; Schaumann, 1957), and it depresses AIB uptake.

A question arises why millimolar concentrations of drugs are necessary to interfere with cholinergic in human placenta. In a preincubated preparation of term placenta the level of ACh is higher than 0.24 mM. This does not include ACh which is continuously synthesized and released. To interfere with the function of such high levels of ACh presents a major problem for studying placental pharmacology. The cholinergic receptor, which is associated with release of ACh from placenta, shares the properties of both muscarinic and nicotinic receptors of innervated tissues and seems to have a low affinity for nicotine (Olubadewo and Sastry, 1978). Similarly, the cholinergic receptor in the plasma membrane of the placental villus exhibits a low affinity for nicotine and atropine (Fant and Harbison, 1981). The opiate receptor in placenta is of a novel type and has a low affinity for morphine (Ahmed et al., 1981). Cocaine is potent for blocking conduction in the nerve but it seems to be weak for blocking Ca^{++} channels. Although nicotine, morphine and cocaine are important drugs of abuse, they are not ideal agents to block cholinergic receptors, opiate receptors and Ca^{++} channels in placenta. In light of the above information, it is not surprising that millimolar concentrations of the above drugs are required to interfere with cholinergic function in placenta.

The effects of nicotine, morphine and cocaine on AIB uptake do not represent general cellular toxicity for a combination of reasons: (a) Except for cocaine at the highest dose used (13 mM), none of the drug concentrations reduced the I/O ratio for AIB uptake lower than unity. (b) More than 90 percent of the effect of morphine and cocaine on AIB uptake was reversed upon washing the tissue with KRB medium. About 84 percent of the effect of nicotine on AIB uptake was reversed by washing. (c) No visible color changes were observed when placental tissues were incubated with these drugs. (d) The depression of the active uptake of AIB by each one of the drugs was concentration dependent.

The extent to which the cholinergic system is involved in regulating amino acid transport can be inferred. With full cholinergic receptor blockade by atropine or ACh, AIB transport is blocked by only 61 percent (Rowell and Sastry, 1978). It may be that basal AIB transport occurs without cholinergic stimulation in the placenta. The cholinergic system may play a facilitative role rather than an initiatative one in regulating this transport. Although high concentrations of cocaine, morphine and nicotine block all active AIB transport, a relatively large inhibition occurs even at lower concentrations. Large effects at lower concentrations may result from altered cholinergic function, whereas at high concentrations the total blockade of AIB transport may be mediated by other actions of the drugs which cannot be explained by the available data.

The present investigations do not exclude the possibility that part of the effect of three drugs of abuse may be due to inhibition of protein synthesis. The ability of a group of compounds related to morphine (in millimolar concentrations) to inhibit the growth of HeLa cells has been correlated with their ability to inhibit protein and RNA synthesis in the intact cell (Noteboom and Mueller, 1969). ACh stimulates protein synthesis in some glandular tissues (Peakall, 1969; Sastry and Sadavongvivad, 1979). Preincubation of placental tissues increases both protein synthesis and ACh levels. The three drugs of abuse may interfere with ACh function in placenta and therefore with protein synthesis.

All of the cholinergic agents at millimolar concentrations studied demonstrate inhibition of amino acid transport. None of the agents used increased transport (Rowell and Sastry, 1978). The in vitro placental preparations may have a maximally stimulated transport system, and any influences on the system manifest as decreased transport.

SUMMARY

Amino acid uptake was measured in vitro in intact human placental villus. Active uptake of α-aminoisobutyric acid (AIB), aspartic acid, isoleucine and lysine was demonstrated. The inhibition of the uptake of these amino acids was studied using the drugs of abuse, cocaine, morphine and nicotine. The uptake of AIB was most sensitive to inhibition by these agents at millimolar concentrations, demonstrating that the different amino acid transport systems may be affected differently by these drugs. The metabolism of aspartic acid, isoleucine and lysine in the placenta may be slightly decreased by these drugs. The inhibition of AIB uptake by these drugs was neither simple competitive nor noncompetitive. The uptake of AIB depends on Ca^{++} in the medium. These findings suggest that the placental cholinergic function by decreasing ACh release may affect amino acid uptake.

ACKNOWLEDGMENTS

This investigation was partially supported by a grant from the Council for Tobacco Research USA, Inc., and by United States Public Health Service Research Grants ES-03172, HD-10607 and RR-05424. One of the authors (SLB) was supported by a predoctoral traineeship from the National Institutes of Health Grant GM0058 from the National Institutes of General Medical Sciences.

REFERENCES

Ahmed, M.S., Byrne, W.L. and Klee, W.A. (1981) Solubilization of opiate receptors from human placenta. *Placenta* (Suppl. 3), 115-122.

Barnwell, S.L. and Sastry, B.V.R. (1982) Influences of nicotine and tobacco gases on the uptake of α-aminoisobutyric acid by isolated human placental villus. *J. Pathol. Environ. Tox. Oncol.* 5, 549-563.

Borghetti, A.F., Piedimonte, G., Tramacere, M., Severini, A., Ghiringhelli, P. and Guidotti, G.G. (1980) Cell density and amino acid transport in 3T3, SV3T3, and SV3T3 revertant cells. *J. Cell. Physiol.* 105,39-49.

Brans, Y. and Cassady, G. (1975) Intrauterine growth and maturation in relation to fetal deprivation. In *The Placenta and Its Maternal Supply Line: Effects of Insufficiency on the Fetus* (ed.) Gruenwals, P., pp. 307-334, Baltimore: University Park Press.

Christensen, H. (1975) *Biological Transport.* Reading, MA: Benjamin, p. 514.

Dancis, J., Money, W., Springer, D. and Levitz, M. (1968) Transport of amino acids by placenta. *Amer. J. Obstet. Gynecol.* 101,820-829.

Dancis, J. and Shafran, M. (1958) The origin of plasma proteins in the guinea pig fetus. *J. Clin. Invest.* 37,1095-1099.

Ellinwood, E.H. and Kilbey, M.M. (1975) Cocaine and other stimulants. In *Advances in Behavioral Biology 21*, Plenum Press.

Enders, R., Judd, R., Donohue, T. and Smith, C. (1976) Placental amino acid uptake. III. Transport systems for neutral amino acids. *Amer. J. Physiol.* 230,706-710.

Fant, M.E. and Harbison, R.D. (1981) Syncytiotrophoblast membrane vesicles: A model for examining the human placental cholinergic system. *Teratology* 24,187-199.

Gazzola, G., Franchi, R., Saibene, V., Ronchi, P. and Guidotit, G. (1972) Regulation of amino acid transport in chick embryo heart cells. I. Adaptive system of mediation for neutral amino acids. *Biochim. Biophys. Acta* 266,407-421.

Gresham, E.L., James, E.J., Raye, J.R., Battaglia, F.C., Markowski, E.L. and Meschia, G. (1972) Production and excretion of urea by the fetal lamb. *Pediatrics* 50,372-379.

Gustke, H. and Kowalewski, S. (1970) Effect of perfusion on the biochemical composition of the human placenta. *Biol. Neonate* 30,116-122.

Harbison, R.D., Olubadewo, J., Dwivedi, C. and Sastry, B.V.R. (1975) Proposed role of a placental cholinergic system in regulation of fetal growth and development. In *Basic and Therapeutic Aspects of Perinatal Pharmacology* (eds.), Morselli, P.L., Garattini, S. and Serini, F., pp. 107-117, New York: Raven Press.

Hasselmeyer, E.G., Meyer, M.B., Catz, C. and Longo, L.D. (1979) Pregnancy and infant health. In *Smoking and Health: A Report of the Surgeon General.* (ed.), Pinney, J.M., pp. 8-1 to 8-93, United States Department of Health, Education and Welfare Publication No. (PHS)79-5006.

Hayter, C., Hutchinson, E., Karvonen, M. and Young, M. (1964) Placental transport of alpha-aminoisobutyric acid in the unanesthetized guinea pig. *J. Physiol.* London: 175,11p-13p.

Hurwitz, L., Battle, F., and Weis, G.B. (1962) Action of the calcium antagonists cocaine and ethanol on contraction and potassium efflux of smooth muscle. *J. Gen. Physiol.* 46,315-332.

Julliard, J.H., Shibaski, T., Ling, N. and Guilemin, R. (1980) High-molecular-weight immunoreactive β-endorphin in extracts of human placenta is a fragment of immunoglobin G. *Science* 208,183-185.

Leventer, S.M., Rowell, P.. and Clark, M.J. (1982) The effect of choline acetyltransferase inhibition on acetylcholine and synthesis and release in term human placenta. *J. Pharm. Exp. Therap.* 322,301-305.

Miller, R.K. and Berndt, W.O. (1974) Characterization of neutral amino acid accumulation by human term placental slices. *Amer. J. Physiol.* 227,1236-1242.

Miller, R.K., Koszalka, T.R., and Brent, R.L. (1976) The transport of molecules across placental membranes. In *The Cell Surface in Animal Embryogenesis and Development*, (eds. Poste G., and Nicolson, G.L., Amsterdam, Elsevier, pp. 145-223.

Nakai, Y., Nakao, K., Oki, S. and Imura, H. (1978) Presence of immunoreactive β-lipotropin and β-endorphin in human placenta. *Life Sci.* 23,2013-2018.

Odagiri, E., Sherrell, B.,. Mount, C., Nicholson, W. and Orth, D.N. (1979) Human placental immunoreactive corticotropin, lipotropin and β-endorphin: Evidence for a common precursor. *Proc. Nat. Acad. Sci. U.S.A.* 76,2027-2031.

Olubadewo, J.O. and Sastry, B.V.R. (1978) Human placental cholinergic system: Stimulation-secretion coupling for release of acetylcholine from isolated placental villus. *J. Pharm. Exp. Therap.* 204,433-445.

Page, E., Glendening, M., Margolis, A. and Harper, M. (1957) Transfer of D- and L-histidine across the human placenta. *Amer. J. Obstet. Gynecol.* 73,589-597.

Paton, W.D.M. (1957) The action of morphine and related substances on contraction and on acetylcholine output of coaxilly stimulated guinea pig ileum. *Brit. J. Pharm. Chemotherapy* 12,119-127.

Peakall, D.B. (1969) Synthesis of silk, mechanism and location. *Amer. Zool.* 9,79.

Riggs, T. and Pan, M. (1972) Transport of amino acids into the oestrogen-primed uterus. Enhancement of the uptake by a preliminary incubation. *Biochem. J.* 128,19-27.

Ring, K., Gross, W., Ehle, H., Foit, B. (1977) Characterization of l-aspartate uptake by Streptomyces hydrogenons. *J. Gen. Microbiol.* 103,307-317.

Rosen, B.P. (1971) Basic amino acid transport in Escherichia coli. *J Biol Chem,* 246,3653-3662.

Rowell, P.P. and Sastry, B.V.R. (1978) The influence of cholinergic blockade on the uptake of α-aminoisobutyric acid by isolated human placental villi. *Tox. Appl. Pharmacol.* 45,79-93.
Rowell, P.P., Chaturvedi, A. and Sastry, B.V.R. (1978) (2- Benzoylethyl)trimethylammonium chloride: A new, selective and stable inhibitor of human placental choline acetyltransferase. *J. Pharm. Exp. Therap.* 205,624- 634.
Rowell, P.P. and Sastry, B.V.R. (1981) Human placental cholinergic system: Depression of the uptake of α-aminoisobutyric acid in isolated human placental villi by cho-line acetyltransferase inhibitors. *J. Pharm. Exp. Therap.* 216,232-238.
Sastry, B.V.R., Olubadewo, J., Harbison, R.D. and Schmidt, D. (1976) Human placental cholinergic system: Occurrence, distribution, and variation with gestational age of acetylcholine in human placenta. *Biochem. Pharm.* 25,425-431.
Sastry, B.V.R., Olubadewo, J. and Boehm, F. (1977) Effects of nicotine and cocaine on the release of acetylcholine from isolated human placental villi. *Arch. Intern. Pharm. Therap.* 229,23-36.
Sastry, B.V.R. and Sadavongvivad, C. (1979) Cholinergic systems in non-nervous tissues. *Pharm. Rev.* 30,65-132.
Sastry, B.V.R., Barnwell, S.L., Tayeb, O.S., Janson, V.E. and Owens, L.K. (1980) Occurrence of methionine enkephalin in human placental villus. *Biochem. Pharm.* 29,475-478.
Sastry, B.V.R., Tayeb, O.S., Barnwell, S.L., Janson, V.E. and Owens, L.K. (1981) Peptides from human placenta: Methionine enkephalin and Substance P. *Placenta* (Suppl. 3), 327-337.
Sastry, B.V.R, Barnwell, S.L. and Moore, R.D. (1983) Factors affecting the uptake of α-amino acids by human placental villus: Acetylcholine, phospholipid methylation, Ca^{++} and cytoskeletal organization. *Troph. Res.* (this volume).
Schaumann, W. (1957) Inhibition by morphine of the release of acetylcholine from the intestine of the guinea pig. *Brit. J. Pharm. Chemotherapy* 12,115-118.
Schneider, H. and Dancis, J. (1974) Amino acid transport in human placental slices. *Amer. J. Obstet. Gynecol.* 120,1092-1097.
Schneider, H., Mohlen, K.-H. and Dancis, J. (1979) Transfer of amino acids across the in vitro perfused human placenta. *Ped. Res.* 13,236-240.
Smith, C.H, Adcock, E.W., Teasdale, F., Meschia, G. and Battaglia, F.C. (1973) Placental amino acid uptake: Tissue preparation, kinetics and preincubation effect. *Amer. J. Physiol.* 224,558-564.
Stone, M., Salerno, L., Green, M. and Zelson, C. (1971) Narcotic addiction in pregnancy. *Amer. J. Obstet. Gynecol.* 109,716-723.
Tuchmann-Duplessis, H. (1975) Drugs acting on the central nervous system. In *Drug Effects on the Fetus*, pp. 142-194, Acton, MA: Publishing Sciences Group, Inc.
Valette, A., Pontonnier, G. and Cros, J. (1979) Evidence for a stereospecific ^3H-etorphine binding in human placenta. *Fed. Europ. Biochem. Soc. Lett.* 103,362-365.
Valette, A., Reme, J.M., Pontonnier, G. and Cros, J. (1980) Specific binding for opiate-like drugs in the placenta. *Biochem. Pharm.* 29,2657-2661.
Welsch, F. (1980) Effects of acetylcholine on the clearance of ^3H-antipyrine in bilaterally perfused lobules of human term placenta. *Gyn. Obstet. Invest.* 11,49-55.
Welsch, F., Wenger, W.C. and Stedman, D.B. (1981) Acetylcholine in human placenta: Tissue levels after in vitro inhibition in intact fragments of choline acetyltransferase and relationship to ^{14}C-α-aminoisobutyric acid uptake. *Placenta* (Suppl. 3), 339- 351.

Trophoblast Research 1:121-134, 1983

TRANSPORT OF NUTRIENTS IN THE EARLY HUMAN PLACENTA: AMINO ACID, CREATINE, VITAMIN B_{12}

Wendy W. Ng and Richard K. Miller[1]

Departments of Obstetrics and Gynecology, Pharmacology and Toxicology
University of Rochester, School of Medicine and Dentistry
Rochester, New York 14642, U.S.A.

INTRODUCTION

The homeostasis of the conceptus is affected by the function of the placenta as early as 1 week of human gestation, and the trophoblast undergoes many changes during gestation. Therefore, when assessments of placental function and its influence on the conceptus are made by using the term placenta, the developmental differences in the placenta need to be taken into consideration.

Due to its availability, the human term placental tissue has been widely used for developmental biology studies in tissue culture, perfusion, in vivo techniques and tissue slice technique (as reviewed by Miller et al., 1976; Stromberg, 1980). With the tissue slice technique, the human term placenta has been shown to concentrate α-aminoisobutyric acid (AIB), a neutral non-metabolizable amino acid (Litonjua et al., 1967; Dancis et al., 1968; Longo et al., 1973; Smith et al., 1975; Miller and Berndt, 1974), creatine (CR) (Miller et al.1977; 1983), and vitamin B_{12} (cobalamin, Cbl) (Ng et al., 1981). In the present study, the transport processes for these 3 compounds were investigated in the early human placenta with the in vitro slice technique. Compromise of transport transport functions in the placenta may be detrimental to the well-being of the conceptus.

Neutral amino acids can be concentrated in both the trophoblast and fetal blood. This concentration is specific and energy dependent as determined by both in vitro tissue slice and perfusion techniques in the human placenta (Litonjua et al., 1967; Dancis et al., 1968; Schneider et al., 1972; Longo et al., 1973; Smith et al., 1973; Miller and Berndt, 1974: Schneider and Dancis, 1974; Enders et al., 1976; Schneider et al., 1979; Wier et al., 1983). The non-metabolized neutral amino acid, α-aminoisobutyric acid, has been a useful marker for the characterization of these amino acid transport processes in the placenta.

Creatine, a glycine molecule with a guanidino group (Figure 1), is also actively concentrated by the term human placenta (Miller et al., 1977; Miller et al., in press) and by the rodent placenta (Davis et al., 1968, Koszalka et al., 1975; Miller et al., 1977). Creatine can be phosphorylated to phosphocreatine, an important high energy source that is found in muscle as well as in the central nervous system and the testes. Both creatine and phosphocreatine are cyclized to creatinine, which is execreted. Creatine is not concentrated by the placenta (Miller et al., 1977).

[1]To whom reprints should be addressed.

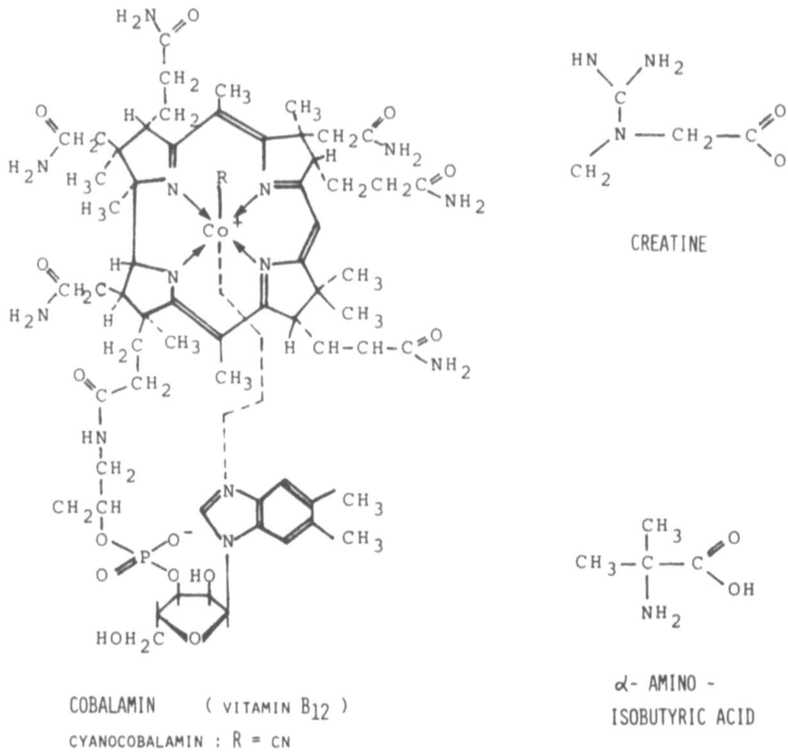

Figure 1. Molecular structures of α-aminoisobutyric acid (AIB), creatine (CR) and vitamin B_{12} (cobalamin, Cbl).

Besides low molecular weight molecules, e.g., AIB and CR, substances greater than 1,000 daltons also can be concentrated in the trophoblast. Among these substrates is vitamin B_{12} (cobalamin, Cbl). Cobalamin is a water-soluble molecule (1355 daltons) and is needed as a coenzyme for lipid metabolism and pyrimidine synthesis (Herbert, 1975). It does not readily diffuse into mammalian cells and its uptake in these cells appears to be mediated by a receptor-mediated endocytosis process in the form of Cbl bound to its plasma carriers: transcobalamin I (TC I,120,000 daltons), transcobalamin II (TC II, 38,000 daltons), and transcobalamin III (TC III, 120,000 daltons) (Meyer et al., 1974; Green et al., 1976; Youngdahl-Turner et al., 1979). Both Cbl and TC II-Cbl are concentrated in the human term placenta (Ng et al., 1981).

The receptor-mediated endocytotic process for specific macromolecule uptake was first described in the placental tissue for the protective materno-fetal transfer of immunoglobulin (Brambell, 1970; Wild, 1981). In the case of materno-fetal transfer of cbl, the human placental tissue possesses a receptor specific for TC II-Cbl but not for other Cbl-protein complexes or free Cbl (Friedman et al., 1977; Seligman and Allen, 1978; Nexø and Hollenberg, 1980).

In the human term placenta, not only is the TC II-Cbl bound by membrane receptors in the proposed process of receptor-mediated endocytosis, but the free Cbl molecule is also concentrated, despite its physical limitations to diffusion. The study of early placental uptake of the Cbl and TC II-Cbl was undertaken to examine the development of this uptake process.

The use of the placental tissue slice technique allows for the direct comparison of the early placental uptake functions with the established values from term placental tissue slice studies (Miller and Berndt, 1974; Miller et al., 1983; Ng et al., 1981).

METHODS

Incubations

Early human placentae (8-20 weeks) were obtained from porrohysterotomies. Term placentae were obtained from normal cesarian or vaginal deliveries. The placentae were transported to the laboratory on ice within 30 minutes of delivery. The early human placental tissue was separated from the uterine tissue. The term placental tissue was cut into chunks of villi without the maternal decidua basalis and the chorionic plate. Both the early and term placental tissue were cut into 100-200 mg chunks, and placed in ice-cold modified Krebs Ringer phosphate (KRP) buffer, pH 7.4 (K^+ = 5 mM, Ca^{++} = 10 mM), until the start of incubations.

Incubations were performed at 37°C, under 100% oxygen. At the start of the incubation, tissue chunks were cut into 30-60 mg segments and placed in 3 ml KRP containing the compound under study, and 10 mM glucose or sodium acetate in 30 ml beakers. Incubations were conducted with 50 µM ^{14}C-AIB (0.01 µCi/ml), 50 µM ^{14}C-1-CR (0.01 µCi/ml), 1 pM ^{57}Co-Cbl or 1 nM ^{3}H-cbl. When present, 30 µl of concentrated solutions of metabolic inhibitors and analogues of AIB and creatine were added directly to the incubation media to result in final concentrations of 0.1 mM 2,4-dinitrophenol, 0.1 mM ouabain, 10 mM L-glycine, 10 mM L-alanine, 10 mM D-alanine, 10 mM AIB, 10 mM creatine, 10 mM N-amidino-alanine (NAA), or 10 mM beta-guanidino-propionic acid (BGPA). The tissue sections were incubated for varying lengths of time with vigorous shaking (120-160 cycles/min) in Dubnoff incubator-shakers (Scientific Products). At the end of the incubation, tissue sections were removed from the media, blotted on student-grade filter paper, and weighed.

The kinetics of early placental uptake for AIB and CR were determined by the methods described previously (Miller and Berndt, 1974). Placental tissue slices were incubated in varying concentrations of AIB or CR (10 - 100 µM) for 30 min at 37°C both in the presence and the absence of 0.1 mM ouabain. The active uptake component of the uptake was determined as the difference between the control and ouabain-treated values. The V_{max} was the maximal rate of the active uptake component and was expressed as µmole of AIB or CR absorbed/100 g tissue/30min. The K_m was expressed as µM AIB or CR.

Except for ^{57}Co-Cbl, the amount of radioactivity in tissues was assayed by scintillation spectroscopy in a Tracor 6881. After weighing, the tissue samples were dissolved in 700 µl NCS (Amersham) at 50-55°C for 3-12 h. Before counting, 10 ml of scintillation fluid (ACS, Amersham or Liquiscint, National Diagnostics) were added and 100 µl of glacial acetic acid were added to reduce chemiluminescence. The radioactivity in the medium was assayed by mixing 100 µl of the post-incubation medium with 10 ml of scintillation fluid and counting by scintillation spectrometry. Samples containing ^{57}Co were analyzed in a Micromedic 5800 gamma counter. Tissue samples and 100 µl aliquots of media were placed in stoppered 12 x 70 mm glass culture tubes for counting.

The results were expressed as ratios of intracellular-to-extracellular water space distribution, which was corrected for the inulin space values (as previously described Miller and Berndt, 1974).

$$(I/E) = \frac{\text{dpm/g tissue} - (\text{dpm/ml medium x inulin space})}{\text{dpm/ml medium (final) x (ml tissue water} - \text{inulin space})}$$

The tissue water, as defined by the tissue distribution of urea, in the placental tissue section was 0.92 ± 0.04; and the inulin space, as defined by the tissue distribution of inulin was 0.52 ± 0.03 for the experiments with Cbl and 0.40 ± 0.04 for the experiments with AIB and CR.

The I/E ratios for creatine reflected the accumulation of creatine, since less than 5% (mostly under 1%) of the ^{14}C creatine was converted to phosphocreatine by the micro-modifications of the Bertel's method (1974).

Gel chromatography

Post-incubation tissues for the Cbl studies were blotted, weighed, quick-frozen in liquid nitrogen, counted and stored at -20°C. Samples were homogenized in 4 ml of gel elution buffer, pH 7.4, 0.75 M NaCl, 0.02% azide, and spun for 1 h at 105,000 x g. Post-incubation media were frozen and stored at -20°C. The cytosol and medium samples (2-ml aliquots) were applied to a 2.6 x 37 cm Sephacryl S-200 (Pharmacia) gel column and eluted at a rate of 52 ml/h with the elution buffer at 0-4°C. Proteins were monitored by UV monitor at 280 nm. Rabbit anti-human transcobalamin II antisera (gift from Dr. C.A. Hall, V.A. Hospital, Albany, NY) were used to determine the nature of the ^{57}Co-peaks eluted at the molecular weight range of 36,000 - 42,000.

RESULTS

The early placenta concentrated AIB and CR to intracellular-to- extracellular water distribution ratios of 8.27 ± 0.81 (n=21) and 3.75 ± 0.16 (n=21), respectively, after 2 h of incubation at 37°C. The ratios increased with the length of incubation to 5 h (Figure 2). The observed I/E ratios were consistently greater than those observed in the term placenta.

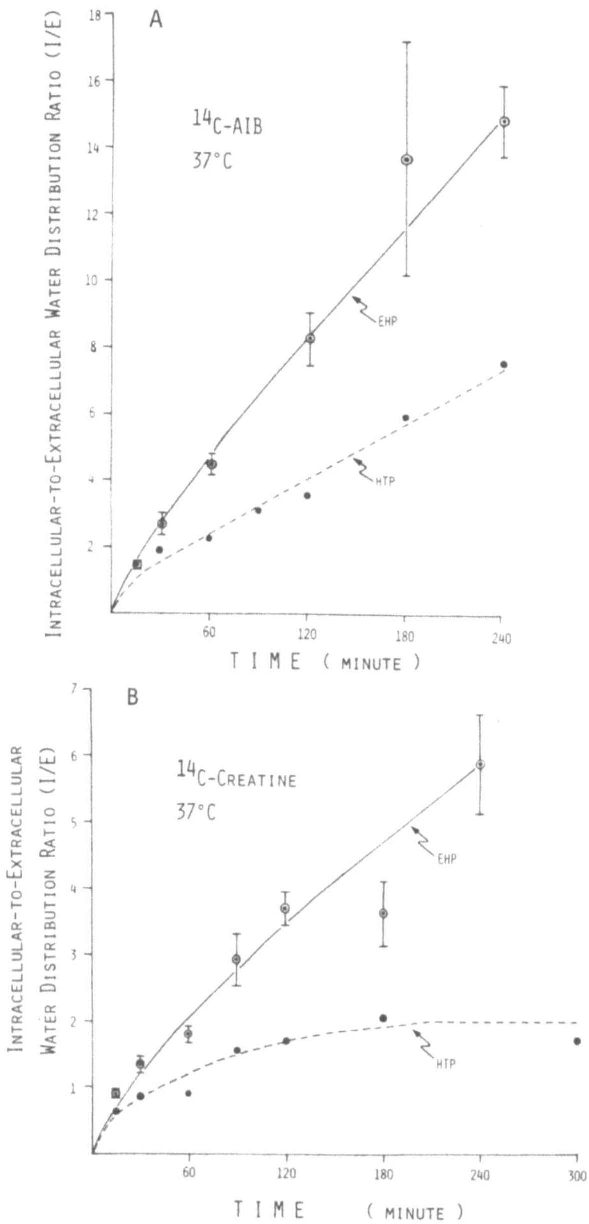

Figure 2. Time course of α-aminoisobutyric acid and creatine uptake in the early and term placental sections. The placental tissue sections were incubated at 37°C in KRP under 100% O_2. The tissue uptake was expressed as I/E and a minimum of three placentae were examined for each point. A. Uptake of ^{14}C-AIB, B. Uptake of ^{14}C-creatine. HTP = human term placenta, EHP = early human placenta.

The early placental accumulations of both AIB and CR were energy-dependent since both processes were reduced by 0.1 mM 2,4-dinitrophenol, and 0.1 mM ouabain (Figure 3). In the presence of sodium acetate as an energy source supplement, the accumulation of AIB by the early placenta was reduced from a control I/E value of 10.13 ± 1.23 (n=9) at 2 h to 4.87 ± 0.63 (n=6) (51.9% reduction) by DNP, and 3.03 ± 0.14 (n=6) (70%) by ouabain. Similarly, the early placental accumulation of CR was reduced from a control I/E value of 3.40 ± 0.16 (n=7) at 2 h to 2.00 ± 0.08 (n=4) (41.2%) by DNP, and 1.54 ± 0.18 (n=4) (55%) by ouabain.

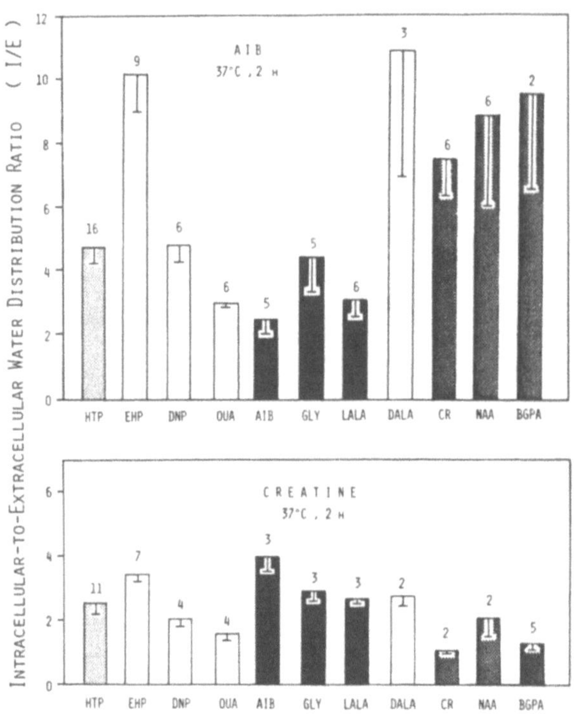

Figure 3. Inhibition of AIB and creatine uptake in the early human placenta. The human placental sections were incubated for 2 h at 37°C in KRP under 100% O_2. The tissue uptake was expressed as I/E ± S.E. The number shown was the number of placentae examined under each condition. HTP = human term placenta, EHP = early human placenta. The metabolic inhibitors, amino acids or guanidino compounds present during incubations of EHP only were: DNP = 2,4 dinitrophenol (0.1 mM), OUA = ouabain (0.1 mM), AIB = α-aminoisobutyric acid (10 mM), GLY = L-glycine (10 mM), LALA = L- alanine (10 mM), DALA = D-alanine (10 mM), CR = Creatine (10 mM), NAA = N- amidino-alanine (10 mM), BGPA = β-guanidino-propionic acid (10 mM).A. Inhibition of AIB uptake, B. Inhibition of Creatine uptake.

The transport of both AIB and CR was specific for those molecules as demonstrated by the inhibition of placental uptake in the presence of analogues. Only L-neutral amino acids depressed AIB uptake, while only guanidino compounds reduced CR uptake (Figure 3). D-alanine did not inhibit either AIB or creatine.

The kinetics of AIB and CR uptake in the early placenta was similar to that of the term placenta. For AIB, the V_{max} of the uptake by the early placenta was 181 ± 75 mmole/100g/30 min, with a K_m of 0.68 ± 0.15 mM (n=4), as compared to the term placental AIB uptake V_{max} of 60 ± 21 μmol/100 g/30 min and K_m of 0.48 ± 0.08 mM (n=10). For CR, the V_{max} of the uptake by the early placenta was 140 ± 49 μmole/100 g/30 min and the K_m was 0.44 ± 0.16 mM (n=4), as compared to the term placental Cr uptake V_{max} of 100 ± 15 μmole/100g/30min and K_m of 0.72 ± 0.09 mM (n=6). All of these transport characteristics for early human placentae were noted for 6-week as well as the 20-week placenta.

For Cbl, it was demonstrated in 11 early human placentae that the capacity to accumulate Cbl is present in porrohysterectomy placental tissue as early as 6 weeks of gestation. After incubation for 2 h at 37°C in 1.01 ± 0.12 pM ^{57}Co-Cbl there were 2.29 ± 0.27 pmole of ^{57}Co-Cbl per gram of tissue, which yielded a I/E ratio of 4.37 ± 0.23 (n=4). When the tissue was incubated in 1.04 ± 0.06 pM plasma protein-bound Cbl, the concentration of ^{57}Co radioactivity was 5.02 ± 3.34 pmole per gram tissue, with a I/E value of 10.77 ± 6.58 (n=2). As with the term placenta, the early human placenta accumulated cbl as well as plasma protein-bound Cbl. No significant difference between the accumulation of 1 nM ^{3}H-cbl by early and term placentae at 37°C was demonstrated during a 4 h time period of incubation.

The early human placental accumulation of Cbl was sensitive to the combined effects of 0.1 mM 2,4-dinitrophenol and iodoacetate, and low temperature at this concentration range. Although the inhibition by the two compounds and low temperature suggests a larger energy-sensitive component in the early human placenta, the effects of iodoacetate on sulfhydryl groups, and hence the intracellular binding changes, prevented definitive conclusions about the energy requirement of Cbl uptake. The tissue content of radioactivity under control incubation conditions was 2.29 pmol Cbl/g tissue and decreased to 1.74 ± 0.26 pmole/g tissue in the presence of 2,4-dinitrophenol plus iodoacetate (n=3). Low temperature alone reduced the tissue content of Cbl to 0.82 pmole/g tissue, in the single placenta examined.

The early human placental accumulation of Cbl was comparable to the uptake of plasma protein-bound Cbl. At a concentration of 1.04 nM bound Cbl, the early human placenta concentrated 5.02 pmol of bound Cbl for each gram of tissue incubated (n=2). Low temperature incubation reduced the tissue concentration of ^{57}Co-Cbl to 1.13 pmol bound Cbl per gram.

The similarity between the early placenta and the term placenta in transport functions was shown also by the intracellular binding and release of the Cbl absorbed from the incubation medium. The early human placental tissue cytosol and medium displayed elution profiles for gel chromatography that were similar to that of the

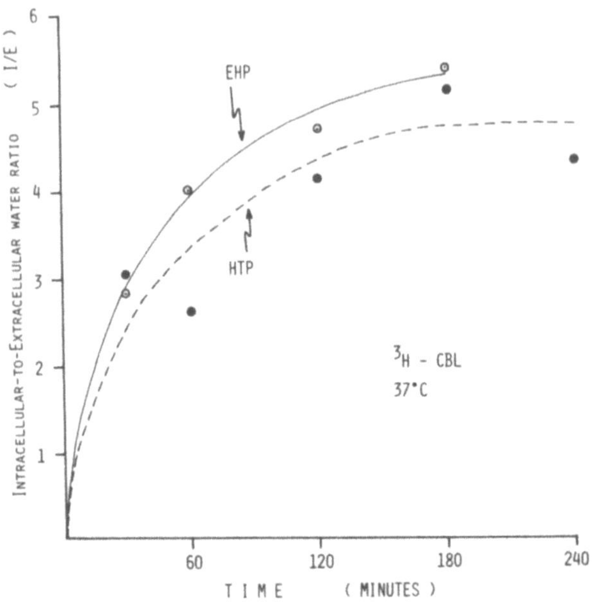

Figure 4. Time course of cobalamin uptake in the early and term placental tissue sections. The placental tissue sections were incubated at 37°C in KRP under 100% O_2 with 1 nM ^{3}H-Cbl. The tissue uptake of cbl was expressed as I/E ratios, which were determined in a minimum of three placentae.

term tissue. Aside from the Cbl peak (infinite volume) which was present in the preincubation media, the postincubation media contained ^{57}Co radioactivity that was associated with a TC I-like protein peak as well as a 38,000 molecular weight peak after 2 h incubation. The cytosolic fractions contained only a single ^{57}Co TC II- Cbl peak (Figure 5). The TC II-Cbl peak identity was identified by the use of anti-TC II-Cbl serum.

DISCUSSION

The human placenta accumulates AIB, CR and Cbl as early as 6-8 weeks of gestation and the concentrative processes persisted to term with modifications only in the amount of the nutrient accumulated per gram of tissue. Despite the limited number of available early placental specimens, it was shown that certain functions of the early and term placental tissue are similar. Under limited experimental conditions, results from term placental tissue may be extrapolated to the early placenta.

The transport processes for AIB and CR in the early placenta are mediated by mechanisms that are similar to those found previously in the term placenta both for their specificity and energy dependence (Miller and Berndt, 1974; Miller et al., 1977).

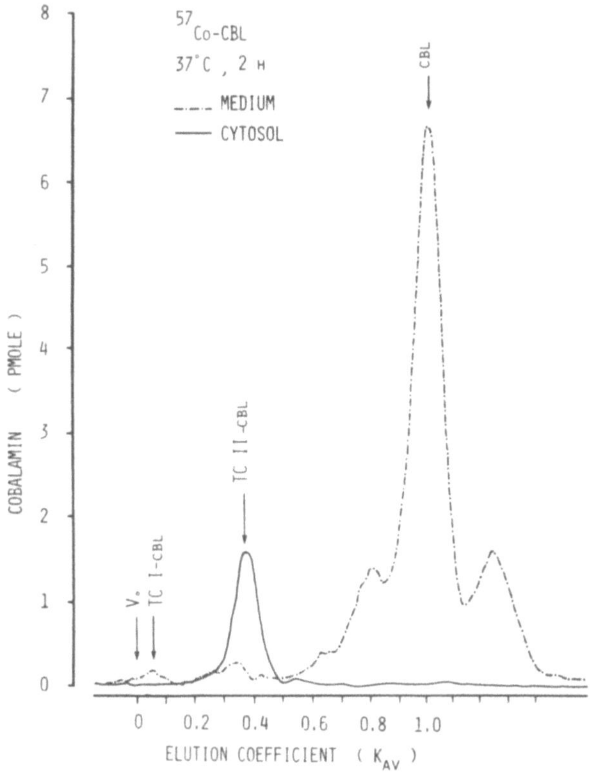

Figure 5. Gel chromatogram of the post-incubation cytosol and medium of Cbl incubations. Early placental tissue sections were incubated with 10 pM ^{57}Co-Cbl for 15 min at 0-4°C under 100% O_2. Aliquots (2 ml) of the post-incubation cytosol and medium were eluted on a Sephacryl S-200 gel column and the elution positions of TC I-cbl and TC II-cbl were indicated by arrows.

The specificity of the uptake of these compounds is indicated by the inhibition by their structural analogues: AIB uptake is decreased by neutral amino acid but not by guanidino compounds or D-amino acids and, similarly, CR uptake is reduced by guanidino compounds but not by neutral L-amino acids. The energy dependence was demonstrated by the inhibition of both AIB and CR uptake in the presence of metabolic inhibitors.

In both the early and term placentae, the depression of AIB and CR uptake by ouabain, a specific Na^+-K^+ATPase inhibitor, was greater than that of oxidative phosphorylation inhibition. This inhibition suggests that the early placenta, as well as the term placental tissue, is dependent on ATP as an energy source. Furthermore, the ATP is not generated solely from the aerobic respiratory processes. The ability to utilize the energy derived from anaerobic respiration exists at least as early as 6 weeks of gestation.

The present report demonstrates that the early human placenta concentrates AIB. This finding is in disagreement with the claims of an earlier study by Harbison et al. (1975) that the early placental uptake of amino acids, as represented by AIB, is depressed (before 20 weeks of gestation) compared to term placental tissue uptake. The difference between the findings of the two studies may be attributed to the viability of the tissues used. The porrohysterotomy specimens used in this current study are obtained immediately after surgery; however, the previous report bases its results from tissues that were obtained after therapeutic abortions. These placentae, following the use of therapeutic agents (e.g., saline and prostaglandins) would have questionable viability due to the delay in obtaining the tissues. Usually the placenta is separated from the uterine wall for a substantial period of time before delivery following such therapeutic interventions. The current study of 32 early human placentae has required eight years, since these tissues are not frequently available.

In the case of the Cbl accumulation, the early placental tissue displays the same ability to concentrate cbl as in the term placenta, and the accumulation is attributable to intracellular binding and subsequent release of the bound Cbl (Ng et al., 1981). Results from this study indicate that the human placenta has specific mechanism for the transport of nutrients and macromolecules and such mechanisms are at least present as early as the sixth week of gestation.

In addition, the uptake processes in the early human placenta may not be developing according to the same pattern as at term. The early placental accumulation of Cbl is the same as that of the term placenta, but the capacity for accumulation of AIB and CR is greater in the early placenta as shown by the amount of the nutrients accumulated per gram of the tissue. Taking into consideration the total mass of the placenta and the demands of the conceptus at the various stages of development, it may be argued that the supply of the nutrients may be tailored to the metabolic needs of the conceptus. Further, it could be argued that at term there is more non-trophoblastic tissues, e.g., fibrin. However, review of histologic sections does not indicate that these differences be accounted for solely by the amount of trophoblastic tissue. The data collected from the various stages of gestation are not complete to allow further speculations.

The early human placental tissue possesses the same uptake processes as the term tissue, although the capacity of these processes may vary (Figures 1, 2, and 3). For these specific uptake processes, the functions of the term placental tissue reflect those of the early placenta. Thus, with the recent interest in the use of the term placenta as an organ for toxicological evaluations (Kelman, 1979; Panigel, 1980; Juchau, 1980 and 1982; Miller et al., 1983), it may be assumed that toxic agents that affect the functioning of the term placenta would interfere with the placenta as early as the first weeks of gestation.

SUMMARY

The ability of the early human placenta to transport selected nutrients was evaluated with an in vitro tissue slice technique. The early human placental sections accumulated α-aminoisobutyric acid (AIB), creatine (CR) and cobalamin (vitamin B_{12}, Cbl). The accumulation of the non- metabolizable AIB and CR was the result of active uptake processes, which were specific and energy-dependent. The characteristics of AIB and CR uptake by the early placenta were similar to those in the term placenta except for greater amounts of AIB and CR accumulated per gram of early placenta examined. In contrast, the early placental accumulation of Cbl was the result of tissue uptake, intracellular binding and release of bound Cbl. The Cbl binders were identified as TC I-like and TC II as detected by gel chromatography and TC II-specific antisera. The early placental uptake of Cbl was similar to the term placental uptake of Cbl in terms of the amount of Cbl accumulated per gram of tissue, intracellular binding patterns and the release of the bound Cbl. Thus, the capability of the early human placenta to accumulate AIB, CR and Cbl was present as early as 6 weeks of gestation. The uptake processes for AIB, CR and Cbl were similar to those of the term placenta in regards to energy requirement, metabolism and specificity, but the early human placenta had an increased capacity for the uptake of AIB and CR.

ACKNOWLEDGMENTS

The authors would like to acknowledge the technical assistance of Kathy Reich. The cooperation of the staffs of the Labor and Delivery floors and Pathology Departments at Strong Memorial Hospital and Highland Hospital, Rochester, New York was greatly appreciated. The study was supported by the Richard W. and Mae Stone Goode Gift and in part by the NIH grant ES02774.

REFERENCES

Bertel, H.H. (1974) Comparative study of various methods for the extraction of free creatine and phosphocreatine from mouse skeletal muscle. *Anal. Biochem.* 60, 347-357.

Brambell, F.W.R. (1970) The Transmission of Passive Immunity from Mother to Young. North-Holland Press, Amsterdam.

Dancis, J., Money, W.L., Springer,D. and Levitz, M. (1968) Transport of amino acids by placenta. *Amer. J. Obstet. Gynecol.* 101, 820-829.

Davis, B.M., Miller, R.K., Brent, R.L. and Koszalka, T.R. (1978) Materno-fetal transport of creatine in the rat. *Biol. Neonate* 33, 43-54.

Enders, R., Judd, R., Donohue, T, and Smith, C. (1976) Placental amino acid uptake III. Transport systems for neutral amino acids. *Amer. J. Physiol.* 230, 706-710.

Friedman, P.A., Shia, M.A. and Wallace, J.K. (1977) A saturable high affinity binding site for transcobalamin II-vitamin B_{12} complexes in human placental membrane preparations. *J. Clin. Invest.* 59, 51-58.

Green, P.D., Savage, C.R., Jr., and Hall C.A. (1976) Mouse transcobalamin: biosynthesis and uptake by L-929 cells. *Arch. Bio. Biophys.* 176, 683-689.

Harbison, R.D., Olubadewo, J., Divivedi, C. and Sastry, B.V.R. (1975) Proposed role of a placental cholinergic system in regulation of fetal growth and development. In: *Basic and Therapeutic Aspects of Perinatal Pharmaclogy* (eds.), Morselli, P.L., Garattini, S. and Serini, F. pp 107- 117, New York, Raven Press.

Herbert, V. (1975) Drugs effective in megaloblastic anemias: vitamin B_{12} and folic acid. In: *The Pharmacological Basis of Therapeutics* (L.S. Goldman and A. Gilman, eds.), 4th ed., pp.1324-1349. Macmillan, New York.

Juchau, M. R. (1980) Drug biotransformation in the placenta. *Pharmacol. Ther.* 8, 501-524.

Juchau, M.R. (1982) The role of the placenta in developmental toxicology. In: *Developmental Toxicology,* (ed.), Snell, K., New York, Praeger Publishers, pp. 187-210.

Kelman, B.J. (1979) Effects of toxic agents on movement of materials across the placenta. *Fed. Proc.* 38, 2246-2250.

Koszalka, T.R., Jensh, R.P. and Brent, R.L. (1975) Placental transport of creatine in the rat. *Soc. Exptl. Biol. Med.* 148, 864-869.

Litonjua, A.D., Canlas, M., Soliman, J. and Paulino, D.Q. (1967) Uptake of alpha-aminoisobutyric acid in placental slices at term. *Amer. J. Obstet. Gynecol.* 99, 242-246.

Longo, L.D., Yuen, P., and Gusseck, D.J. (1973) Anaerobic, glycogen-dependent transport of amino acids by the placenta. *Nature* 243, 531-533.

Meyer, L.M., Gams, R.A., Ryel, E.M., Miller, I.E., and Kuman, S. (1974) Delivery of $^{57}Co-B_{12}$ to lymphoblasts derived from mice with transplanted 1210 ascites tumor cells by transcobalamin I, II and IIV. *Proceeding of the Society of Exp. Biol. Med.* 147, 679-680.

Miller, R.K. and Berndt, W.O. (1974) Characterization of neutral amino acid accumulation by human term placental slices. *Amer. J. Physiol.* 227(6), 1236-1242.

Miller, R.K., Davis, B.M., Brent, R.L. and Koszalka, T.K. (1977) Creatine transport by rat placentas. *Amer. J. Physiol.* 233, E308-E315.

Miller, R.K., Koszalka, T.R., and Brent, R.L. (1976) The transport of molecules across placental membranes. In: *The cell surface in Animal Embryogenesis and development* (eds.), Poste, G. and Nicholson, G.L., Amsterdam; Elsevier North Holland Biomedical Press, pp. 145-223.

Miller, R.K., Ng, W.W. and Levin, A.A. (1983) The placenta: relevance to toxicology. In: *Reproductive and Developmental Toxicity of Metals* (eds.), Clarkson, T., Nordberg, G. and Sager, P., Plenum Press, New York, pp. 569- 605.

Miller, R.K., Reich, K.A., Fox, H.E., Davis, B.M., Brent, R.L., and Koszalka, T.R. (1977) creatine transport and energy metabolism by the human placenta. *The Seventh Rochester Trophoblast Conference Transcripts* 7, 80- 83.

Nexø, E. and Hollenberg, M.D. (1980) Characterization of the particulate and soluble acceptro of transcobalamin II from human placenta and rabbit liver. *Biophys. Biochem. Acta* 628(2), 190-200.

Ng, W.W., Catus, R.G. and Miller, R.K. (1981) Macromolecule transfer in the human trophoblast: transcobalamin II-vitamin B_{12} uptake. *Placenta* (Suppl. 3), 145-160.

Panigel, M. (1981) Placental Function: Toxicology and pathology. In: *Placenta: Receptors, Pathology and Toxicology.* (eds.), Miller, R.K. and Thiede, H.A., London, W.B. Saunders, pp. 275-287.

Seligman, P.A. and Allen, R.H. (1978) Characterization of the receptor for TC II isolated from human placenta. *J. Biol. Chem.* 253(6), 1766-1772.

Schneider, H. and Dancis, J. (1974) Amino acid transport in placental slices. *Amer. J. Obstet. Gynecol.* 120, 1092-1098.

Schneider, H., Panigel, M., and Dancis, J. (1972) Transfer across the perfused human placenta of antipyrine, sodium, and leucine. *Amer. J. Obstet. Gynecol.* 114, 822-828.

Schneider, H., Mohlen, K.H., and Dancis, J. (1979) Transfer of amino acids across the in vitro perfused human placenta. *Ped. Res.* 13, 236-240.
Smith, C.H., Enders, R.H. and Judd, R.M. (1975) Placental transport systems for neutral amino acids. *Pediat. Res.* 9, 280.
Stromberg, K. (1980) The human placenta in cell and organ culture. In: *Methods in cell biology*, Vol. 21B, Chapt. 10, Academic Press, pp.117-252.
Wier, P.J., Maulik, D. and Miller, R.K. (1983) Bidirectional transfer of alpha-aminoisobutyric acid by the perfused human placental lobule. *Trophoblast Research* (this volume).
Wild, A.E. (1981) Endocytic mechanisms in protein transfer across the placenta. *Placenta* (Suppl. 1), 165-186.
Youngdahl-Turner, P., Mellman, I.S., Allen, R.H., and Rosenbereg, L.E. (1979) Protein mediated vitamin uptake. Absorptive endocytosis of the transcobalamin II-cobalamin complex by cultured human fibroblasts. *Exp. Cell Res.* 118, 127-134.

STUDIES ON THE PLACENTAL HYDROLYSIS AND TRANSFER OF LIPIDS TO THE FETAL GUINEA PIG

Chris R. Thomas, Clara Lowy, R. Jim St. Hillaire[1] and John D. Brunzell [2]

Departments of Medicine and Chemical Pathology
St. Thomas Hospital, London, SE1 7EH, United Kingdom

INTRODUCTION

Early studies on the placental transfer of lipids using the sheep (James et al., 1971) and the rat (Koren and Shafrir, 1964) suggested that very little fat was transferred from mother to fetus. The majority of fetal lipids were assumed to be formed from transferred maternal glucose (Coltart, 1972). However, investigations in species such as rabbit (Elphick et al., 1975), guinea pig (Hershfield and Nemeth, 1968; Bohmer and Havel, 1975), primate (Portman et al., 1969) and more recently in the rat (Hummel et al., 1974) indicated that not only did free fatty acids (FFA) readily cross the placenta, but that they did so in amounts exceeding those required to fulfill lipid storage requirements (Jones, 1976).

Less is known about other lipid moieties. The placenta, of all those species investigated, appears to be virtually impermeable to esterified lipids (McBride and Korn, 1964; Kayden et al., 1969) although FFA derived from maternal triglyceride (TG) have been shown to cross the placenta in rabbit and man (Elphick and Hull, 1977; Elphick et al., 1978). These studies, however, have used a TG emulsion (Intralipid, Vitrium, Stockholm), and this may not be a good substrate for investigating the contribution of esterified maternal lipids to the fetus. Hummel et al. (1976) found that FFA from chylomicron TG did not cross the rat placenta whilst FFA from very low density lipoprotein (VLDL) did. Since Intralipid has a composition akin to chylomicrons, we decided to investigate the clearance and placental transfer of a bolus of endogenously prepared VLDL in the pregnant guinea pig. We compared this with the results of a bolus of radioactively labeled palmitic acid to resolve whether VLDL and/or the FFA resulting from its hydrolysis were transferred across the guinea pig placenta in the same way as administered FFA. The results we obtained implied the hydrolysis of VLDL within the placenta itself, and we have subsequently investigated the presence and distribution of heparin elutable lipoprotein lipase (HELPL) (EC 3.1.1.3) within the guinea pig placenta.

Present Addresses:
[1] G.I. Research Laboratory, Veterans Hospital,
San Francisco, California, U.S.A.
[2] Department of Medicine RG-20, University of Washington, Seattle, Washington, 98195, U.S.A.

METHODS

Preparation of ^{14}C-VLDL

A Dunkin-Hartley guinea pig in late gestation (60 to 65 days assessed by the method of Thomas and Lowy, 1982) was anesthetized with sodium pentobarbital (15 mg/kg body weight intravenously). A polyethylene cannula was inserted and tied into one carotid artery, and the animal partially immersed in a supine position, in a saline bath at 37°C. Approximately 0.2 mCi of (1 - ^{14}C) palmitic acid (Radiochemical Centre, Amersham) complexed to 30 g/l of human serum albumin (Blood Products Labs., Herts.) was infused over a 3 hour period using a syringe pump. Following laparotomy, blood was collected for the umbilical vein of each fetus, placed in EDTA tubes at 0°C, centrifuged at 1500 g from 10 minutes at 4°C, and aspirated. The plasma was centrifuged at 105,000 g for 16 hours in a sucrose solution of density 1.06, and the VLDL separated by cutting the centrifuge tube. Purity of the VLDL labeling was assessed by running chloroform-methanol extracts on thin-layer chromatography (solvent mixture, hexane 70: ether 30: acetic acid 1; V/V) and scanning for radioactivity using a 2 dimensional scanner (Tracerlab, N.Y.). It was found that approximately 90% (range 88.8 - 91%) of the label was associated with TG in these extracts.

Bolus injections of VLDL or palmitic acid

The experimental model was a modification of that described by Reynolds and Young (1971). A pregnant guinea pig (gestational age range 48 - 65 days) was anesthetized; each carotid artery and an external jugular vein were cannulated. The lines were kept patent by a slow infusion of 0.9% (W/V) NaCl since the use of heparin, which enhances TG hydrolysis, had to be avoided. The animal was placed in a saline bath, a laparotomy performed, and the umbilical vessels of a fetus cannulated using two 22 gauge and one 18 gauge Medicut cannulae (Sherwood Medical Industries, St. Louis, U.S.A.). Human serum albumin at 30 g/l which had been dialysed overnight against 10 volumes of a Ringer solution, was perfused through the placenta via the umbilical arteries at 1 ml/minute by a peristaltic pump. The albumin solution (termed perfusate) was collected, after a single passage through the placenta, from the umbilical vein. Perfusion pressure and maternal blood pressure were monitored continuously.

Two milliliters of VLDL or palmitic acid complexed to albumin were injected as a bolus over 10s into the left carotid artery, perfusate collections were made and maternal blood collected into chilled EDTA tubes at various time intervals for up to 1.5 h. Blood samples were centrifuged (1500 g, 10 min.), the plasma aspirated and aliquots of perfusate and maternal plasma immediately extracted and separated into FFA and TG by the method of Dole and Meinertz (1960). The extracts were dried under air, scintillation fluid added and the radioactivity counted and corrected to disintegrations/min.

To monitor efficiency of 'exchange' between maternal and fetal circulations, antipyrine was infused into the maternal circulation. Antipyrine measurements were made in plasma and perfusates by the method of Meschia (1964).

Lipoprotein lipase assay

Placentae were obtained by laparotomy from anaesthetized pregnant (52 - 65 days) guinea pigs and were sectioned vertically on ice. The central sections were rinsed in Krebs Ringer phosphate buffer, pH 7.4 and cut into 1 mm cubes. The HELPL content of 70 - 100 mg of placenta was immediately estimated in triplicate by the method of Pykalisto et al. (1975), and expressed as nEq FFA released/g/min. Control incubations using 1M NaCl or omission of plasma from the TG substrate were performed, and interassay variability was checked against a post-heparin plasma standard.

Heparin boluses on maternal and fetal sides of the placenta

The internal iliac arteries of 2 pregnant guinea pigs (approx. 52 days) were ligated and a bolus injection of 2 ml of 0.9% (W/V) NaCl containing 5 IU heparin sulphate was administered anteriorly into the dorsal aorta on a level with the renal arteries. Blood was sampled simultaneously from the aorta and left ovarian vein, centrifuged and aspirated.

In a further 3 animals, the fetal side of the placenta was perfused at 1 ml/min. with 0.9 (W/V) NaCl containing 2 IU/ml heparin. The perfusate was collected over 0 - 4, 4 - 6, 6 - 8 minutes after a single passage through the placenta.

Plasma and perfusate samples were immediately assayed for HELPL content as above.

Calculation of metabolic clearance rate (MCR) and half lives ($t_{1/2}$)

The MCR of maternal TG was estimated by fitting two exponentials by least square methods to the logarithms of the data, calculating the area under the first exponential and dividing this by the dose administered. The $t_{1/2}$ for the maternal TG, FFA and perfusate FFA were calculated using the log values for the first exponential of the respective data.

RESULTS

Status of the experimental animal

The perfusate/maternal ratio for antipyrine had a mean value of 0.86 $\pm$ 0.03 (SEM) for the twelve FFA, VLDL bolus experiments indicating 'satisfactory' placental function. Maternal blood pressure remained within 35 - 60 mm Hg in all the experiments, and placental perfusion pressure, at a flow rate of 1 ml/min., remained stable at 11 mm Hg. At the end of the experiments, the maternal blood pH had a mean value of 7.36 $\pm$ 0.02 (SEM) the PO_2 a mean value of 98 $\pm$ 7.3 (SEM) and the PCO_2 a mean value of 35 $\pm$ 1.5 (SEM).

Bolus injection of (1 - ^{14}C) palmitate

Maternal plasma radioactivity rapidly declined (mean $t_{1/2}$ = 2.40 ± 0.21 (SEM) min., Table 1) following a bolus injection of (1-^{14}C) palmitic acid into four sows, and was closely followed by the appearance of radioactive FFA in the perfusate. From 2.5 min the radioactive FFA declined in the perfusate in parallel with the disappearance in the mother (perfusate FFA $t_{1/2}$ = 2.41 ± 0.15 (SEM) min.) but with a mean delay time of 1.59 ± 0.10 (SEM) minutes. The areas under the (^{14}C) disappearance-time curves for 0 to 30 minutes had a mean perfusate/maternal ratio of 0.81 ± 0.02 (SEM), and these ratios were not found to relate to gestational age or the weight of fetuses remaining intact within the uterus.

Bolus injection of (1 - ^{14}C) VLDL

A rapid fall ($t_{1/2}$ range 0.7 to 8.9 min.) in labeled maternal plasma TG was found following a bolus injection of (1 - ^{14}C) VLDL to eight sows (Table 2), and the (1 - ^{14}C) TG MCR was found to be very variable. It was not found to be correlated ($0.1 > p > 0.05$) with gestational age, but was significantly correlated ($n=8$, $r=0.79$, $p<0.02$) with the weight of fetuses remaining within the uterus. In all experiments, virtually no labeled TG was found to enter the perfusate (0.08 ± 0.03% (SEM) of dose by 30 min.).

Maternal plasma (1 - ^{14}C) FFA derived from injected VLDL (termed (^{14}C) TG-FFA) rose from the time of injection to approximately 5 minutes and then declined with a $t_{1/2}$ of 13.05 ± 2.76 (SEM) min. A similar rise and fall of (^{14}C) TG-FFA was seen in the perfusate samples, where the $t_{1/2}$ (12.34 ± 2.63 (SEM) min.) was not significantly different from the maternal plasma (^{14}C) TG-FFA $t_{1/2}$ by paired t-test.

In half of the experiments, concentrations of perfusate (^{14}C) TG-FFA were higher than in the corresponding maternal blood sample (Figure 1). The areas under the (^{14}C) TG-FFA disappearance-time curves for 0 to 30 minutes had perfusate/maternal ratios which correlated significantly ($n=8$, $r=0.77$, $p<0.05$) with gestational age and from the computed regression line the ratio exceeds unity from 55 days of gestation.

Placental HELPL content

Preliminary results obtained on 11 placentae indicate that whilst placental weight does not substantially increase in late gestation (Kaufman and Davidoff, 1977), there is a rapid and dramatic rise in HELPL content, especially after a mean fetal weight of 50 g, or a gestational age of 55 days (Table 3). By 60 days, levels of HELPL per gm are 5 fold higher than at 55 days and by approximately 65 days they are increased 11 fold.

Table 1

Results obtained after the bolus injection of (1 - ^{14}C) palmitate into four pregnant guinea pigs.

Guinea-Pig	Gestational age (days)	Weight of fetuses in utero (gm)	Antipyrine ratio *	Maternal (^{14}C) FFA $t\frac{1}{2}$ (min.)	Perfusate (^{14}C) FFA $t\frac{1}{2}$ (min.)	Perfusate Maternal (^{14}C) FFA ratio +
1	60	187	0.80	2.43	2.33	0.85
2	60	261	0.90	2.51	2.35	0.74
3	62	252	1.01	2.84	2.85	0.86
4	65	240	0.86	1.84	2.12	0.79
Mean	62	235	0.89	2.40	2.41	0.81

*Perfusate antipyrine value divided by corresponding maternal antipyrine level. Mean given of at least 5 points throughout each experiment.

+Values for perfusate/maternal areas for (^{14}C) FFA for 0 to 30 minutes (calculated by least squares fit of log data).

Table 2
Results obtained following a bolus injection of (1 - ^{14}C) VLDL into eight pregnant guinea pigs.

Guinea-pig	Gestational age (days)	Weight of fetuses in utero (gm)	Antipyrine Ratio*	Maternal (1-^{14}C) TG $t_{\frac{1}{2}}$ (min.)	Maternal (1-^{14}C) TG-FFA $t_{\frac{1}{2}}$ (min.)	Perfusate (1-^{14}C) TG-FFA $t_{\frac{1}{2}}$ (min.)	Maternal (1-^{14}C) TG MCR (min.)	Perfusate/ Maternal (1-^{14}C) TG-FFA ratio +
1	48.0	0++	0.81	8.94	13.42	20.46	1.0	0.06
2	50.5	97	0.85	1.13	27.23	14.61	6.5	0.79
3	52.5	0++	0.70	2.06	22.98	26.12	5.3	0.40
4	55.5	300	0.76	0.71	8.25	7.24	24.5	0.44
5	58.0	163	0.76	1.74	8.80	9.96	9.7	1.93
6	58.5	181	0.86	1.31	9.83	8.38	9.4	2.68
7	59.0	60	1.06	1.03	5.69	5.96	17.3	1.33
8	65.0	251	0.94	0.90	8.26	6.03	20.1	2.01
Mean	56.0	-	0.84	2.22	13.05	12.34	-	-

*Perfusate antipyrine value divided by corresponding maternal antipyrine level. Mean given of at least 5 points throughout each experiment.
+Values for perfusate/maternal areas for (^{14}C) TG-FFA for 0 to 30 minutes (calculated by least squares fit of log data).
++There was only one fetus, which was removed when the placenta is perfused in this preparation.

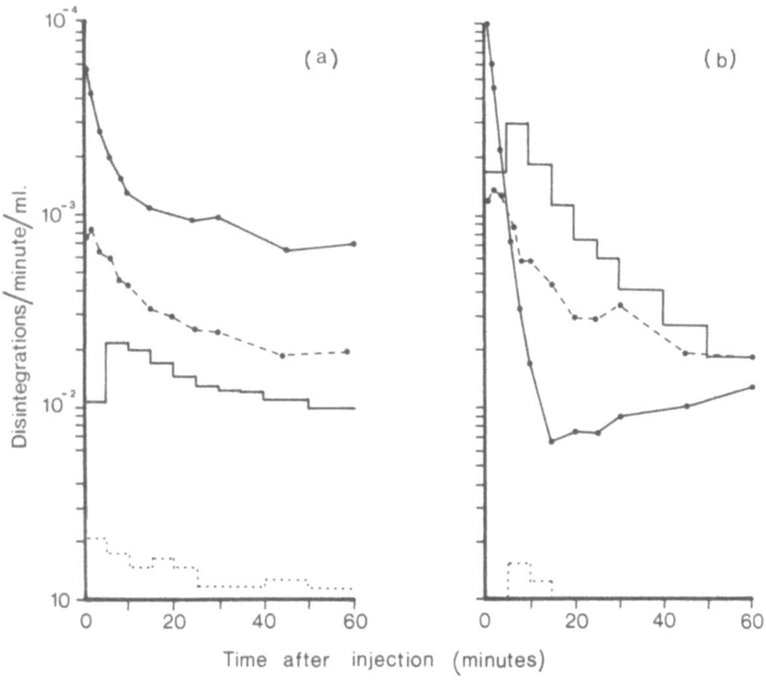

Figure 1. Values for (^{14}C) label associated with maternal TG (●—●)and FFA (●-----●) and perfusate TG (-----) and FFA (—)on a log scale versus time in minutes following a bolus injection of (1 - ^{14}C) VLDL at time 0. Results are shown for two animals (a) at 52.5 days gestation (guinea pig 3) and (b) at 58.5 days gestation (guinea pig 6).

Release of HELPL on the maternal and fetal sides of the placenta

Following the heparin bolus, there was a substantial increase in the LPL content of the blood in the left ovarian vein in both experiments (Figure 2) where levels rose 6 fold over basal levels in 2 to 3 minutes. In experiment 2, a three fold rise in LPL content was seen in the sample taken between 15 and 30 seconds, which must reflect release of the enzyme from the uterine contents (circulation time in the guinea pig is approximately 25 seconds, Bissonnette et al. 1979). A similar but less pronounced rise in the LPL content of the aorta was found, indicating release of LPL from extrauterine sites and dilution in the total maternal blood volume. The values for the ovarian vein samples will be contaminated with this extrauterine LPL after one circulation time, and may account for the biphasic response seen in experiment 2.

In all 3 experiments which involved the perfusion of the fetal side of the placenta with heparin, there was no change found in LPL content (Table 4) which was very low in all experiments.

Table 3
Placental heparin elutable lipoprotein lipase in the guinea pig.

Gestational age (days)	Fetal weight (g)	Mean Placental weight (g)	LPL* / g	LPL Placenta	Number of samples
52 - 55	40 - 49	3.3	43	141	7
56	51	4.3	47	201	1
60	62	2.9	231	685	1
62 - 65	72 & 79	3.4	501	1689	2

*LPL measured, after incubation of 70 - 100 mg of placenta with heparin, by the method of Pykalisto et al. (1975) and expressed as nEq FFA/min/g placenta.

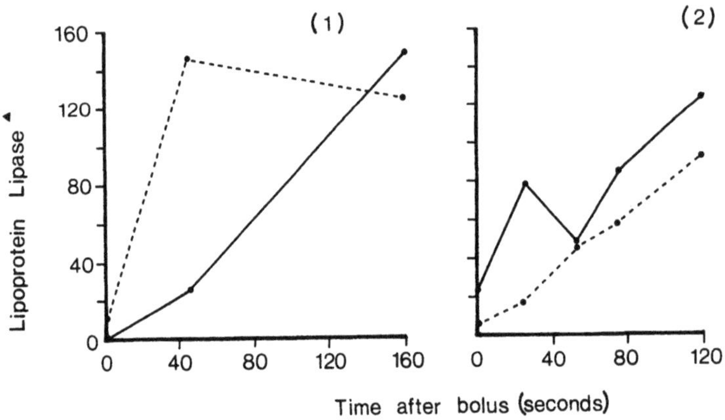

Figure 2. Levels of lipoprotein lipase in aorta and ovarian venous blood following a bolus of 5 IU heparin into the maternal circulation of two pregnant guinea pigs. LPL expressed as nEqFFA/min/ml. in blood from the dorsal aorta (●-----●) or left ovarian vein (●——●).

Table 4
Lipoprotein lipase released by heparin from the fetal side of the guinea pig placenta.

Sample	Time (mins.)		LPL*		
		EXPT	1	2	3
1	0 - 4		0.56	1.06	4.7
2	4 - 6		0.50	0.99	4.5
3	6 - 8		0.54	0.98	4.5

*LPL measured by the method of Pykalisto et al. (1975) in samples of perfusate collected over the times indicated and expressed as nEq FFA/min/ml.

DISCUSSION

The mean plasma $t_{1/2}$ of 2.4 minutes found for a (^{14}C) palmitate bolus in this study is similar to the corresponding $t_{1/2}$ of 1.3 minutes reported by Hershfield and Nemeth (1968). A number of workers have reported rapid placental transfer of FFA in the guinea pig (Hershfield and Nemeth, 1968; Bohmer and Havel, 1975; Jones, 1976) although precise figures have not been published. The mean lag time reported here of 1.59 min. and the similarity in decay profiles of (1 - ^{14}C) FFA in maternal plasma and perfusate (2.4 and 2.41 min. respectively) reaffirm that the guinea pig placenta is readily traversed by FFA.

This does not appear to be the case with esterified fats, only very small amounts of labeled TG were found to cross the placenta intact in this study, the figures being within the error of the method of extraction. This lack of TG transport agrees with findings of other studies in the guinea pig (Hershfield and Nemeth, 1968; Kayden et al., 1969) the rabbit (Elphick and Hull, 1977), rat (Hummel et al., 1978) and human (Elphick et al., 1978). The rapid disappearance of labeled TG from the maternal plasma is similar to the value of 3.56 min. found in the rat by Humphrey et al. (1980) and in the sheep by Shand and Noble (1979).

The rise in labeled maternal FFA accompanying the decline of labeled maternal TG, after the injection of VLDL, implies that hydrolysis of the lipoprotein occurs in capillary beds within the sow's body (Robinson, 1970; Scow et al., 1976). The $t_{1/2}$ of this TG-FFA in the maternal plasma of approximately 13 minutes was considerably longer than that found for the bolus of palmitate. One explanation for this may be the continued appearance of FFA from the hydrolysis of TG at the same time as FFA clearance from the plasma. However, since the half life of VLDL is shorter than the half life for the corresponding TG-FFA in each experiment, levels of label associated with maternal FFA are 2 to 3 fold higher than levels associated with TG from about 5 min. onwards. It is thus unlikely that TG-FFA is released immediately into the maternal plasma. This delayed appearance may be due to short term uptake and then release of FFA from the tissues at the site of hydrolysis.

As with the palmitate bolus studies, the perfusate $t_{1/2}$ for TG-FFA had a similar value to that in the maternal plasma (12.34 and 13.05 respectively), but in the VLDL studies there was a transplacental lag time of 9.38 min. in the experiments where TG was contributing large amounts of FFA to the perfusate (i.e., where the perfusate/maternal TG-FFA ratio > 1). This implies that whilst FFA per se cross the guinea pig placenta very rapidly, TG- FFA is handled differently by the tissue prior to release into the fetal circulation and may again be evidence of a short term store for hydrolysis products.

When the total TG-FFA in the perfusate is corrected for umbilical flow (Shepherd and Whelan, 1951) and litter size, a mean value of 7.95% ($\pm$ 1.88%, SEM) of the injected VLDL dose would be transferred as FFA to the fetuses in the first 30 minutes.

The significant correlation found between the MCR of maternal TG and the weight of fetuses in utero indicates, perhaps, that the uterine content has a considerable role in TG uptake. This uptake must be mediated via LPL, which fits with the dramatic rise in placental HELPL content as gestation proceeds (uterine HELPL levels remain about a mean value of 14 nEqFFA/g/min - R.J. St. Hillaire - unpublished observations). The observations that in the experiments performed in later gestation (after 55 days) the perfusate/maternal TG-FFA ratio exceeds unity also confirms the presence and action of placental HELPL since the perfusate/maternal FFA ratio following a (1 - ^{14}C) palmitate bolus had a mean value of only 0.81 despite a mean gestational age of 62 days.

That this LPL is localized on the maternal side of the placenta is interesting, and explains the exceptionally high levels of TG in guinea pig fetal plasma (Bohmer et al., 1972). FFA transported to the fetus are rapidly taken up and esterified by the fetal liver (Bohmer and Havel, 1975; Jones, 1976; Thomas et al., 1977) and released into the circulation as VLDL. Whilst transfer of FFA occurs readily from fetus to mother in many species (Portman et al., 1969; Dancis et al., 1973; Elphick et al., 1975; Noble et al., 1979) it is unlikely that intact TG will transfer, although we are unaware of any published data which confirms this. The virtual absence of HELPL on the fetal side of the placenta will tend to minimize fetal TG hydrolysis and the lowering of fetal adipose tissue LPL activity as gestation proceeds (Jones, 1976) means that once FFA from the mother is converted to VLDL in the fetus, it cannot be transferred back (preliminary results of 3 experiments in which labeled VLDL was recycled through the fetal side of the placenta tend to substantiate this; no radioactivity was found in the maternal plasma - Thomas and Lowy, unpublished observations).

In conclusion, separate mechanisms have been described by which maternal lipids in the form of FFA or TG can give rise to FFA in the fetal circulation. After esterification of these FFA's by the fetal liver, a mobile fat store in the form of VLDL circulates within the fetus. This store is not available to the mother due to the absence of LPL on the fetal side of the placenta. This fat may be important as a fuel store during the first few days of postnatal life, since after birth the hyperlipemia subsides rapidly (Bohmer et al., 1972).

SUMMARY

Following a bolus injection of (1 - ^{14}C) palmitate into 4 pregnant guinea pigs, the label disappeared with a half-life of 2.4 minutes. Labeled palmitate crossed the placenta which was being perfused in situ, with a lag time of 1.6 minutes and had a half-life in the perfusate of 2.41 minutes.

In a further eight guinea pigs, levels of (1 - ^{14}C) triglyceride declined rapidly (half-life 0.7 to 9.8 minutes) following an injection of endogenously labeled very low density lipoprotein. No (1 - ^{14}C) triglyceride crossed the placenta intact but hydrolysis products appeared in maternal plasma and perfusate where they subsequently declined in parallel but at a slower rate (13.05 and 12.34 minutes respectively) than after palmitate injections. The time lag across the placenta was also longer (9.4 minutes) for the triglyceride derived free fatty acid.

Placental heparin elutable lipoprotein lipase was found to rise 11 fold over the last sixth of gestation and was found to be localized specifically on the maternal side of the placenta. In guinea pigs over 55 days of gestation, concentrations of labeled free fatty acids were higher in the perfusate than in the maternal plasma, which implies intraplacental hydrolysis of triglyceride.

REFERENCES

Bissonnette, J.M., Cronan, J.Z., Richards, L.L., and Wickham, W.K. (1979) Placental transfer of water and nonelectrolytes during a single circulatory passage. *Amer. J. Physiol.* 236, C47-C52.

Bohmer, T. and Havel, R.J. (1975) Genesis of fatty liver and hyperlipemia in the fetal guinea pig. *J. Lipid Res.* 16, 454-460.

Bohmer, T., Havel, R.J. and Long, J.A. (1972) Physiological fatty liver and hyperlipemia in the fetal guinea pig: Chemical and ultrastructural characterization. *J. Lipid Res.* 13, 371-382.

Coltart, T.M. (1972) Effect on fetal liver lipids of ^{14}C glucose administered intravenously to the mother. *J. Obstet. Gynaecol. Brit. Commonw.* 79, 639-643.

Dancis, J., Jansen, V., Kayden, H.J., Schneider, H. and Levitz, M. (1973) Transfer across perfused human placenta II. Free fatty acids. *Pediat. Res.* 7, 192-197.

Dole, V.P. and Meinertz, H. (1960) Micro determination of long chain fatty acids in plasma and tissues. *J. Biol. Chem.* 235, 2595-2599.

Elphick, M.C., Filshie, G.M. and Hull, D. (1978) The passage of fat emulsion across the human placenta. *Brit. J. Obstetr. Gynaecol.* 85, 610-618.

Elphick, M.C., Hudson, D.G. and Hull, D. (1975) Transfer of fatty acids across the rabbit placenta. *J. Physiol.* 252, 29-42.

Elphick, M.C. and Hull, D. (1977) Rabbit placental clearing-factor lipase and transfer to the fetus of fatty acids derived from triglycerides injected into the mother. *J. Physiol.* 273, 475-487.

Hershfield, M.S. and Nemeth, A.M. (1968) Placental transport of free palmitic and linoleic acids in the guinea pig. *J. Lipid Res.* 9, 460-468.

Hummel, L., Schirrmeister, W., Zimmerman, T. and Wagner, H. (1974) Studies on the lipid metabolism using ^{14}C-1-palmitate in fetal rats. *Biol. Neonate 24*, 298-305.

Hummel, L., Schwartze, A., Schirrmeister, W. and Wagner, H. (1976) Maternal plasma triglycerides as a source of fetal fatty acids. *Acta Biol. Med. Ger.* 35, 1635-1641.
Hummel, L., Zimmerman, T., Schenk, H., Schwartz, A., Schirrmeister, W. and Wagner, H. (1978) Studies on the hypertriglyceridemia in the pregnant rat. *Acta Biol. Med. Ger.* 37, 259-266.
Humphrey, J.L., Childs, M.T., Montes, A. and Knopp, R.H. (1980) Lipid metabolism in pregnancy. VII. Kinetics of chylomicron triglyceride removal in fed pregnant rat. *Amer. J. Physiol.* 239, E81-E87.
James, E., Meschia, G. and Battaglia, F.C. (1971) A-V differences of free fatty acids and glycerol in the ovine umbilical circulation. *Proc. Soc. Exper. Biol. Med.* 138, 823-826.
Jones, C.T. (1976) Lipid metabolism and mobilization in the guinea pig during pregnancy. *Biochem. J.* 156, 357-365.
Kaufmann, P. and Davidoff, M. (1977) The guinea pig placenta. *Advances in Anat. Embry. Cell Biol.* 53, 1-91.
Kayden, H.J., Dancis, J. and Money, W.L. (1969) Transfer of lipids across the guinea pig placenta. *Amer. J. Obstet. Gynaecol.* 104, 564-572.
Koren, Z. and Shafrir, E. (1964) Placental transfer of free fatty acids in the pregnant rat. *Proc. Soc. Exper. Biol. Med.* 116, 411-414.
McBride, O.W. and Korn, E.D. (1964) Uptake of free fatty acids and chylomicron glycerides by guinea pig mammary gland in pregnancy and lactation. *J. Lipid Res.* 5, 453-458.
Meschia, G. (1964) *Proceedings Technicon International Symposium on Automation in Analytical Chemistry*, Chauncey, N.Y.: Technicon Instruments Corp.
Noble, R.C., Shand, J.H. and Bell, A.W. (1979) Fetal to maternal transfer of palmitic and linoleic acids across the sheep placenta. *Biol. Neonate* 36, 113-118.
Portman, O.W., Behrman, R.E. and Soltys, P. (1969) Transfer of free fatty acid across the primate placenta. *Amer. J. Physiol.* 216, 143-147.
Pykalisto, O.J., Smith, P.H. and Brunzell, J.D. (1975) Human adipose tissue lipoprotein lipase: Comparison of assay methods and expressions of activity. *Proc. Soc. Exper. Biol. Med.* 148, 297-300.
Reynolds, M.L. and Young, M. (1971) Transfer of free amino nitrogen across the placental membrane in the guinea pig. *J. Physiol.* 214, 583-597.
Robinson, D.S. (1970) The function of the plasma triglyceride in fatty acid transport. In *Comprehensive Biochemistry* (eds.), Florkin, M. and Stotz, E.H., vol. 18, Amsterdam: Elsevier, pp. 51-116.
Scow, R.O., Blanchette-Mackie, E.K. and Smith, L.C. (1976) Role of capillary endothelium in the clearance of chylomicrons. A model for lipid transport from blood by lateral diffusion in cell membranes. *Circul. Res.* 39, 149-162.
Shand, J.H. and Noble, R.C. (1979) The role of maternal triglycerides in the supply of lipids to the ovine fetus. *Res. Vet. Sci.* 26, 117-119.
Shepherd, J.T. and Whelan, R.F. (1951) The blood flow in the umbilical cord of the fetal guinea pig. *J. Physiol.* 115, 150-157.
Thomas, C.R. and Lowy, C. (1982) The assessment of gestational age and litter size in the guinea pig using a radiographic method. *Placenta* 3, 91-98.
Thomas, C.R., Lowy, C., Bacchus, R.A. and Yeoman, D.K. (1977) Transfer of free fatty acid across the guinea pig placenta. *Diabetologia* 13, pp. 436.

DISCUSSION

ILLSLEY (Harrow): Is there any specificity to the transfer of free fatty acids? And was there any specificity in the breakdown of the triglycerides during your perfusions? We have been studying in the human placenta, organic acid chromatograms from our perfusates. We believe we note a large peak of glycerol in this chromatogram. We are still trying to confirm this. We were not sure where it is coming from because there was no obvious pathway whereby glycerol could be produced under these conditions. If there is a large amount of triglyceride in the placenta, perhaps this is the source for the glycerol that we may be seeing. Have you noticed the same observations?

THOMAS (London): We have only evaluated ^{14}C-palmitate for nonesterified free fatty acid and tripalmitate for the esterfied fatty acids. We have not examined the breakdown products per se; however, when we have chromatographed the eluates, it appears they are the same fats. The triglyceride store within the placenta is considerable and perhaps could account for the appearance that you see.

VAN KREEL (Rotterdam): In the development of the hypothesis concerning the transfer of free fatty acids, have you labelled the glycerol part of the triglyceride with one radioisotope and labeled the free fatty acid with another? This would perhaps help to answer the questions posed.

THOMAS (London): That is an interesting idea. We could determine whether there was a directionality in the metabolism and release of these components.

MOORE (Manchester): Do you suggest that lipids have a possibly unrecognized role in maintaining the fetus rather than just our consideration of carbohydrates and proteins as such sources? Do you have any observations along these lines?

THOMAS (London): No. I am not suggesting that lipids should be thought of as replacing carbohydrates. Our suggestion is that not all of the fetal lipids come originally via fetal lipogenesis, i.e., are derived from maternal glucose. Fetal lipids may be of maternal origin rather than just of fetal origin, and may be complementary to glucose and amino acids in maintaining the fetus.

WINICK (New York): How important are the essential fatty acids in the guinea pig compared with the human? It is conceivable that there is a fetal need for essential fatty acids in both.

THOMAS (London): Certainly the fetal guinea pig does require essential fatty acids as does the human; however, the nature of the transport of essential fatty acids appears to be more rapid than for nonessential fatty acids. This certainly needs to be evaluated in greater depth. We have only examined the nonessential fatty acid, palmitate.

DANCIS (New York): We have studied the transfer of free fatty acids across guinea pig placenta using the in situ perfusion technique (Kayden et al., 1969, Transfer of lipids across the guinea pig placenta, *Amer. J. Obstet. Gynecol.* 104,564-572). We did not find a difference in transfer rates between essential and non-essential fatty acids. More significantly, the transfer rates of the free fatty acids across the perfused guinea pig placenta was much more rapid than across human perfused placenta (Dancis et al., 1973, Transfer across perfused human placenta II. Free fatty acids, *Pediat. Res.* 7, 192-197). Transfer of fatty acids in the human appears to be insufficient to provide for the fetal fat deposition that occurs in the last trimester. Conversion of carbohydrates is probably necessary. The same may not be true for the guinea pig.

THOMAS (London): Hull in Nottingham (Elphick et al., 1978, The passage of fat emulsion across the human placenta, *Brit. J. Obstet. Gynaecol.* 85, 610-618) has evaluated the effect of giving intralipids to mothers prior to birth. He has found that the fetal plasma is highly enriched with those fatty acids present in the intralipid. Thus, in their in vivo experiments, they found the transfer of fats from triglycerides. These data in the human would be supportive of our observations in the guinea pig.

Trophoblast Research 1:149-158, 1983

DOPPLER ASSESSMENT OF FETOPLACENTAL CIRCULATORY DYNAMICS

Debabrata Maulik,[1] Vasant D. Saini,[1,2] and Navin C. Nanda[3]

Departments of Obstetrics/Gynecology,[1] Electrical Engineering[2] and Medicine [3]
Division of Cardiology, Univ. of Rochester, School of Medicine and Dentistry
Strong Memorial Hospital, Rochester, NY 14642, U.S.A.

INTRODUCTION

The recent development of Doppler Ultrasonic Flowmetry has substantially contributed to non-invasive assessment of hemodynamics in humans (Shatumora, 1957; Franklin et al., 1961; Baker, 1970; Peronneau et al., 1974). This technique has been successfully applied to investigate human peripheral circulation (Woodcock, 1972; Light and Cross, 1972; Fronek et al., 1973; Blackshear et al., 1980). More recently, preliminary studies have demonstrated the feasibility of its application in the assessment of human fetal hemodynamics (Fitzgerald and Drumm, 1977; McCallum et al., 1978, Gill et al., 1980; McCallum 1981; Maulik et al., 1982a,b). The present study evaluates the Doppler-derived flow-velocity indices for characterizing human fetoplacental hemodynamics. The first phase of this study was accomplished in a simplified in-vitro model of the fetoplacental circuit. This allowed the effects of upstream and downstream circulatory impedence on various blood flow indices to be studied. The second phase extended this investigation to a population of pregnant patients to evaluate its clinical applicability.

METHODS

In-vitro phase

A pulsatile roller pump (Manostat, Varistaltic) was used to pump heparinized human blood (40 percent hematocrit) through silastic tubing which had an internal diameter of 5 mm. A variable constriction was inserted in the flow circuit so the effect of flow impedance on upstream and downstream flow velocity characteristics could be studied. Figure 1 depicts the in-vitro model schematically. An IREX Pedof Doppler ultrasonic flowmeter was used to measure the blood flow velocity at different points in the upstream circuit, as well as downstream from the constriction. Operating at 2 MHz., this instrument was used in the continuous wave mode in order to avoid problems related to aliasing and range ambiguity. A Doppler shift of 2.55 KHz. corresponds to blood flow velocity of 1 m/sec. A constant flow rate (180 ml/min) was used throughout this experiment. The Doppler Frequency Shift signal, as well as the pressure drop across the constriction, was recorded on FM-tape for different measurement sites and constrictions. A Precision Instruments FM tape recorder (Model PI-6204) was used for this purpose. A recording speed of 37.5 inches/sec was used, providing an upper 3-db. cut-off frequency of 10 KHz. The flow meter had a calibration factor of 2.55 KHz. per m/sec velocity; therefore, velocities up to 3.9 m/sec could be recorded by this arrangement.

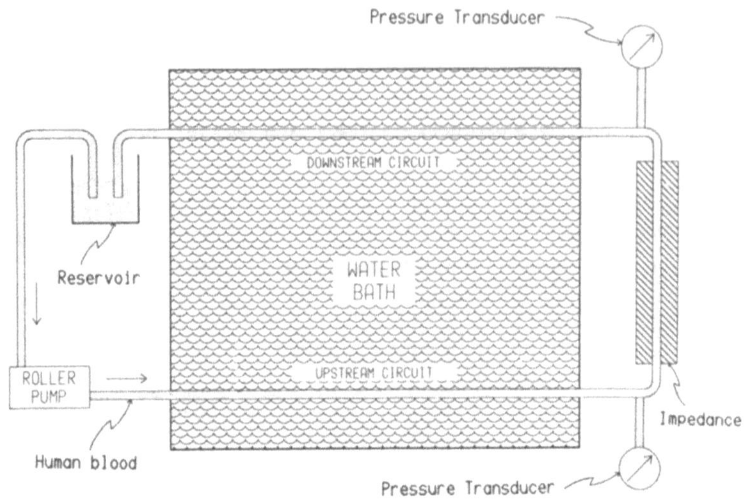

Figure 1. Schematic of in-vitro setup.

The recorded FM signals were then digitized using a Perkin-Elmer Model 7/32 minicomputer having a general purpose analog interface. The analog tapes were played back at 0.375 inches/sec and digitized at a sampling rate of 0.4 KHz., providing an effective signal sampling frequency of 40 KHz. The digitized Doppler Shift Frequency and pressure drop signals were written onto 9-track digital tape for subsequent processing.

The Doppler Frequency Shift signal was analyzed by first computing its Fourier Transform using the Fast Fourier Transformation Algorithm. The Fourier spectra of the Doppler Frequency Shift signal were computed using a 512-point FFT resulting in a frequency resolution of 78.125 Hz., with each spectrum representing a time window of 0.0128 sec. In order to reduce the spectral variance of the frequency spectra, each such time window was multiplied with a cosine window prior to computation of the FFT (Bingham et al., 1967). Spectral variance was further reduced by averaging together 16 spectra computed over overlapping time windows for every 50 milliseconds of recording. This resulted in 20 spectral representations of the Doppler Frequency Shift signal for every second of recording.

Several measures of blood flow were computed from the Frequency Shift spectra obtained. First, the maximum significant frequency in each spectrum was computed. This resulted in a waveform proportional to the spatially peak flow velocity with a digitization rate of 20 samples/sec. Computation of this frequency was based on the amplitude as well as the high-end trail-off characteristics of the spectra. Next, centoid frequency of the spectra was computed, using the previously derived maximum significant frequency as the upper cut-off point. This procedure minimized the effect of high-frequency noise on the calculated centroid frequency, and resulted in a waveform proportional to the spatially mean flow velocity. Finally, the First Moments of the Fourier Spectra around the zero-frequency axis were computed, again using the maximum significant frequency as the upper cut-off point, resulting in the First Moments waveform. The First Moment is the summation of the amplitude-frequency products in the frequency spectrum. The amplitude component is proportional to the population density of back-scattering blood cells within the insonated target volume, and the frequency is proportional to the velocity of blood cells producing the Doppler shift. Therefore, the First Moment is proportional to the volume flow rate. This relationship is dependent on the assumption that the entire vessel lumen is being uniformily insonated.

For each of the waveforms obtained by the above procedure, a Pulsatility Index was computed. Over one pump cycle, let V_p represent the peak value of a waveform, V_t represents the minimum (trough) value, and V_m the mean value. Then, the pulsatility index, PI, is defined as

$$PI = (V_p - V_t)/V_m$$

i.e., it is the magnitude of the temporal swing of the waveform over one pump cycle normalized by the mean value of the waveform during that cycle. As its name suggests, this index quantitates the temporal variations in the waveform. It is used to assess the effect of hemodynamic parameters such as blood vessel elasticity or impedance to flow caused by vessel constrictions. In the in-vitro model, this index was observed as a function of the location of the measurement point with respect to the constriction, as well the magnitude of the constriction. The latter was quantitated by the temporal average of the pressure drop across the constriction, since flow rate was constant.

In-vivo phase

The study population consisted of 48 pregnant women with gestational ages ranging from 29 to 42 weeks. An ATL Mark-V duplex real-time system, and an IREX Pedof Doppler Flowmeter (2 MHz frequency) with an ADR real-time scanner (Model 4000S, 3.5 MHz transducer) were used. A preliminary scan established the spatial orientation of the fetus, placental insertion, and distribution of the umbilical cord in the amniotic cavity. In the duplex system, a moving cursor localized the target area of the cord. An immediate change of mode into Doppler produced flow velocity waveforms which were displayed in real-time as well as recorded on a Panasonic video recorder (Model 8950). With the second system, real-time scanning was performed with the ADR system. The target area was located and its depth measured. The Pedof Doppler flow probe was then used in the pulsed mode to obtain Doppler frequency shift signals which were recorded on FM tape. This was further analysed by FFT to produce the flow-velocity waveform. Details of this and the technique of computation of PI have previously been described in the in- vitro section.

RESULTS

In-vitro phase

Figure 2 shows the PI of the spatially peak flow velocity and the first moments of the Fourier spectra at three different measurement points upstream from the flow constriction. It was observed that when the measurement point was closer to the point of impedance, PI was reduced by increasing the impedance to flow. However,

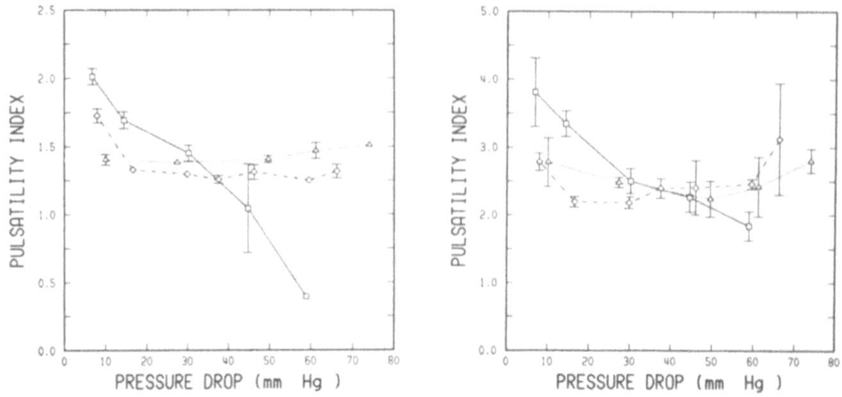

Figure 2. Effect of changes in flow impedance downstream from the measurement point (measured by pressure drop across the constriction) on PI of the Peak Velocity (a) and First Fourier Moment (b) waveforms. The three curves correspond to measurement points 350 cm (Δ), 270 cm (◇) and 110 cm (□) from the pump.

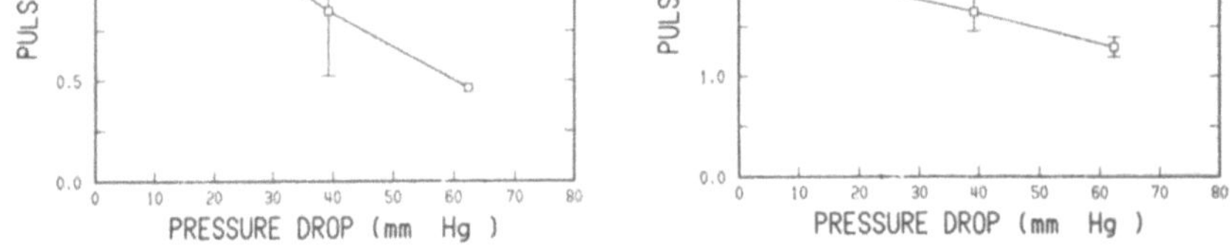

Figure 3. Effect of changes of flow impedance upstream from the measurement point (measured by pressure drop across the constriction) on PI of the Peak Velocity (a) and First Fourier Moment (b) waveforms.

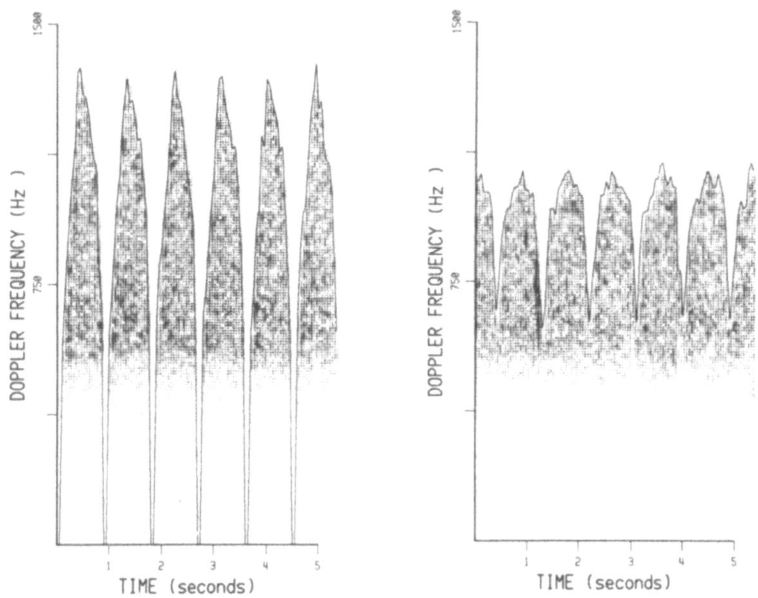

Figure 4. This figure illustrates the effect of flow impedance upstream from the measurement point. (a) shows the signal with minimal constriction (pressure drop = 10 mm Hg), while (b) shows the signal obtained from the same point with constriction introduced (pressure drop across constriction = 62 mm Hg) Note the reduced flow pulsatility.

this effect was not observed as the point of measurement was moved closer to the pumping source. Figure 3 demonstrates the variation in PI with changing flow impedance when flow was measured downstream from the constriction. A definite fall in flow pulsatility is observed as flow impedance is increased.

Variations in the PI of the spatially mean velocity were identical to those in the PI of the spatially peak velocity. The results for the First Fourier Moment waveform (Figures 2(b) and 3(b)) showed considerable variation in the values of PI at any given measurement point and constriction. Since the First Moments of the Fourier Spectra are sensitive not only to the velocity of the travelling blood cells but also to their population density within the target volume, this increased variability may have been due to variations in the population density of these cells. However, the trend in the variation of the PI of the First Moments waveform was seen to be similar to that observed for the PI of the spatially peak flow velocity.

As a matter of illustration, Figures 4(a) and 4(b) describe the Doppler Frequency Shift signals measured upstream from the constriction for low and high values of flow impedance respectively. The marked reduction in flow pulsatility was obvious.

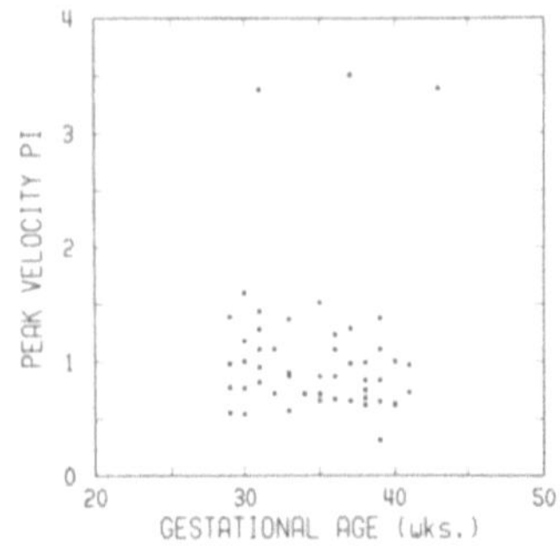

Figure 5. Scattergram of PI values as a function of gestational age.

The results seem to indicate that whereas the PI is indicative of impedance to flow imposed by cardiovascular parameters, factors such as the location of the point of measurement with respect to the region of flow impedance must be considerd. If the region of impedance is upstream from the measurement point, PI is reduced as flow impedance is increased; if the region of impedance is downstream of the measurement point, the behavior of PI as a function of the impedance depends on the location of the measurement point.

In-vivo phase

Figure 5 shows the scattergram of the PI from the peak velocity waveform obtained during different gestational ages. The mean value of PI was 1.09 ± 0.667 illustrating the wide distribution of PI in umbilical arterial circulation during the last trimester of human pregnancy. A linear regression on PI vs. Gestational age (measured in weeks) produced a slope coefficient of 0.007313 (coefficient of determination = 0.001812). No significant change in the PI was observed as the gestation advanced towards term.

Three of the 48 patients showed umbilical arterial PI values more than two standard deviations above the mean. Figure 6 shows a typical umbilical arterial flow velocity waveform. It should be noted that forward flow continued through the diastole indicating a low impedance in the fetoplacental circulation. Figure 7 is a

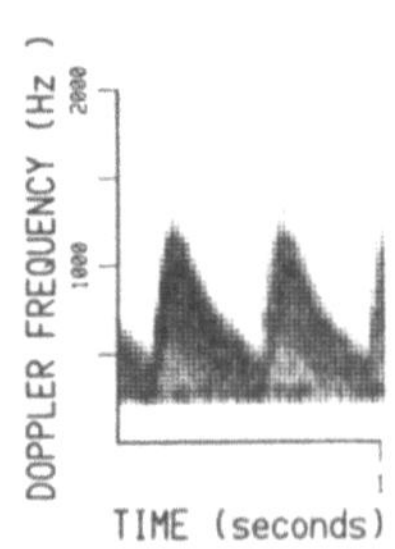

Figure 6. Typical umbilical arterial flow velocity waveform.

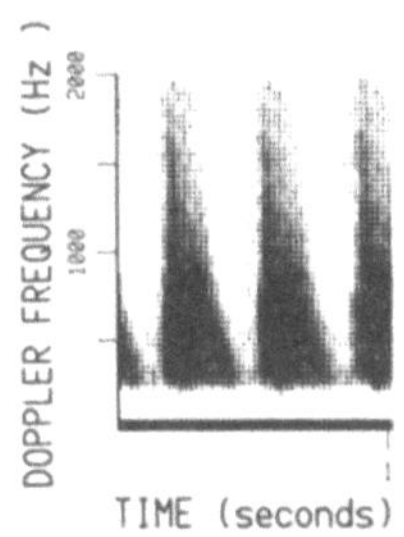

Figure 7. Umbilical arterial flow waveform in association with oligohydramnios.

waveform typical of the three patients with high PI. It is noteworthy that in this case, forward flow virtually stopped during diastole. All three patients suffered from oligohydramnios. One of them also had premature rupture of membranes. More research into the significance of these abnormal waveforms is warranted.

DISCUSSION

The technique of Doppler Flowmetry has been successfully used to measure human fetal blood flow, but it has become quite apparent that any attempts at accurately measuring volumetric flow in deep-lying vessels are fraught with serious limitations. An error range of $\pm 30\%$ can be made in measuring flow in the human fetal aorta (Reid et al., 1980); greater error is likely with umbilical and other fetal circulations. Deep location, unfavorable beam-vessel angle, and difficulty in precisely measuring the vessel dimension are the main sources of error.

McDonald (1974) and others have shown that the blood flow velocity waveform is dependent on multiple hemodynamic parameters such as vessel compliance, impedance to flow, and the force of ventricular contraction. Analysis of the waveform therefore can potentially yield information on these characteristics on a circulation. This realization has led to the development of indices such PI (Gosling, et. al., 1971), and the peak-trough ratio (Stuart et al., 1980) which are independent of beam-vessel angle and vascular dimension. These indices have been used in assessing peripheral circulation (Humphries et al., 1980) and umbilical circulation (Stuart et al., 1980; McCallum, 1981). However, there is a dearth of their verification under controlled experimental conditions. The present study offered such an opportunity by designing an in-vitro circulatory system with pulsatile blood flow in which experimentally produced variations in impedance could be accurately measured by observing the pressure decline across the impedance. The primary limitation of such an in-vitro system is that it can never fully reproduce the complex hemodynamic features of an in-vivo circulation. Within this context, the results presented here indicate that the PI is indicative of impedance to flow imposed by cardiovascular parameters. However, factors such as location of the point of measurement in relation to the region of impedance must also be taken into consideration. If the region of impedance is located upstream from the measurement point, the PI is a reliable indicator of variations in the impedance. If the location of impedance is downstream from the measurement point, the behavior of PI as a function of impedance depends on the site of measurement.

The above trend remained valid irrespective of whether the PI was based on the peak frequency, mean frequency or the first moment or the Fourier spectra around the zero-frequency axis. As mentioned earlier, assuming full insonation of the target vessel, the first moment represents the integrated cell count - velocity product within the Doppler target volume, and thus is indicative of total flow. We have shown elsewhere that under in vitro conditions, the first moment is a more linear measure of volume flow rate than the peak or mean flow velocities (Saini et al., 1982). In a preliminary clinical study, it has also been shown that the first moment is a more sensitive indicator of changes in the umbilical flow during a cardiac cycle than peak or mean velocities (Maulik et al., 1982a).

The in-vivo phase of the study demonstrates preliminary clinical applicability of this technique. Our data do not demonstrate any significant change in the PI during the last trimester of pregnancy. Additionally, for each gestational age, there was a wide distribution of the PI values. Stuart et al. (1980) showed a progressive decline in peak-trough ratio of the velocity waveform with advancing gestational age. It should be noted that in their study steepest decline in the peak-to-trough ratio was observed during the second trimester of pregnancy, which was excluded from our population. A much larger population needs to be studied before such characteristics of PI can be defined.

The three high PI values noted in association with oligohydramnios offer the interesting possibility of an increased impedance to fetoplacental blood flow. However, it is premature to make any such definitive conclusion, particularly in view of our in-vitro findings on the behavior of PI for changes in the downstream impedance.

In conclusion, the PI seems to be a reliable indicator of changes in the circulatory impedance, when the relationship between the location of the impedance and the site of measurement are taken into account. Moreover, other factors such as vascular compliance need to be considered in relation to their contribution to flow pulsatility. Further work is needed in this area before these indices can be transformed into reliable clinical tools.

SUMMARY

This investigation consisted of an in-vitro and in-vivo assessment of computer-assisted Doppler ultrasound flowmetry for the evaluation of fetoplacental hemodynamics. The in-vitro study demonstrated that an increase in flow impedance upstream of the measurement point reduced flow pulsatility. It was also shown that the effect of changes in impedance downstream from the measurement point was dependent on the location of the measurement point in the circuit. The in-vivo study extended the above technique to a pregnant population with gestational ages ranging from 29 to 42 weeks, using pulsed Doppler ultrasound systems. No significant change in the PI was observed with advancing gestation. An increase in the PI greater than two standard deviations was observed in conjunction with oligohydramnios, suggesting possible changes in the fetoplacental circulatory impedance. This study demonstrates the potential utility of Doppler Flowmetry for evaluating fetoplacental hemodynamics, and justifies further work in this area to transform these indices into reliable clinical tools.

ACKNOWLEDGMENT

This research was partially supported by a gift from the estate of Richard W. Goode and Mae Stone Goode.

REFERENCES

Baker, D.W. (1970) Pulsed Ultrasonic Doppler blood-flow sensing. *IEEE Trans. on S. and US.*, SU17, 170-185.

Bingham, C., Godfrey, M.D., and Tukey, J.W. (1967) Modern Techniques of Power Spectrum Estimation, *IEEE Trans. Audio Electroacoust.*, AU-15, 56-66.

Blackshear, W.M., Jr., Phillips, D.J., Chibos, P.M., Harley, J.D., Thiele, B.L., and Strandress, D.E., Jr. (1980) Carotid artery velocity patterns in normal and stenotic vessels. *Stroke* 11, 67-71.

Fitzgerald, D.E., and Drumm, J.E. (1977) Non-invasive measurment of the fetal circulation using ultrasound: A new method. *Br. Med. J.* 2, 1450-1451.

Franklin, D.L., Schlegal, W.A., and Rushmer, R.F. (1961) Blood flow measured by Doppler frequency shift of backscattered ultrasound. *Science* 134, 564- 565.

Fronek, A., Johansen, K.H., and Dilley, R.B. (1973) Non-invasive physiologic tests in the diagnosis and characterization of peripheral occlusive disease. *Amer. J. Surg.* 126, 204-214.

Gill, R.W., Kossoff, B.J., Trudinger, G.J., and Warren, P.S. (1980) Flow velocity in the venous return from the placenta. In: *Recent Advances in Ultrasound Diagnosis* 2 (ed.), A. Kurjak, pp. 229- 232, Amsterdam: Excerpta Medica.

Gosling, R.G., Dunbar, G., King, D.H., Newman, D.L., Side, C.D., Woodcock, J.P., Fitzgerald, D.E., Keates, J.S. and MacMillan, D. (1971) The quantitative analysis of occulsive peripheral arterial disease by a non-intrusive ultrasonic technique. *Angiology* 22, 52-55.

Humphries, K.N., Hames, T.K., Smith, S.W.J., and Cannon, V.A. (1980) Quantitative assessment of the common femoral to popliteal arterial segment using continuous wave Doppler ultrasound. *Ultrasound in Med.* and *Biol.* 6, 99- 105.

Light, L.H., and Cross, G. (1972) Cardiovascular data by transcutaneous aorta velography. In *Blood Flow Measurement* (ed.), Robert, C., London: Sector Publishing Ltd.

Maulik, D., Saini, V.D., Nanda, N.C., and Rosenzweig, M.S. (1982a) Doppler evaluation of fetal hemodynamics. *Ultrasound in Med. Biol.* 705-710.

Maulik, D., Saini, V.D., and Nanda, N.C. (1982b) Computerized Doppler evaluation of umbilical hemodynamics. *Proc. 2nd. Annual. Symp. on Computers in Perinat. Med.* 138-140.

McCallum, W.D. (1981) Fetal cardiac anatomy and vascular dynamics. *Clin. Obstet. Gynec.* 24, 837-849.

McCallum, W.D., Williams, C.S., Napel, S., and Daigle, R.E. (1978) Fetal blood velocity waveforms. *Amer. J. Obstet. Gynecol.* 132, 425-429.

McDonald, D.A. (1974) *Blood Flow in Arteries.* 2nd. Ed. London: Edward Arnold Publishers.

Perronneau, P.A., Bugnon, A., Bervinat, J.P., Xhaard, M., and Hinglais, J. (1974) Instantaneous bidimensional blood velocity profiles in the major vessels by a pulsed ultrasonic Doppler velocimeter. In: *Ultrasonics in Medicine* (ed.), DeVlieger, M., et al., pp. 259-266, Amsterdam: Excerpta Medica/Amercian Elsevier.

Reid, M.H., Mackay, R.S., and Lantz, B.M.T., (1980) Noninvasice measurement of fetal and neonatal blood flow. *Acta Radiol.* (Stockholm) 21, 197-212.

Saini, V.D., Maulik, D., and Nanda, N.C. (1982) Computerized evaluation of Fetal Blood Flow indices, *abstr. Xth. World Congr. of Gynecol. and Obstet.* Oct., 1982, Abst. 1939, p. 481.

Shatumora, S. (1957) Ultrasonic Doppler Method for the inspection of cardiac functions. *J. Acoust. Soc. Amer.* 29, 1181-1185.

Stuart, B., Drumm, J., Fitzgerald, D.E., and Duignan, N.M. (1980) Fetal blood velocity waveform in normal pregnancy. *Br. J. Obstet. Gynaec.* 81, 780-785.

Woodcock, J.B., Gosling, R.G., and Fitzgerald, D.E. (1972) A new non-invasive technique for assessment of superficial femoral artery obstruction. *Br. J. Surg.* 59, 226-231.

Trophoblast Research 1:159-166, 1983

FINE STRUCTURE OF THE HUMAN CHORION LAEVE

Tzuneng Wang and Dieter Hemann Albert Maas

Frauenklinik der Medizinischen Hochschule
Hannover, 3000 Hannover 51, Federal Republic of Germany

INTRODUCTION

Many morphologcial studies on the human amnion have indicated that the intercellular spaces of the amniotic epithelium may represent a paracellular route for protein transfer between the amniotic cavity and the maternal circulation (Hempel, 1976; Franke and Estel, 1978; King, 1982; Wang and Schneider, 1982a). Since the fetal membranes consist of reflected amnion and chorion laeve, the structural characteristics of the chorion laeve are equally important as those of the amnion in terms of the non- placental protein transfer.

The object of this paper is to describe the ultrastructure of the chorion laeve following normal pregnancy. The findings will be compared with other studies on the chorion laeve known to date (Bourne, 1962; Lister, 1968; Anderson and McKay, 1969; Thliveris and Speroff, 1977; Nehemiah et al., 1981).

MATERIALS AND METHODS

Chorion laeve was taken, immediately after delivery, from the placentae of 10 patients following normal pregnancies. The membrane was dissected into small pieces and fixed in a mixture of glutaraldehyde (2.5 percent) and formaldehyde (2.0 percent) in 0.1 M sodium-cacodylate buffer (pH 7.3) for one hour at 4°C. After a brief rinsing in the same buffer, it was fixed once again in 1 percent phosphate buffered osmium-tetroxide solution for one hour at room temperature.

All specimens were then dehydrated in graded alcohols and embedded in Epon. Thin sections were prepared with an LKB-4800 III ultrotome, stained with uranyl acetate and lead citrate. The electron microscope was a Siemens Elmiskop Ia.

RESULTS

The epithelium of the human chorion laeve consisted partly of a single layer and partly of multiple layers (up to 4 layers) of trophoblastic cells. The surface of the cells displayed numerous microvilli as well as cell processes. The processes were rarely connected by desmosomes to similar processes of the adjacent cells (Figure 1). Besides desmosomes, gap junctions and occluding junctions were also occasionally found, where the cell processes were in close contact with each other or with cell bodies (Figures 2 and 3). Within the intercellular spaces, flocculent material and microfibrils were observed. The plasma membrane often showed deep folds followed closely by a thin layer of basement membrane. Hemidesmosomes were recognized along the plasma membrane. The nuclei of trophoblastic cells were polygonal with folded surface. The mitochondria were regularly distributed in the cytoplasm. Rough endoplasmic reticulum was seldom found. Golgi complexes were often observed in the vicinity of the nucleus. Near the desmosomes and hemidesmosomes, bundles of filaments could clearly be seen. Lipid and glycogen particles were also commonly found. The basement membrane was stratified and showed many breaks (Figure 4). Numerous microfibrils were found adjacent and between the layers of the basement membrane. Necrotic trophoblastic cells were rarely observed.

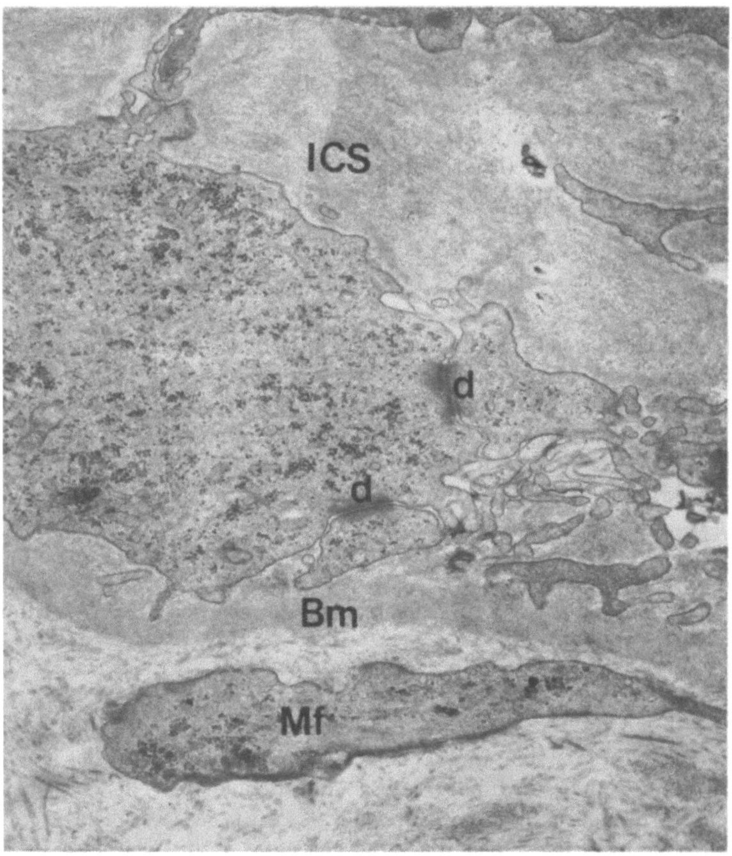

Figure 1. The adjacent trophoblastic cells are connected by desmosomes (d). Numerous microfibrils are present within the intercellular spaces (ICS). Bm: Epithelial basement membrane; Mf: Myofibroblast. x 16,000.

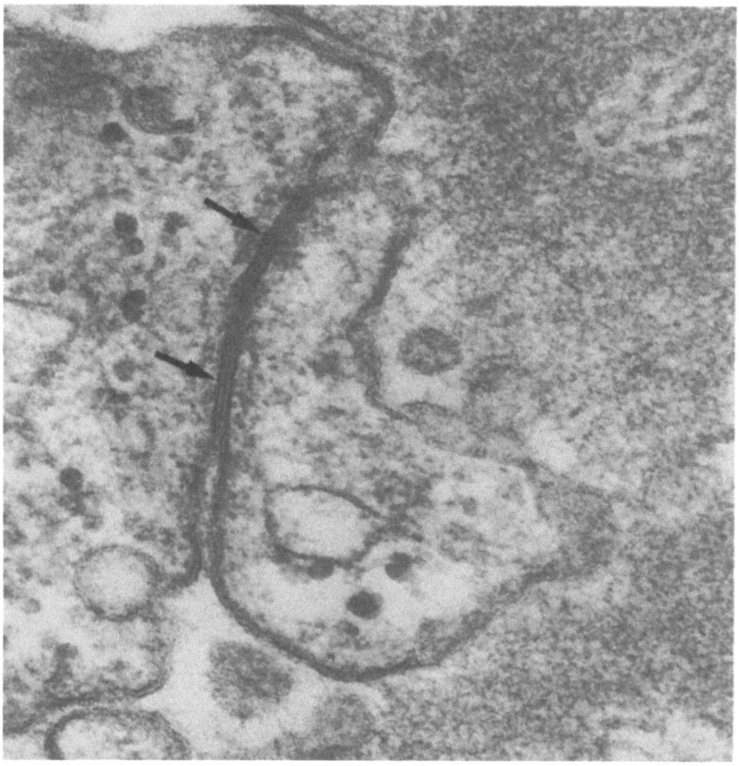

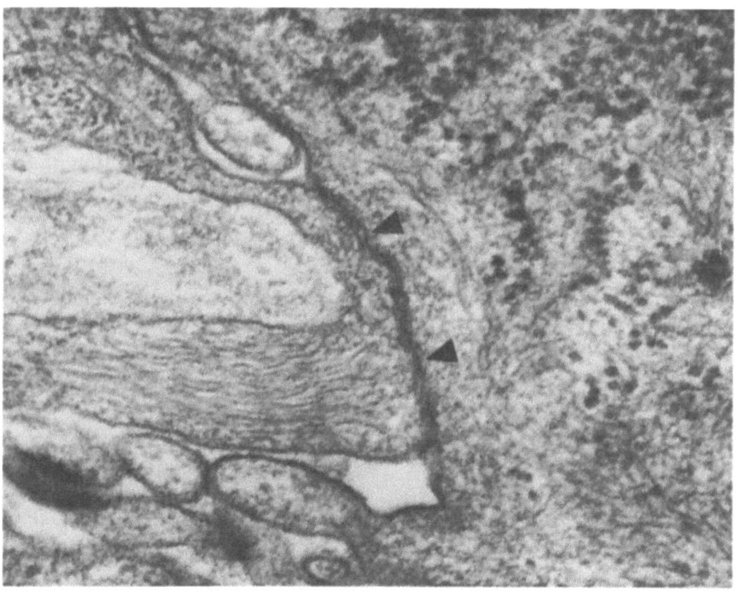

Figures 2 (above) and 3 (below). Gap junctions (arrow) and occluding junctions (Δ) are occasionally found between the adjacent trophoblastic cells. (Figure 2) x 60,000 and (Figure 3) x 80,000.

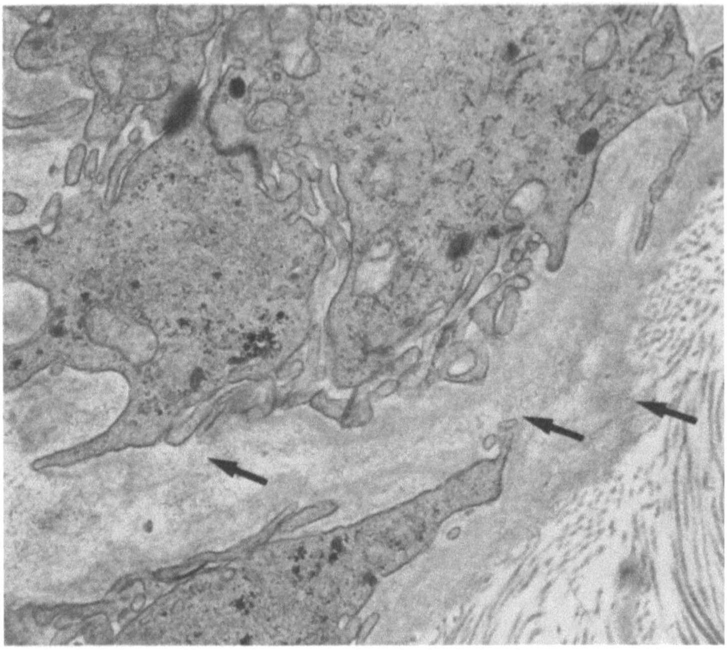

Figure 4. The basement membrane of the chorionic epithelium is stratified and discontinuous (arrrows) x 16,000.

In addition to typical fibroblasts and macrophages, the connective tissue of the human chorion laeve contained numerous myofibroblasts (Figure 1). These cells were often connected to similar cells by desmosomes. Their nuclei were elongated and frequently indented. Numerous bundles of 5 nm thick filaments with dense bodies were observed in the cytoplasm (Figure 5). The plasma membrane often had hemidesmosome-like zones of thickening. Basement membrane-like material was visible at some places on the cell surface (Figure 6).

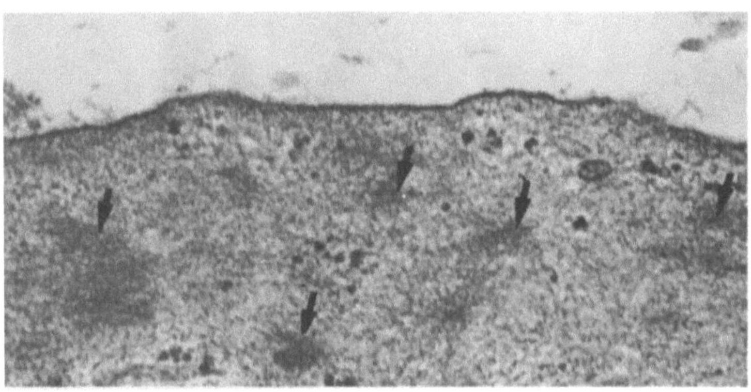

Figure 5. The cytoplasm of myofibroblasts contains numerous bundles of filaments with dense bodies (arrows) x 40,000.

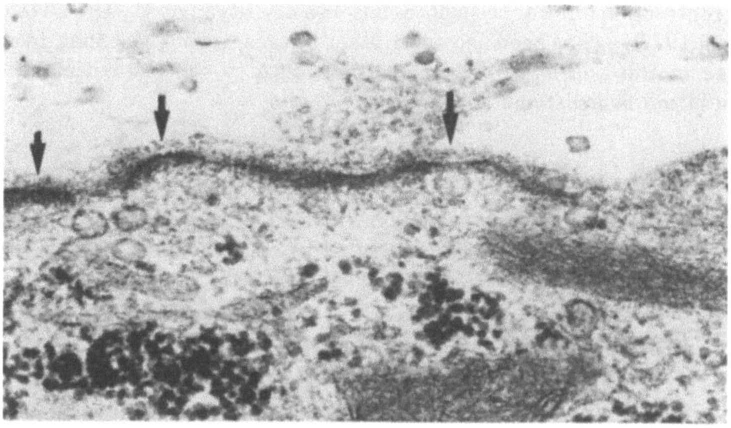

Figure 6. Basement membrane-like material (arrows) is visible at some places on the cell surface of myofibroblasts x 67,500.

DISCUSSION

In comparison to studies on the human chorion laeve known to date, our findings show the following new morphological aspects:

1. The cellular junctions of adjacent trophoblast cells consist not only of desmosomes but also gap junctions and occluding junctions.

2. The epithelial basement membrane is stratified and discontinuous.

3. Besides the fibroblasts and macrophages, the chorion laeve contains myofibroblasts.

Between the adjacent trophoblastic cells, we found desmosomes, gap junctions and occluding junctions forming cellular junctions. Physiologically, it is known that desmosomes play an important role in adhesion, and gap junctions in electronic and metabolic coupling of adjacent cells (McNutt and Weinstein, 1973; Staehelin, 1974). They do not present a diffusion barrier for proteins (Farquhar and Palade, 1963; Brightman and Reese, 1969). Functionally, belt-like occluding junctions (zonulae occludentes) prevent diffusion of proteins through epithelia (McNutt and Weinstein, 1973; Staehelin, 1974). Since the occluding junctions are only seldom present in the chorion laeve and could clearly be classified as maculae or fasciae occludentes in freeze-fracture replicas (Bartels and Wang, 1983), they are apparently not significant for the paracellular protein transfer. The basement membrane of the human chorion laeve is discontinuous and can therefore hardly function as a barrier. These structural characteristics indicate that the intercellular spaces and the discontinuous basement membrane of the chorionic epithelium could represent a paracellular route for the non-placental protein transfer.

As in the human amnion (Wang and Schneider, 1982b), myofibroblasts could be found in the connective tissue of the human chorion laeve. Since they possess the ability of contraction similar to smooth muscle cells (Ryan et al., 1974; Gabbiani and Montandon, 1977), as has been shown in other tissues, we suggest that, in connection with those in the amnion, they may contribute to the protection of the fetal membranes from overdistension.

SUMMARY

Human chorion laeve at full term of normal pregnancy was examined by electron microscopy. In comparison with other known studies of human chorion, our findings show the following new morphological aspects:

1. The intercellular junctions between adjacent trophoblastic cells consist of not only of desmosomes but also of gap junctions and occasional occluding junctions.

2. The epithelial basement membrane is stratified and discontinuous.

3. In addition to fibroblasts and macrophages, the connective tissue of the human chorion contains numerous myofibroblasts.

The occluding junctions are rarely found in the chorionic epithelium, which means that they may have little significance in terms of the non- placental transfer. Similar to the amniotic epithelium, the intercellular spaces and the discontinuous basement membrane of the chorionic epithelium could represent a paracellular route for the non-placental protein transfer. Since the myofibroblasts are able to contract similarly to smooth muscle cells, we suggest that they could contribute, along with the myofibroblasts in the amnion, to the protection of fetal membranes from overdistension.

REFERENCES

Anderson, W. and McKay, D.G. (1969) Electron microscope study of the trophoblast in normal and toxemic placentas. *Amer. J. Obstet. Gynecol.* 95,1134-1148.

Bartels, H. and Wang, T. (1983) Intercellular junctions in the human membranes. A freeze-fracture study. *Anat. Embryol.* 166,103-120.

Bourne, G. (1962) *The Human Amnion and Chorion.* London: Lloyd-Luke.

Brightman, M.W. and Reese, T.S. (1969) Junctions between intimately opposed cell membranes in the vetebrate brain. *J. Cell. Biol.* 40,648-677.

Farquhar, M.G. and Palade, G.E. (1963) Junctional complexes in various epithelia. *J. Cell. Biol.* 17,375-412.

Franke, H. and Estel, C. (1978) Untersuchungen über die Ultrastruktur und Permeabilität des Amnions unter besonderer Berücksichtigung mikrofilalmentärer und mikrotubulärer Struktur. *Arch. Gynäk.* 225,319-338.

Gabbiani, G. and Montandon, D. (1977) Reparative processes in mammalian wound healing. The role of contractile phenomena. *Int. Rev. Cytol.* 48,187-219.

Hempel, E. (1976) Ultrastrukturelle Untersuchungen über die Durchlässigkeit des Amnionepithels fur Peroxidase und Ferritin. *Zbl. Gynäk.* 98,1565-1572.

King, B.F. (1982) Cell surface specializations and intercellular junctions in human amniotic epithelium. An electron microscopic and freeze-fracture study. *Anat. Rec.* 203,73-82.
Lister, U.M. (1968) Ultrastructure of the human amnion, chorion and fetal skin. *J. Obstet. Gynaecol. Brit. Cwlth.* 75, 327-341.
McNutt, N.S. and Weinstein, R.S. (1973) Membrane ultrastructure at mammalian intercellular junctions. In: *Progress in Biophysics and Molecular Biology.* (eds.) Butler, J.A.V. and Noble, D., 26,47-101. Oxford, New York, Toronto, Sydney, Braunschweig: Pergamon Press.
Nehemiah, J.L., Schnitzer, J.A., Schulman, H. and Novikoff, A.B. (1981) Human chorionic trophoblasts, decidual cells and macrophages. A histochemical and electron microscopic study. *Amer. J. Obstet. Gynecol.* 140,261-268.
Ryan, G.B., Cliff, W.J., Gabbiani, G., Irle, C., Montandon, D., Statkov, P.R. and Majno, G. (1974) Myofibroblasts in human granulation tissue. *Human Pathol.* 5,55-67.
Staehelin, L.A. (1974) Structure and function of intercellular junctions. *Int. Rev. Cytol.* 39,191-283.
Thliveris, J.A. and Speroff, L. (1977) Ultrastructure of the placenta ville, chorion laeve, and decidua parietalis in normal and hypertensive pregnant women. *Amer. J. Obstet. Gynecol.* 129, 492-498.
Wang, T. and Schneider, J. (1982a) Location of anions in human amnion. Evidence for a non-placental route for the transfer of proteins into amniotic fluid. *Arch. Gynecol.* 231, 269-277.
Wang, T. and Schneider, J. (1982b) Myofibroblasten im Bindegewebe des menschlichen Amnions. *Z. Geburth. u. Perinat.* 86, 164-168.

Trophoblast Research 1:167-172, 1983

NUTRITION REPORTS

Nutrition Related Teratogenicity: Rat Embyro Culture Using Human Serum from Epileptics

(Chatot and Klein, 1982)

Embryo cultures using early rat implantation sites have provided new approaches to the evaluation of the extraembryonic membranes and their relationship to nutrition and toxicity. Norman Klein presented an exciting, detailed evaluation of rat embryos grown in culture on serum from patients treated with anticonvulsants. These embryo culture technics are based upon the original work of New (1966) and modified as presented by Carey et al. (this volume).

Serum samples from 128 different epileptics who either received or did not receive anticonvulsant therapy were tested for embryonic abnormalities, serum drug levels and supplementation with vitamins and amino acids. When the embryos cultured in serum specimens were evaluated for the frequency of abnormalities, sera from untreated and phenobarbital-treated epileptics were lower than sera from carbamazepine, valporic acid, or phenytoin-treated patients. However, the drug levels in the serum were not correlated with the abnormalities in the embryos. The background incidence for embyronic abnormalities in the control population was approximately 20 percent. In 53 serum specimens, which produced malformations and were then supplemented with both amino acids and vitamins, the teratogenicity was overcome in 32 cases. This result was reflected in improved embryo morphology and increases in embryonic protein content. Only sera from patients (6) treated with valporic acid were unresponsive to supplementation with amino acids and vitamins.

The control incidence of malformations in this system implies that even in this in vitro model not all parameters are known or are controlled. Such environmental impact on the conceptus and its nutritional implication certainly warrant further investigations, which directly involve placenta, whether yolk sac or chorioallantoic.

Iron and Transferrin in the Isolated Perfused Placenta of the Guinea Pig

(van Dijk and Heeren, 1982)

In 1981, Hans van Dijk reviewed in depth the proposed mechanisms involved with iron transport across the placenta. He and Dr. Heeren have further developed these models by studying the passage and intracellular binding/distribution of ^{125}I-transferrin bound with either ^{59}Fe or ^{56}Fe given in a bolus injection into either the maternal or fetal circulations of an isolated perfused placenta preparation from the guinea pig. They compared their transfer of these molecules with the movement of ^{125}I- albumin. It was found that there was very little uptake of albumin but that the uptake of ^{125}I-transferrin was substantial and was bound to receptors. This binding was not displaced by non-labeled transferrin. Further studies demonstrated that there was no significant difference in binding for either guinea pig or human transferrin in the guinea pig perfusion preparation. Within five to seven minutes of the bolus injection on the maternal side, the fetal concentration of iron increased and then decreased in a steady one exponential decline. It appears that there is a placental compartment which becomes filled with iron after its detachment from transferrin. This all apparently occurs during the short period in which the bolus is passing through the placenta. The authors calculated a fetal clearance from this tissue compartment of approximately 0.05 ± 0.02 ml/min in ten experiments. The cytosol from these 55 day placental preparations were chromatographed on S6B and resulted in three iron peaks: 1) ferritin, 2) a low molecular weight fraction of approximately 6,000 daltons and 3) transferrin, which also contained the ^{125}I. These investigators proposed that this low molecular weight fraction represented the assumed transit pool for iron in the placenta. The data were not conclusive but were most suggestive that following multiple bolus injections of both ^{59}Fe or ^{55}Fe, there was a slow incorporation of iron into ferritin. Thus, this small placental iron compartment appeared to have an important role in the transfer of iron across the placenta. This turnover of iron in the ferritin fraction may be coupled with the maintenance of this low molecular weight iron fraction. These studies represent renewed interest in the transfer of this important nutrient, iron, and further indicate the complexity of the transfer processes for these protein bound nutrients.

Transfer of Calcium across the Isolated Perfused Placenta of the Guinea Pig

(van Kreel and van Dijk, 1982)

Drs. van Kreel and van Dijk presented a most informative presentation on their continuing studies of calcium transport across the isolated perfused placenta of the guinea pig. As has been previously noted, there is a large electrochemical potential gradient for calcium towards the trophoblast cell, and calcium uptake into the trophoblast results in a depolarization of the cell potential. These investigators examined the movement of ^{45}calcium into the trophoblast. They noted that when sodium chloride in the medium was exchanged with potassium chloride or choline chloride, the uptake of ^{45}calcium was increased. This increasing calcium uptake can also be achieved by using potassium cyanide. In addition, magnesium was found to enhance the uptake of calcium but was not central to calcium uptake. In evaluating these observations and experiments, these investigators proposed that there is a sodium-calcium antiporter located in the trophoblast membrane. In further studies, they found they could not increase sodium release after increasing the calcium concentrations. Thus, they conclude that calcium pumps do exist in the trophoblast membrane, and most likely there is unequal distribution of these sites between the maternal and fetal surfaces of this tissue. Perhaps this is the reason that a calcium gradient is generated from the fetus to the mother.

IUGR and the Placenta: A Histomorphometric Evaluation

(Teasdale, 1982)

A substantial amount of discussion always follows a morphologic review of a placenta because of the wide variations within a given placental unit whether for the lobule, cotyledon, or entire placenta. Francois Teasdale from the University of Montreal has performed detailed morphometric studies of placentae from normal and idiopathic IUGR pregnancies. Dr. Teasdale cannot determine what came first, placental alterations, maternal compromise or fetal deficits, but he did beautifully demonstrate large differences in parenchymal tissue and in surface area. Five placentae (256 g) from small for gestation age infants (1611 $\pm$ 336 g) were compared with placentae (462 g) from normal term infants (3195 $\pm$ 140 g). Parenchymal and non-parenchymal tissues were significantly reduced by approximately 50 to 60 percent in the placentae from IUGR pregnancies when compared with control placentae; however, the actual distribution of parenchymal tissue within the placentae from IUGR pregnancies was similar to control values. The surface area in terms of peripheral capillary, villous, and intervillous space volumes found in the placentae of intrauterine growth retarded pregnancies were all significantly reduced by approximately 50 percent when compared with control placentae. The total number of cells and cellular content were also reduced by 50 percent in the IUGR placentae.

Thus, Dr. Teasdale demonstrated that through these morphometric evaluations, there are many similarities between gross placental evaluations, fetal weight, and morphometry. With a 50 percent reduction in parenchymal tissue and surface area for exchange, Dr. Teasdale concluded that fetal growth retardation certainly would be expected. As in rodent models, this rather uniform relationship between placental weight and fetal weight as well as morphometry leads one to ponder the intricate balance between fetus and the trophoblast as related to nutritional supply, metabolism, and fetal growth.

Ultrasound Evaluation of the Placenta from Normal and Abnormal Gestations

(Sharma, 1982; Sharma and Anderson, 1982)

Ultrasonography has become an important and relatively commonly used clinical tool in Obstetrical care. However, only recently has the placenta been evaluated with relationship to parameters such as size, thickness, echogenicity and cystic changes. Shashi Sharma and Virginia Anderson presented such a study correlating ultrasonographic observations with histology and fetal karyotypic analysis. In thirty-nine patients undergoing genetic amniocentesis; thirty-two for abnormal fetal karyotype, and seven for elevated alpha-feto-protein in the amniotic fluid, ultrasonographic two-dimensional gray scale imaging of the placenta was performed. In twenty-four of the patients, histologic evaluation of the placenta was reported.

Ultrasound reveals decreased placental thickness (less than 2.0 cm) in 43 percent of trisomies, 50 percent of translocations, and in 33 percent of anneploidies. Increased placental thickness (greater than 3.5 cm) was found in 12 percent of trisomies, 66 percent of translocations, 66 percent of triploidies, 33 percent of anneploidies and in 28 percent with elevated AFP. Multiple 0.5 to 1.5 cm size cysts were seen in 12 percent of trisomies, 66 percent of triploidies, and 13 percent with elevated AFP. Histology revealed villous fibrosis in 10 percent of the trisomies. The placenta was available only in 1 mosaicism, 1 translocation, and 1 anneploidy and each showed villous fibrosis. More severe fibrosis was associated with severe phenotypic stigma of Down's Syndrome. 100 percent of the triploid placenta showed proliferating syncytiotrophoblast (molar areas) and intravillous cysterns. These findings could account for cystic areas and increased placental thickness found on ultrasound. The fetal survival varies with the extent of placental involvement. 13 percent of trisomy placentae had hypovascular secondary villi with central cystic degeneration that were perceived by ultrasound as cystic areas. The placental findings in triploidies may be diagnostic. This placental fibrosis may be a cause for decreased placental thickness and account for high abortion rate in chromosomal errors.

Placental to Fetal Weight Relationship in a Porcine Model

(Michael et al., 1982)

Many factors have been associated with intrauterine growth retardation. Among these factors has been the size of the placenta. Dr. Moore presented a fascinating paper concerning placental and fetal size in a porcine model. In particular, they evaluated the influence of small placentae on fetal size. Their studies utilized large White/Landice cross sows in the third or fourth pregnancy. Placental macroscopic surface area, weight, and fetal weights were determined following hysterectomy between gestational ages 70 and 112 days (term approximately 115-120 days).

These authors documented that the placental weight and microscopic surface area are closely correlated with fetal weight throughout the second half of gestation of the pig. As gestation advances, the limiting effect of placental size on the fetal weight becomes even more obvious. If one evaluates the light-weight placentae within the individual litters, it was determined that up to 150 percent more macroscopic surface area per unit placenta was noted than in normal weight placentae. These observations in the pig certainly give further support and evidence to the significance of placental growth to low birth weight and overall fetal development.

REFERENCES

Chatot, C.L. and Klein, N.W. (1982) Demonstration of nutrition related teratogenicity in sera from anticonvulsant treated and untreated human epileptics using rat embryo cultures. *9th Rochester Trophoblast Conference Abstracts*, p. 16.

Michael, K., Ward, B.S, Moore, W.O. (1982) Relationship of fetal to placental size: the pig model. *9th Rochester Trophoblast Conference Abstracts*, p. 18.

New, D. A. T. (1966) Development of rat embryos cultured in blood sera. *J. Reprod. Fertil.* 12, 509-524.

Sharma, S. (1982) Ultrasound evaluation of placenta, *9th Rochester Trophoblast Conference*, p. 35.

Sharma, S. and Anderson, V. (1982) Ultrasound evaluation of placenta in abnormal gestations, *9th Rochester Trophoblast Conference Abstracts*, p. 34.

Teasdale, F. (1982) Histomorphometry of the human placenta in cases of idiopathic intrauterine growth retardation. *9th Rochester Trophoblast Conference Abstracts*, p. 17.

Teasdale, F. (1983) Idiopathic intrauterine growth retardation. Histomorphometry of the human placenta, *Placenta* (in press).

van Dijk, H.P. and Heeren, J.W.A. (1982) Uptake and transfer of iron by the isolated and perfused guinea pig placenta. *9th Rochester Trophoblast Conference Abstracts*, p. 13.

van Dijk, H.P. (1981) Active transfer of the plasma bound compounds calcium and iron across the placenta. *Placenta* (Suppl. 1), 139-164.

van Kreel, B.K. and van Dijk, J.P. (1982) Mechanisms involved in the transfer of calcium across the isolated guinea pig placenta. *9th Rochester Trophblast Conference Abstracts*, p. 14.

METABOLISM

Trophoblast Research 1:175-184, 1983

ENZYMES, RECEPTORS, METABOLISM AND PLACENTAL FUNCTION

-A Review-

Claude A. Villee

Department of Biological Chemistry and
Laboratory of Human Reproduction
and Reproductive Biology
Harvard Medical School
Boston, Massachusetts 02115, U.S.A.

The placenta is a complex and interesting organ which carries out for the fetus during gestation many of the functions performed after birth by the lungs, digestive system, liver and kidneys. It also fulfills a number of important endocrine functions during pregnancy, producing hormones that in the adult are produced by the adrenals, the gonads, the pituitary and the hypothalamus. Studies of placental function are of interest not only to reproductive physiologists, who are interested in the placenta for its important role in reproduction, but also to investigators studying problems in general physiology and endocrinology for whom they provide a useful alternative model.

The previous time I was invited to serve as a moderator at one of these Rochester Trophoblast Conferences was in 1965. At that time there was considerable excitement concerning the development, by Kermit Krantz and by Ernest Page among others, of methods for simultaneously perfusing entire term human placentae from both the fetal and maternal circulations. Quite a few investigators, including our own laboratory (Charreau et al., 1968), have taken advantage of these methods to conduct a variety of studies on placental metabolism and function. At the present time improvements in the techniques of perfusing organs, together with advances in biochemical methods of dealing with hormones, have served to renew interest in studies of human placental function at term by methods of perfusion.

All of the oxygen and nutrients that the fetus obtains are transferred to it from the maternal compartment via the placenta. The placenta facilitates the entry of some of these and limits the transfer from mother to fetus of other compounds. In addition, the placenta disposes of a variety of metabolic waste products from the fetus such as carbon dioxide, urea and bilirubin. The subject of placental transport is being explored in the Nutrition Section, and here we will concentrate on some aspects of the cellular biochemistry of the trophoblast.

Over the years the placenta has served as a unique source of tissue for the isolation and characterization of human enzymes and the elucidation of human metaboblic pathways. With the development of Human Studies Committees, other types of human tissues have become increasingly difficult to obtain and, as a consequence, the importance of the placenta for studies of human biochemistry has greatly increased. We have recently reported the preparation of glucose-6-phosphatase from term placentae using affinity chromatography with glucose-6-

phosphate as the bound ligand to purify the enzyme (Reczek and Villee, 1982). The pure enzyme is now being used to produce an antibody to the enzyme. As new fields of biomedical science have appeared, developed and blossomed, the placenta has continued to serve as the substrate for the investigation of these fields in the human.

With the development of endocrinology, the placenta was shown to produce chorionic gonadotropin (hCG) and placental lactogen (hPL) as well as the steroids, progesterone and estradiol. The placenta needs a bit of help from the fetal adrenal and liver to produce the latter. Continuation of these investigations has shown that the placenta produces a whole battery of protein hormones, a chorionic thyroid stimulating hormone (TSH), chorionic ACTH (cACTH) and chorionic FSH (cFSH) (Villee, 1977). In addition, the placenta has been shown to produce a compound similar to the LRH secreted by the hypothalamus; it produces melanocyte stimulating hormone (MSH), relaxin, oxytocin, vasopressin and renin, as well as heat stable alkaline phosphatase and several globulins that are found only in the blood of pregnant women. Thus the placenta is a versatile protein synthesizing organ, one that provides unique opportunities to study the mechanisms of protein synthesis and their controls in human tissues.

Although both hCG and hPL are synthesized by the placenta, their patterns of production are markedly different. Human chorionic gonadotropin, a glycoprotein composed of α- and β-subunits, is produced by the embryo as early as the morula stage. The hormone begins to appear in maternal blood as soon as the blastocyst has been imbedded in the endometrium. It serves as a signal to maintain the maternal corpus luteum and prevent menstruation, and is the basis of our pregnancy tests. The production of chorionic gonadotropin rises rapidly and reaches a peak at 8 to 10 weeks of gestation, then decreases some five-fold and remains at a low level throughout the rest of gestation (Braunstein et al., 1976). In contrast, the production of placental lactogen rises steadily throughout gestation and is maximal at term.

Placental lactogen is a single polypeptide chain of 191 amino acids with an amino-terminal valine and a carboxyterminal phenylalanine; it has no carbohydrate constituents and is not a glycoprotein. It is produced as a prohormone with a signal sequence of 25 hydrophobic amino acids at the N-terminal end. The similarity in the amino acid sequence of placental lactogen and pituitary growth hormone is striking; both have 191 amino acids with two intrachain disulfide bridges. Both hPL and hGH have growth-promoting and lactogenic properties which differ only in degree. Pituitary prolactin, which has lactogenic but not growth-promoting properties, also is a single polypeptide chain with considerable homology to both hPL and hGH.

The synthesis of the placental peptide hormones has been studied in cell free protein synthesizing systems prepared from placenta. The synthesis of proteins by placental polysomes can be greatly increased by adding soluble cell fractions from rat liver which have an abundance of transfer RNA's and initiation factors (Hubert et al., 1974). Specific messenger RNA's have been extracted from placental polysomes and translated by incubation with cell free systems derived from wheat germ embryos, from ascites tumor extracts or from reticulocyte lysates (Hubert and Cedard, 1975). The hormonal peptides produced in the cell free system can be isolated by immunoprecipitation with an antibody specific to the peptide.

Chatterjee et al. (1976) showed that some 11 percent of all of the nascent peptides on polysomes from placentae of first trimester pregnancies were hCG, whereas only 2 percent of the nascent peptides from the polysomes of term placentae were hCG. The decline in the fraction of polysomes synthesizing hCG is paralleled by the decline of hCG in the plasma and urine. This finding implies that the amount of hCG made by the placenta is determined by the availability of its specific messenger RNA. Chatterje and Munro (1977) then extracted messenger RNA from placental polysomes and translated it in a cell free protein synthesizing system from wheat germ embryos. They measured the relative rates of synthesis of the α- and β-subunits of hCG at varying stages in pregnancy by specific immunoprecipitation of the subunits. The amount of a chains on the polysomes declined from 4.9 to 1.3 percent of total peptides synthesized and the synthesis of β-chains fell from 3.9 to 0.6 when first trimester and term placentae were compared. Both early and term placentae produced more α- than β-chains, which agrees with the observation of increasing amounts of free α-chains in the plasma of pregnant women as pregnancy progresses. The production of the two subunits appears not to be coordinated, and the amount of complete hCG secreted into the plasma is limited by the availability of the β-subunit.

It appears that the rate of production of hCG and hPL is regulated somehow at the transcriptional level, for the amount of messenger RNA coding for chorionic gonadotropin that can be recovered from the placenta reaches a peak early in gestation; much less is present in term placentae. In contrast, there is relatively little messenger RNA for placental lactogen in the placenta early in gestation but a great deal is present later on, at term. In early pregnancy, chorionic gonadotropin stimulates the maternal corpus luteum and maintains the high level of progesterone needed to maintain pregnancy. Later in gestation the placenta itself synthesizes an adequate amount of progesterone to maintain pregnancy. Chorionic gonadotropin may also play a role in stimulating the fetal testis to grow and produce androgens.

The placenta has been shown to have receptors for LRH (Currie et al., 1981) for gonadotropins (Page et al., 1981) and for steroids (McCormack and Glasser, 1976). Adding exogenous LRH to placental explants increases the production and release of gonadotropins. Adding exogenous gonadotropins increases the production and release of progesterone and other steroids. It is quite possible that there may be feedback control of the releasing hormones by the steroids, and the placenta may actually be a self-contained, self-regulated endocrine system.

LRH itself is synthesized by the placenta and has been shown to stimulate the secretion of chorionic gonadotropin in some placental systems. It is known, of course, that LRH regulates the production and secretion of luteinizing hormone (LH) by the pituitary. Since LRH also regulates the production of chorionic gonadotropins in the placenta, the question arises whether the control by LRH pituitary LH secretion and of placental hCG secretion is similar. In the pituitary system, the release of both FSH and LH is influenced by the activity of the receptor for LRH. The amount of LRH receptors present in the pituitary is modulated by LRH and by steroid hormones such as estradiol, progesterone and testosterone (Clayton and Catt, 1981). The production of chorionic gonadotropin (Gaspard et al., 1980) and of both progesterone and estrogens in the placenta has been localized to the placental syncytiotrophoblast (Chard, 1976).

The secretion of chorionic gonadotropin by trophoblast tissue can be stimulated by cyclic AMP and its derivatives and also by phosphodiesterase inhibitors (Hussa, 1980). This suggests that the effect of LRH on chorionic gonadotropin secretion may be mediated by cyclic AMP. Progesterone and pregnenolone both inhibit the secretion of chorionic gonadotropin by trophoblast cells in vitro (Pattillo et al., 1974) and by placental explants (Wilson and Jawad, 1980). The major precursor for the placental synthesis of progesterone is the cholesterol present in the low density lipoprotein, LDL, of maternal plasma (Simpson and Burkhart, 1980).

An interesting study was reported recently by Haning et al. (1982) of the effects of LRH, dibutyryl cyclic AMP, dehydroepiandrosterone sulfate, LDL, and the aromatase inhibitor, 4-hydroxy-androst-4-ene-3, 17-dione on the synthesis of chorionic gonadotropin, progesterone and 17β-estradiol.

In their system, adding LRH increased the output of chorionic gonadotropin by the placental explants, but it had no effect on the production of either progesterone or estradiol. The addition of LDL cholesterol had no effect on the production of either progesterone or estradiol or, incidentally, on the production of chorionic gonadotropin. This suggests that the amount of cholesterol available is not rate limiting for the process. In marked contrast, the addition of dehydroepiandrosterone sulfate increased the production of estradiol some twenty-fold, but did not affect the production of progesterone or of chorionic gonadotropin. This is to be expected since dehydroepiandrosterone sulfate is the immediate precursor of estradiol and it is well known that the placenta has a very active sulfatase and aromatase system for converting DHAS first to dehydroepiandrosterone and then, by way of androstenedione, to estradiol. In their system the addition of dibutryl cyclic AMP increased the output of human chorionic gonadotropin. The aromatase inhibitor, 4-hydroxy-andros-4-ene-3, 17-dione decreased the production of estradiol as expected, but it also decreased the production of chorionic gonadotropin. The results of the experiments suggest that the inhibition of hCG output by the aromatase inhibitor is not the result of a diminished estrogen production, but is by some other as yet unknown mechanism.

The concentration of hCG in the serum of women bearing male fetuses is less than that in women bearing female fetuses. Hobson and Wide (1975) reported that placentae of male children have only half as much hCG as those of female children at term. In twin pregnancies the placentae of male and female fetuses contain similar amounts of hCG, which indicates that the sex difference in hCG content is not due to a direct effect of the sex chromosomes on placental peptide synthesis. This difference appears to be mediated by fetal sexual development and may reflect a negative feedback effect on placental function by testosterone secreted by the male fetus during the second trimester in response to stimulation by hCG.

The regulation of hPL synthesis remains to be clarified. Human placental lactogen has a relatively short half-life of 16 to 30 minutes; the placenta at term produces one or more grams of hPL per day. Several reports have suggested that the concentration of hPL in maternal serum decreases when glucose is administered to the pregnant woman and rises during hypoglycemia.

The placenta has joined the group of tissues that have been shown to produce those fascinating derivatives of polyunsaturated fatty acids, the prostaglandins, prostacyclins and thromboxanes. The production of these compounds in the placenta is controlled in part by estrogens (Cane and Villee, 1975) The physiological function of these compounds in the placenta is not yet completely clear.

The placenta has also played a role in studies of human molecular biology, for it is a fine source of human genes to be used in recombinant DNA technology. The placenta has a genome identical to that of the fetus, for they both develop from the same fertilized egg. It is becoming clear that a surprisingly large number of these genes is transcribed and translated in the placenta. An entire library of human genes has been prepared from human term placenta. The messenger RNAs for hCG and hPL prepared from human placenta have been used to produce the corresponding proteins in cell-free, protein-synthesizing systems derived from wheat germ or rabbit reticulocyte lysate.

One of the recurring problems in toxicological studies is to find a suitable system in which to test potentially toxic material. It requries a considerable amount of extrapolation to infer from a demonstrated mutagenic property of a compound in a bacterial system that the compound is either carcinogenic or teratogenic in the human. Testing the toxicity of a new compound in the rat, dog, or Rhesus monkey is time-consuming and exceedingly expensive. The suggestion that perfused placentae or explants of placentae may be a suitable system for the testing of toxicological compounds was explored in a symposium that I chaired at Harvard nearly two years ago. The possibility of developing methods to use term placentae in such tests is an ongoing project in several laboratories. The perfused placental lobules remain viable and metabolize substrates at a uniform rate for periods of considerably more than four hours. Explants of trophoblast maintained in cultures survive for a week or more, as do individual cells maintained in the cell culture. Each of these protocols is a potential system for studies in toxicology.

An interesting finding was reported by Welch and his coworkers (1969) who demonstrated that placental aryl hydrocarbon hydroxylase (AHH) was elevated when the mother had smoked cigarettes during pregnancy. This is an enzyme that oxidizes polycyclic aromatic hydrocarbons such as benzo-(α)-pyrene, a compound present in cigarette smoke. This finding has been confirmed by several other laboratories (Nebert et al., 1969; Juchau, 1971; Pelkonen et al., 1972), but the studies showed that the amount of enzyme induction in placentae of different women was quite variable. The induction of AHH was a function of the duration of the exposure to cigarette smoke, being minimal in placentae from early pregnancy and greatest in term placentae. There was considerable variation in the activity of the enzyme in the placentae of different women even when they smoked comparable numbers of cigarettes. The induction of aryl hydrocarbon hydroxylase activity could be demonstrated in the fetal lymphocytes if the mother had been smoking cigarettes during gestation.

Experiments with inbred strains of mice suggest that there is a significant genetic component which influences the induction of placental aryl hydrocarbon hydroxlase (Nebert, 1976). By culturing lymphocytes obtained from the cord blood of twins, and measuring the aryl hydrocarbon hydroxylase in these cells the investigators showed that both maternal cigarette smoking and the genetic composition of the offspring played a role in determining the induction of the enzyme (Paigen et al., 1978; Pelkonen et al., 1981). In inbred mice a clear relationship has been demonstrated between the inducibility of the aryl hydrocarbon hydroxylase and susceptibility to cancer (Thorgeirsson and Nebert, 1977). It is claimed that human lung cancer and other cancers linked to smoking are associated with a high degree of inducibility of AHH as measured in lymphocytes (Pelkonen et al., 1980).

Exposure to cigarette smoke causes a number of other toxic manifestations in the fetus reflected in reduced birth weight and increased morbidity and mortality. When polycyclic hydrocarbons are metabolized they may be converted into much more reactive intermediates; these bind to specific molecules in the cell and result in toxic effects (Nebert and Atlas, 1977). Further metabolism of these reactive toxic intermediates can convert them into non-toxic products. The conversion of polycyclic hydrocarbons such as benzo-(α)-pyrene into reactive components is catalyzed mainly by aryl hydrocarbon hydroxylase. Large amounts of reactive metabolites are produced in vitro from benzo-(α)-pyrene when it is incubated with placental microsomes from mothers who have smoked and whose placentae have elevted AHH activity (Pelkonen and Saarni, 1980). In studies such as this, as in many other studies, it would be very useful to have a method for culturing term placental trophoblast cells so that the effects of exogenous influences on genetic traits could be studied under controlled conditions.

Sometime in the future it may be possible to identify and isolate cells from specific human term placentae that would be analagous to the especially sensitive strains of Salmonella typhimurium that are used for testing mutagenicity. It might be possible to find placentae which genetically resemble D2 mice in that they are not responsive to polycyclic hydrocarbons. Other placentae might be very sensitive to polycyclic hydrocarbons and thus resemble the B6 strain of mice. If the assorted technical problems could be solved, human placentae could be used for screening and monitoring in toxicological research.

Studies in several laboratories have shown that the rabbit placenta contains enzymes to metabolize compounds such as hexobarbitone and zoxazolamine (Dixon and Wilson, 1968). These enzymes are induced by environmental agents such as phenobarbitol and chlordane. Further studies have shown that these enzymes that metabolize compounds from the environment are induced by a wide variety of chemical and biological factors (Juchau, 1973; Mirkin, 1975; Nebert et al., 1977). The ability of the placenta to carry out the repair of DNA is an important factor in the toxicity of these compounds. Studies of DNA synthesis in cultures of cytotrophoblast and fibroblast cells from placentae, both mature and immature, have shown that the induction of DNA repair by ultraviolet light is dependent on the type of cell and is relatively independent of gestational age (Lefkowitz et al. 1979). Thus, fibroblasts showed a three-fold greater ability to repair DNA than did cytotrophoblast cells from the same placenta whether these were taken at 11 weeks, early in gestation or at term.

The teratogenic effects of ethyl alcohol have been demonstrated in laboratory animals and in humans (Streissguth, 1980). Ethanol is readily transported across the placenta and the concentration of ethanol in fetal blood is about as high as in the maternal circulation. Alcohol abuse by pregnant women can lead to malformations, growth retardation, abnormalities of the central nervous system, and behavioral deficits in the offspring. Ethyl alcohol is a teratogen and its effects range from the fetal alcohol syndrome, evident in some offspring of women who are chronic alcoholics, to women who have a moderate consumption of alcohol and whose offspring may show reduced birth weight. Behavioral deficits range from mental retardation in children with fetal alcohol syndrome to less extensive behavioral effects in infants born to women who are social drinkers. Exposure of laboratory animals during gestation to ethanol results in fetal malformations and deaths, growth retardation, and behavioral abnormalities.

The fetus, of course, depends completely on the placenta and maternal blood for all of the necessities of life. Because of this, chemicals may affect fetal nutrition by having effects on the vasculature of the placenta or by affecting the panoply of enzymes present in the placenta.

Various metabolic uncouplers and inhibitors have been shown to alter placental metabolism and, secondarily, to alter placental transport processes (Miller et al., 1976; Kelman, 1979). Inhibitors of glycolysis such as iodo-acetic acid secondraily decrease the uptake of glycine and other amino acids by human placental slices. Inhibitors of adenosine triphosphatase such as ouabain can affect the transport of ions by the placenta (Miller and Berndt, 1975). The activity of a number of placental enzymes has been correlated with the concentration of trace heavy metals such as cadmium, mercury and lead. The activity of carnitine-palmityl transferase, steroid sulfatase, benzo-(α)-pyrene hydroxylase, isocitric dehydrogenase and glucose-6-phosphate dehydrogenase were found to be inversely correlated with concentrations of cadmium, mercury and lead in the environment (Karp and Robertson, 1977).

The placenta remains a gold mine as yet largely untapped by biochemists, molecular biologists and toxicologists. It is a prime source of human enzymes and human genes for study and an attractive alternative system for the testing of the toxicity, mutagenicity and carcinogenicity of compounds in human tissues.

REFERENCES

Braunstein, G.D., Rason, J., Adler, D., Danzer, H. and Wade, M.E. (1976) Serum human chorionic gonadotropin levels throughout normal pregnancy. *Amer. J. Obstet. Gynecol.* 126, 678-688.

Cane, E.M. and Villee, C.A. (1975) The synthesis of prostaglandin F by human endometrium in organ culture. *Prostaglandins* 9, 281-286.

Chard, T. (1976) Assessment of fetoplacental function by biochemical determinations, *J. Clin. Pathol.* (Suppl.) 10, 18-35.

Charreau, E., Jung, W., Loring, J. and Villee, C.A. (1968) Biosynthesis of estrogens by perfused full-term placentae. *Steroids* 12, 29-40.

Chatterjee M., Baliga, B.S. and Munro, H.N. (1976) Synthesis of hPL and hCG by polysomes and mRNAs from early and full- term placentae. *J. Bio. Chem.* 251, 2945-2951.

Chatterjee, M. and Munro, H.N. (1977) Structure and biosynthesis of human placental peptide hormones. *Vitamins and Hormones* 35, 149-208.

Clayton, R.N. and Catt, K.J. (1981) Gonadotropin-releasing hormone receptors: characterization, physiological regulation, and relationship to reproductive function. *Endocrinology Reviews* 1, 186-197.

Currie, A.J., Fraser, H.M. and Sharpe, R.M. (1981) Human placental receptors for luteinizing hormone releasing hormone. *Biochem. Biophys. Res. Commun.* 99, 332-339.

Dixon, R.L. and Wilson, V.J. (1968) Metabolism of hexobarbital and zoxazolamine by placental and fetal liver supernatant fraction and response to phenobarbital and chlordane treatment. *Archives International Pharmacodynamics* 172, 453-462.

Gaspard, U.J., Hustin, J. Reuter, A.M., Lambotte, R. and Franchimont, P. (1980) Immunofluorescent localization of placental lactogen, chorionic gonadotropin and its alpha and beta subunits in organ cultures of human placenta. *Placenta* 1, 135-144.

Haning, R.V., Choi, L., Kiggens, A.J., Kuzma, D.L. and Summerville, J.W. (1982) Effects of dibutyryl adenosine 3',5'-monophospohate, luteinizing hormone releasing hormone, and aromatase inhibitor on simultaneous outputs of progesterone, 17β-estradiol and human chorionic gonadotropin by term placental explants. *J. Clin. Endo. Metabol.* 213-218.

Hobson, B.M. and Wide, L. (1975) Relationship of the sex of the fetus to the amount of human chorionic gonadotropin in placenta. *J. Endo.* 64, 117-124.

Hubert, C., Baliga, B.S., Villee, C.A. and Munro, H.N. (1974) Protein synthesis in a cell-free system prepared from human placenta. *Biochem. Biophys. Act.* 374, 359-374.

Hubert, C. and Cedard, L. (1975) Isolation and in vitro translation of human placental lactogen messenger RNA from human term placenta. *Nucleic Acid Research* 2, 1903-1910.

Hussa, R.O. (1980) Biosynthesis of human chorionic gonado- tropin. *Endo. Rev.* 1, 269-285.

Juchau, M.R. (1971) Human placental hydroxylation of 3,4- benzopyrene during gestation and at term. *Toxicol. Appl. Pharm.* 18, 665-672.

Juchau, M.R. (1973) Placental metabolism in relation to toxicology. *CRC Critical Reviews in Toxoicology* 2, 125- 139.

Karp, W.B. and Robertson, A.F. (1977) Correlation of human placental enzymatic activity with trace metal concentration in placentae from three geographical locations. *Environmental Research* 13, 470-476.

Kelman, B.J. (1979) Effects of toxic agents on movements of materials across the placenta. *Fed. Proc.* 38, 2246-2252.

Lefkowitz, D.M., Johnson, R.C., Faulk, W.P. and Vincent, R.A., Jr. (1979) Unscheduled DNA synthesis in primary cultures of human placentae. *Exp. Cell Res.* 121, 153-157.

McCormack, S.A. and Glasser, S.R. (1976) A high affinity estrogen binding protein in rat placental trophoblast. *Endocrinology* 99, 701-712.

Miller, R.K. and Berndt, W.O. (1975) Mechanism of transport across the placenta. *Life Sciences* 16, 7-30.

Miller, R.K., Koszalka, T.R. and Brent, R. (1976) The transport of molecules across placental membranes. In *The Cell Surface in Animal Embryogenesis and Development* (eds.), Poste, G. and Nicholson, G.L. p. 145-223 New York: Elsevier/North Holland.

Mirkin, B.L. (1975) Perinatal pharmacology: placental transfer, fetal localization and neonatal disposition of drugs. *Anesthesiology* 43, 156-16.
Nebert, D.W. (1976) Use of fetal cell cultures as an experimental system for predicting drug metabolism in the intact animal. *Clin. Pharmacol. Therap.* 14, 693-702.
Nebert, D.W. and Atlas, S.A. (1977) Aryl hydrocarbon hydroxylase induction (Ah locus) as a possible genetic marker for cancer. *In Genetics of Human Cancer* (eds.), Davis, W., Harrap, K.R. and Stathopoulso, G. p. 301. New York: Raven Press.
Nebert, D.W., Levitt, R.C., Jensen, N.M., Lambert, G.H. and Felton, J.S. (1977) Birth defects and aplastic-anemia-differences in polycyclic hydrocarbon toxicity associated with Ah locus. *Arch. Toxicology* 39, 109-118.
Nebert, D.W., Winker, J. and Gelboin, B.V. (1969) Aryl hydrocarbon hydroxylase activity in human placenta from cigarette smoking and nonsmoking women. *Cancer Research* 29, 1763-1771.
Page, W.E., Villee, C.A. and Villee, D.B. (1981) *Human Reproduction.* 4th Ed. Philadelphia: W.B. Saunders Co., p. 233.
Paigen, B., Ward, W., Steenland, K., Houten, L., Gurtoo, H.L. and Minowada, J. (1978) Aryl hydrocarbon hyroxylase in cultured lymphocytes of twins. *Amer. J. Human Genetics* 30, 561-569.
Patillo, R.W., Rinke, M.L. and Hussa, R.O. (1974) Effects of pregnenolone cyanoketone and equilenin on the human malignant trophoblast in vitro. *In Vitro* 10, 77-83.
Pelkonen, O, Karki, N.T. and Sotaniemi, E. (1980) Determination of carcinogen-activating enzymes in the monitoring of high-risk groups. *In Human Cancer: Its Characterizations and Treatment* (eds.), Davis, W., Harrap, K.R. and Stathopoulos, G. Amsterdam: Excerpta Medica, p. 48.
Pelkonen, O. and Sarni, H. (1980) Unusual patterns of benzo-(α)-pyrene metabolites and DNA-benzo-(α)-pyrene adducts produced by human placental microsomes in vitro. *Chemical-Biological Interactions* 30, 287-295.
Pelkonen, O., Karki, N.T. and Tuimala, R. (1981) A relationship between cord blood and maternal blood lymphocytes and term placenta in the induction of aryl hydrocarbon hydroxylase. *Cancer Letters* 13, 103-108.
Pelkonen, O., Jouppila, P. and Karki, N.T. (1972) Effect of maternal smoking on 3,4-benzpyrene and N-methylaniline metabolism in human fetal liver and placenta. *Toxicol. Appl. Pharmacol.* 23, 399-407.
Reczek, P.R. and Villee, C.A. (1982) A purification of microsmal glucose-6-phosphatase from human tissue. *Biochem. Biophys. Res. Communications* 107, 1158-1165.
Simpson, E.R. and Burkhart, M.F. (1980) Regulation of cholesterol metabolism by human choriocarcinoma cells in culture: effect of lipoproteins and progesterone on cholesteryl ester synthetase. *Arch. Biochem. Biophys.* 200, 86-93.
Streissguth, A.P. (1980) Teratogenic effects of alcohol in humans and laboratory animals. *Science* 2029, 353-359.
Thorgeirsson, S.S. and Nebert, D.W. (1977) The Ah locus and the metabolism of chemical carcinoigens and other foreign compounds. *Advances in Cancer Research* 25, 159-166.
Villee, C.A. (1977) Synthesis of proteins in the placenta. *Gynecological Investigations* 8, 145-161.

Welch, R.M., Harrison, Y.E., Commi, B.W., Poppers, P.J., Finster, M. and Conney, W. (1969) Stimulatory effect of cigarette smoking on the hydroxylation of 3,4-benzpyrene and the N-demethylation of 3-methyl-4-monoethylamino azobenzene by enzymes in the human placenta. *Clin. Pharmacol. Therapeutics* 10, 100-109.
Wilson, E.A. and Jawad, M.J. (1980) Luteinizing hormone- releasing hormone suppression of human placental progesterone production. *Fertility and Sterility* 33, 91-98.

Trophoblast Research 1:185-196, 1983

cAMP-DEPENDENT PROTEIN KINASE AND cAMP, cGMP AND CALCIUM STIMULATED PHOSPHORYLATION IN HUMAN PLACENTA: COMPARISON OF CYTOSOL AND MEMBRANE FRACTIONS

John J. Moore[1,2], Jeffrey V. Baker[2], and Jeffrey A. Whitsett[2]

[1]Newborn Division, Department of Pediatrics, Case Western Reserve University School of Medicine, Metropolitan General Hospital, 33095 Scranton Road, Cleveland, Ohio 44109, U.S.A.
[2]Children' Hospital Research Foundation, Newborn Division, Department of Pediatrics, University of Cincinnati, College of Medicine, 231 Bethesda Avenue, Cincinnati, Ohio 45276, U.S.A.

INTRODUCTION

Many effects of 3'5'-cyclic adenosine monophosphate (cAMP) on placental metabolism have been described. Human chorionic gonadotropin, estrogen and lactate synthesis are increased in human placental explants by cAMP analogs (Cedard et al., 1970; Ginsburg and Jeacock, 1964). Placental explants exposed to epinephrine show increased glycogenesis and progesterone production, and decreased human placental lactogen synthesis (Ginsburg and Jeacock, 1968; Satoh and Ryan, 1971; Demers et al., 1973; Coritis and Zeleznik, 1980). These effects of catecholamines on placental metabolism are presumably mediated by cAMP which is produced following hormone stimulation of placental β-adrenergic receptors coupled to catecholamine sensitive adenylate cyclase (Whitsett et al., 1980; Moore and Whitsett, 1981). In liver and skeletal muscle the effect of cAMP is mediated through its binding to the regulatory subunit of cAMP dependent protein kinase and the resultant activation of the catalytic subunit of this enzyme. The activated catalytic subunit then facilitates the phosphorylation of cell proteins resulting in changes in metabolism (Krebs and Beavo, 1979). In addition to cAMP, cGMP and calcium, in association with the calcium dependent regulator protein, calmodulin, have been shown to activate specific protein kinases resulting in phosphorylation of cell proteins of some tissues (Nishizuka et al., 1979).

Recently two isozymes of cAMP-dependent protein kinase have been demonstrated in human placental cytosol (Moore et al., 1983). The cGMP- and calcium-dependent kinases have not been described in placenta but both guanyl cyclase and calmodulin have recently been reported in placental fractions. The purpose of this study was to compare cAMP-dependent protein kinase isozymes, and cAMP-, cGMP- and calcium-stimulated phosphoproteins in human placental cytosol and microsomal membranes. A single isozyme of cAMP-dependent protein kinase was demonstrated in microsomal membrane fractions while two isozymes were found in the cytosol. Phosphoprotein substrates stimulated by cAMP, cGMP and calcium were also demonstrated in both cytosol and membrane placental fractions.

MATERIALS AND METHODS

[^{3}H]cAMP (36.4 Ci/mmol) and [^{32}P]ATP (35 Ci/mmol) were purchased from New England Nuclear Corporation (Boston, Massachusetts). cAMP-dependent protein kinase inhibitor, cAMP, cGMP, 3'5'-dibutyryl cAMP [$(BU)_2$ cAMP] and other reagents were purchased from Sigma Chemical Co. (St. Louis). DEAE-cellulose was obtained from Whatman Inc. (Clifton, New Jersey). Cellulose acetate filters were from Millipore Corp (Bedford, Massachusetts). All other reagents were obtained from Fisher Scientific Company. Calmodulin was a generous gift of Dr. James Potter (University of Cincinnati).

Tissue preparation

Placentae from uncomplicated term pregnancies were obtained at delivery and placed immediately on ice. The placentae were perfused with approximately one liter of normal saline, and cotyledons which were blanched white and demonstrated no grossly visible calcifications, clots or irregularities were chosen for dissection. Decidual tissue and large blood vessels were removed by sharp dissection. The remaining tissue was washed in iced buffer containing 250 mM sucrose and 10 mM Tris-HCl (pH 7.2). Approximately 50 g of washed tissue was then homogenized with a Tekmar Tissuemizer (Tekmar Co., Cincinnati, Ohio) in 300 ml of the sucrose buffer (3 x 5 seconds at high setting). The homogenate was poured through four layers of cheesecloth and centrifuged at 3000 x g for 10 minutes. The supernatant was centrifuged at 40,000 x g for 20 minutes. The pellet obtained was resuspended by gentle homogenization in the same amount of iced buffer and centrifuged again at 40,000 x g for 20 minutes. This washed pellet was then resuspended in 250 mM sucrose and 10 mM Tris-HCl (pH 7.2) to a final membrane protein concentration of 5-10 mg/ml as determined by the method of Lowry et al. (1951). This membrane preparation was used as the placental microsomal membrane. The supernatant of the first 40,000 x g centrifugation (above) was centrifuged again at 100,000 x g for 60 minutes and the final supernatant used as the placental cytosol preparation.

Samples were assayed on the day of preparation or after freezing in a dry ice-acetone bath and storage at -70°C.

Solubilization

Membranes prepared as above were solubilized by the method of Reitherman et al. (1981). The membranes were placed in 0.1% Triton X-100 for 16 hours at 4°C. They were then centrifuged at 100,000 x g for 90 minutes. The clear supernatant was used as solubilized membrane.

[3H]cAMP binding assay

cAMP binding activity was determined by a method similar to that of Gilman (1970) as previously described (Moore et al., 1983). Triplicate samples containing approximately 90 µg protein were incubated at 4°C for 1.5 hours in 100 mM sodium acetate buffer (pH 4.0) with [^{3}H]cAMP. Under these conditions, equilibrium binding of [^{3}H]cAMP to the receptor is achieved. The 200 µl assay volume was then precipitated with 0.5 ml saturated $(NH_4)_2SO_4$ and filtered through 0.45 millipore filters. The filters were washed with 30 ml (3 x 10ml) of 20 mM phosphate buffer (pH 7.0), dried and counted by standard scintillation techniques. Non-specific binding was assessed in identical assays containing 1 mM unlabeled cAMP. Non-specific binding was less than 1% of total binding.

Displacement studies were performed at 2 x 10^{-7}M [^{3}H]cAMP with various concentrations of cAMP, cGMP, $(BU)_2$ cAMP or other nucleotides added to the incubation mixture. The percent displacement of [^{3}H]cAMP binding by an agent was calculated from the binding in the presence of the agent, binding in the absence of the agent (100%) and the binding in the presence of 1 mM cAMP (0%). The dissociation constants (KD) were determined from the ED_{50} by the method Cheng and Prusoff (1973).

Protein kinase assay

Protein kinase activity was measured by a modification of the method of Gill and Walton, (1979). The reaction mixture (total volume 0.2 ml) consisted of the protein sample (50-150 µg), 10 mM $MgCl_2$, 10 mM NaF, 0.5 mM EGTA, and 50 mM potassium phosphate (pH 6.8), 5 mM theophylline, histone II A, 1 mg/ml, 0.5 mM [γ^{32}P]ATP (5-20 cpm/pmole) with or without cAMP (1.0 x 10^{-6}M). Incubations were for 10 minutes at 30°C and the reaction terminated by the addition of 50 µl of 2.5% bovine serum albumin (BSA) in 0.02% deoxycholate followed by 2.5 ml of 2.5% trichloracetic acid at 4°C. The mixture was then filtered through glass fiber filters (GF/F) which had been presoaked in 10% trichloracetic acid and 2.5% sodium pyrophosphate. The filters were washed with an additional 7.5 ml of 2.5% trichloracetic acid, dried and counted by standard scintillation techniques. Under these conditions, protein phosphorylation was nearly linear with respect to incubation time and to placental protein concentration.

DEAE - cellulose chromatography

DEAE - cellulose chromatography (DE-52, Whatman Inc., Clifton, New Jersey) was performed on a column equilibrated with 10 mM potassium phosphate (pH 7.0). Samples were placed on the column which was then washed with 1000 ml of phosphate buffer. The column was developed with a continuous gradient of NaCl at a buffer flow rate of 0.5-1 ml/min. Fractions were assayed for conductivity, protein concentration, [^{3}H]cAMP binding and protein kinase activity. Fractions were stored and frozen and used within 2 months without appreciable change in activity.

The relative amounts of the regulatory subunits (Types I and II) of cAMP-dependent protein kinase were determined by plotting specific [^{3}H]cAMP binding per ml eluant and comparing the areas of the two resultant peaks.

Gel electrophoresis and autoradiography

Phosphorylation substrates were identified by incubation of placental cytosol or solubilized membranes with [γ^{32}P]ATP followed by gel electrophoresis and autoradiography. In these experiments the reaction mixture (total volume 0.2 ml) consisted of the protein sample (5-10µg), 5 µM [γ^{32}P]ATP (5-20 cpm/pmole), 20 mM Tris-HCl (pH 7.2), 5 mM $MgCl_2$, 1 mM EGTA, 10 mM NaF, and 5 mM theophylline plus added cAMP (1.0 x 10-6M), cGMP (1.0 x 10-6M), or $CaCl_2$. The amount of $CaCl_2$ required to give specific free Ca^{++} concentrations was calculated by a computer program according to the method of Sillen and Martell (1964). cAMP-dependent protein kianse inhibitor (0.2mg/ml), calmodulin (40µg/ml and trifluoperazine (10^{-5}M) were also added to specific assays. The assays were initiated by the addition of

[^{32}P]ATP and incubated for 6 minutes at 30°C in a water bath. The reaction was terminated by the addition of 100µl of 12% trichloroacetic acid at 4°C. The protein was the precipitated and the pellet washed twice with 350µl H_2O. The pellet was then dissolved in a solution (60µl) containing 2% SDS, 10% glycerol, 5% B-mercaptoethanol and 0.001% bromophenol blue and boiled for 5 minutes. The samples were loaded on an SDS polyacrylamide gel (4.3% stacking, 10% running) for electrophoresis according to the method of Laemmli (1970). The gels were fixed overnight in 50% methanol and 7.5% acetic acid, stained with Commassie Blue and destained. Gels were dried on Whatman grade 3 filter paper, autoradiographed on Kodak XR film and developed after various periods (24 hours-2 wks) to demonstrate the phosphorylated proteins.

RESULTS

cAMP-dependent protein kinase

DEAE cellulose chromatography was performed on human placental cytosol, and solubilized microsomal membranes. [^{3}H]cAMP binding and cAMP-dependent kinase activity were determined in the fractions obtained. Two coincident peaks of [^{3}H]cAMP binding and cAMP-dependent kinase activity were present in the cytosol (Figure 1a) corresponding to the Type I and Type II cAMP-dependent protein kinase isozymes described in other tissues (Dosdeland and Ogried, 1981). Single peaks of [^{3}H]cAMP and cAMP-dependent protein kinase activity were present in the microsomal membranes (Figure 1b). The conductivity at which the peaks from solubilized placental membranes eluted corresponded to that of the Type II cAMP dependent protein kinase seen in placental cytosol.

Peak fractions of kinase activity separated by DEAE-cellulose chromatography of human placental cytosol and solubilized microsomal membranes were tested for specificity of [^{3}H]cAMP binding by competition studies. Competition for [^{3}H]cAMP binding followed the order of potency cAMP > cGMP > $(BU)_2$ cAMP (Figure 2). Adenosine, AMP, ADP, ATP and GTP did not compete for the binding. The binding affinities for cyclic nucleotides which compete for the [^{3}H]cAMP binding site were similar in the two placental fractions studied (Table I).

Protein Phosphorylation

Autoradiographs of polyacrylamide gel electrophoresis of human placental cytosol protein incubated with [γ^{32}P]ATP under phosphorylation conditions show 20-25 phosphate-labeled proteins. Six proteins (MW = 25,000, 27,000, 39,000, 45,000, 52,000 and 73,000) are cAMP-dependent as determined by increased labeling with cAMP (10^{-6}M) which was inhibited by cAMP-dependent kinase inhibitor (Figure 3). cGMP (10^{-4}M) but not cGMP (10^{-6}M) also increased phosphate incorporation into these six proteins (Data not shown). One protein of 97,000 MW showed increased phosphorylation in the presence of calcium and calmodulin (Figure 3). Trifluoperazine (10^{-4}M) suppressed this phosphorylation. (Data not shown)

Autoradiographs of polyacrylamide gels of placental microsomal membranes under the same conditions demonstrate only 2-3 phosphorylated proteins (Figure 4). The phosphorylation of a 66,000 molecular weight protein is enhanced by cAMP, cGMP and calcium. cAMP-dependent protein kinase inhibitor strongly inhibits phosphorylation of this protein. A phosphorylated protein of 66,000 daltons is present in the cytosol fraction but does not exhibit cAMP- or calcium-dependence.

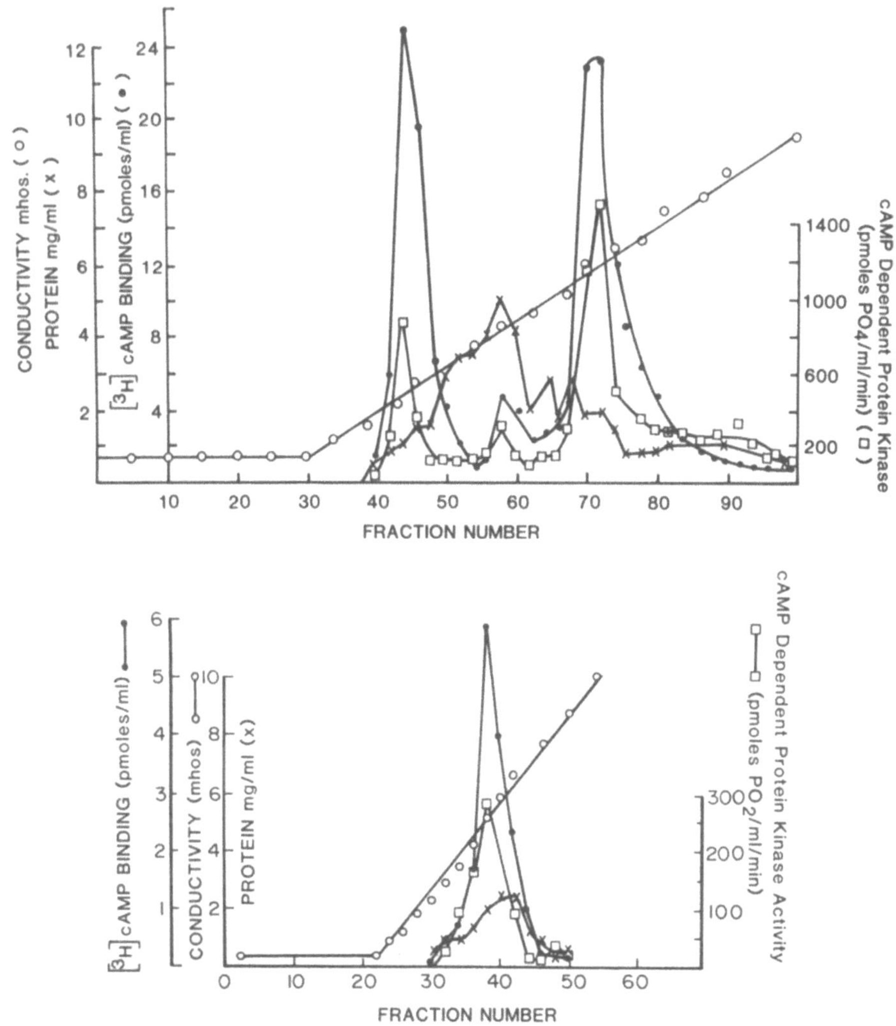

Figure 1. DEAE - Cellulose Chromatography of Placental Cytosol (a-above), and Solubilized Plasma Membranes (b-below). These placental fractions were prepared as described in Methods. Chromatography was performed as described in Methods but each placental fraction was chromatographed on a different column: a) Placental cytosol - 200 ml of 3.5 mg/ml cytosol protein was placed on a 2 x 30 cm column, washed and developed (0-400 mM; 200 ml each) with a continuous NaCl gradient at 0.5-1.0 ml/min. Four-ml fractions were collected. b) Solubilized placental microsomal membranes - 40 ml of 2.0 mg/ml solution was placed on a 2 x 10 cm column, washed and developed with a continuous NaCl gradient (0-400 mM, 50ml each). Two-ml fractions were collected. In each case (a, b) protein kinase activity in the presence of 10^{-6}M cAMP, protein, [^{3}H]cAMP binding and conductivity are shown on the vertical axis. Fraction number is indicated on the horizontal axis. The designation I and II refer to protein kinase isozymes I and II. The results shown are representative of four chromatography experiments done with each of the placental fractions. Each experiment utilized preparations from a different placenta.

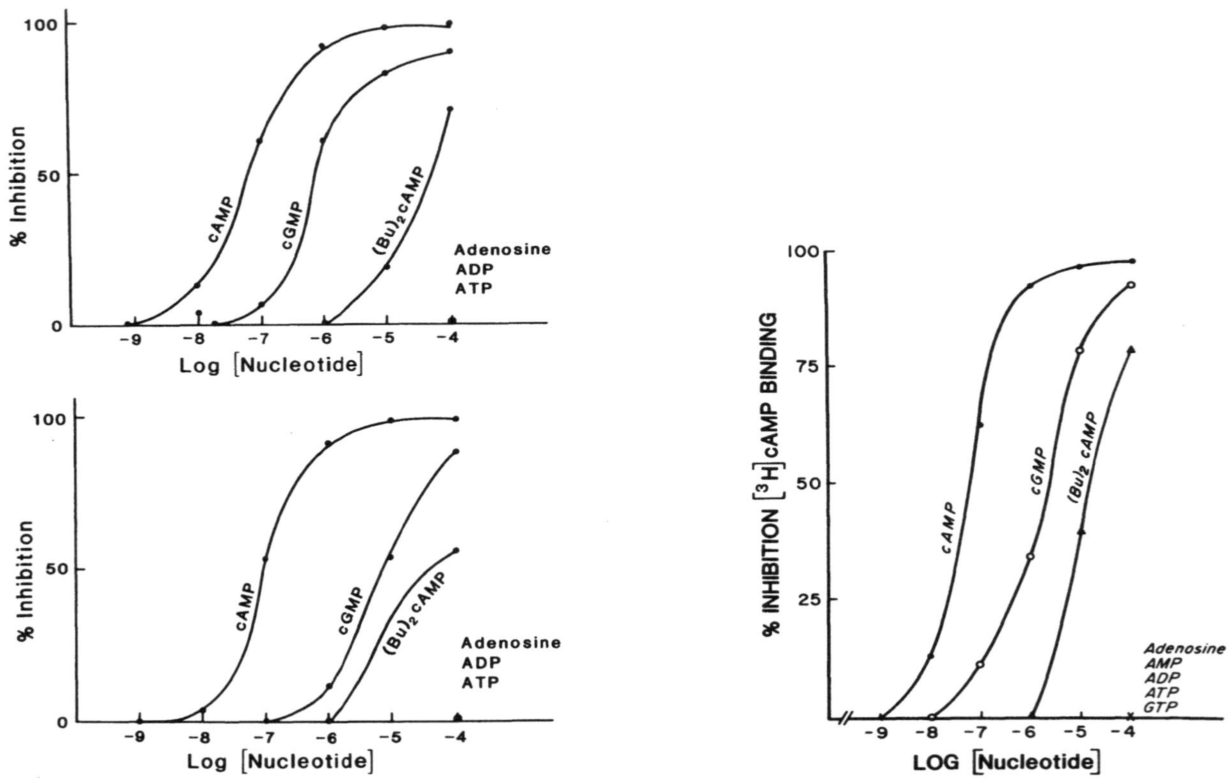

Figure 2 (a,b,c). Nucleotide Inhibition of [^{3}H]cAMP Binding to Placental Cytosol and to Solubilized Microsomal Membranes. Specificity of cAMP binding in fractions demonstrating peak cAMP-dependent protein kinase activity was determined by competition studies as detailed in Methods. Placental cytosol peak I (a-above left), peak II (b-below left), or solubilized microsomal membranes (c-above) (70µg protein/tube) were incubated with [^{3}H]cAMP [2 x 10^{-7}M]. The concentrations of the inhibiting nucleotides are indicated on the horizontal axis and the percent inhibition of [^{3}H]cAMP binding on the vertical axis. These results are representative of four binding experiments done on each peak fraction. Each experiment utilized preparations from a different placenta.

Table 1. Cyclic nucleotide binding to cAMP-dependent protein kinase isozymes

	cAMP	cGMP	$(BU)_2$ cAMP
Cytosol Isozyme I	$1.3 \pm 0.3 \times 10^{-8}$	$1.3 \pm 0.4 \times 10^{-7}$	$1.0 \pm 0.2 \times 10^{-5}$
Cytosol Isozyme II	$1.1 \pm 0.4 \times 10^{-8}$	$9.5 \pm 0.6 \times 10^{-7}$	$2.5 \pm 0.5 \times 10^{-5}$
Plasma Membrane Isozyme	$8.9 \pm 0.5 \times 10^{-9}$	$1.5 \pm 0.3 \times 10^{-7}$	$1.5 \pm 0.4 \times 10^{-6}$

The dissociation constants (KD) of cyclic nucleotide binding to the cAMP-dependent protein kinase isozymes separated by DEAE-cellulose chromatography (Figure l) were determined from the IC50s of competition experiments with $[^3H]$ cAMP (Figure 2) by the method of Cheng and Prusoff (1973). The units are moles/liter(M). Each value is the mean ± SEM from competition experiments done on peaks of cAMP-dependent kinase activity from four different chromatography runs.

DISCUSSION

Cyclic 3',5'-adenosine monophosphate-dependent protein kinase, and cAMP and calcium-dependent phosphoproteins of human placental cytosol and placental membrane fractions were compared in this study. Human placental cytosol contains both Type I and Type II cAMP-dependent protein kinases while the placental membrane fractions contained only the Type II isozyme. The ratio of Type I to Type II cAMP-dependent protein kinase varies between organs (Dosdeland and Ogried, 1981) and in different phases of the growth cycle (Costa et al., 1976). Predominance of Type I relative to Type II has been reported in the cytosol from cells from growing tissues: neonatal rat testis (Lee et al., 1976), neonatal mouse heart (Malkinson et al., 1978), neonatal rat uterus (Eppenberger et al., 1979), various human tumors (Fossberg et al., 1978; Handschin and Eppenberger, 1979) and 3T3 cells after viral transformation (Gharrett et al., 1976). Type II predominance has been associated with inhibition of cell growth in a mammary tumor cell line (Cho-Chung et al., 1979).

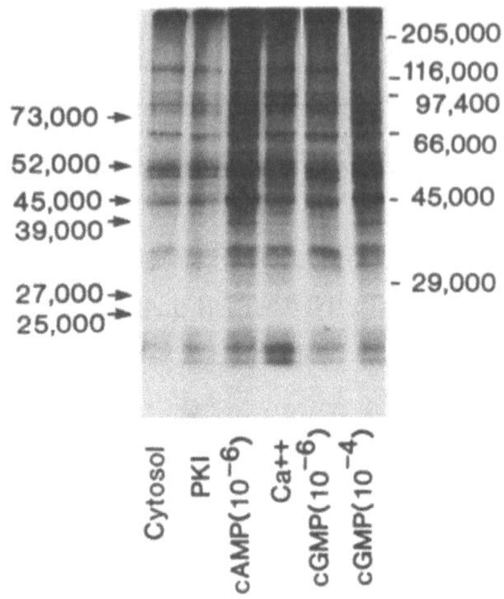

Figure 3. Autoradiograph of Phosphorylated Proteins in Placental Cytosol Separated by SDS-Polyacrylamide Gel Electrophoresis. Placental cytosol (5 μg) was incubated as described in Methods with cAMP-dependent protein kinase inhibitor (0.2 mg/ml), cAMP (10^{-6}M), Ca^{++} (10^{-6}M) or cGMP (10^{-6}M or 10^{-4}M). Arrows indicate the differentially phosphorylated proteins. The positions of marker proteins are also indicated to the right. The results shown are representative of 8 gels of placental cytosol from eight placentae.

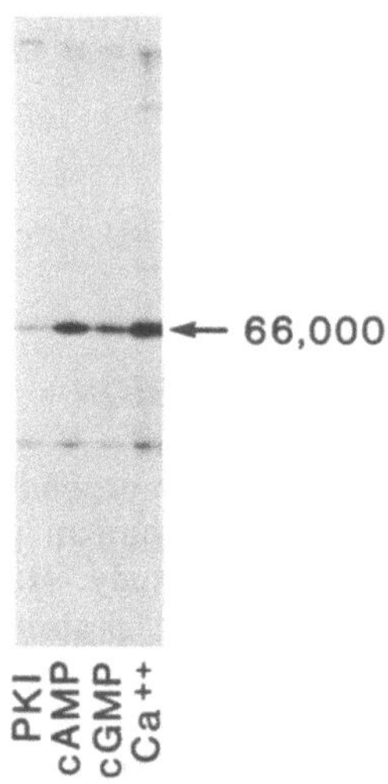

Figure 4. Autoradiograph of Phosphorylated Proteins in Solubilized Placental Microsomal Membranes. Solubilized placental plasma membrane (5 μg) was incubated as described in Methods with cAMP-dependent protein kinase inhibitor (0.2 mg/ml), cAMP (10^{-6}M), cGMP (10^{-6}M) or Ca^{++} (10^{-6}M)/calmodulin (40μg/ml). The arrow indicates the major phosphorylated protein of 66,000 daltons. The results are representative of gels from placental membranes of five placentae.

This has led to the hypothesis that cAMP dependent protein kinase Type I is a positive effector of growth, while Type II is a growth inhibitor (Russel, 1978). Human placental cytosol showed a predominance of Type II kinase activity in studies of term gestation placentae in which growth has become minimal. This is consistent with the hypothesis. Since the study was done in tissue homogenates, however, it is not possible to determine which of the placental cell types contains Type II cAMP-dependent protein kinase. Microsomal membrane fractions of brain, heart and adrenal cortex, like microsomal membranes from human placenta show significant amounts of Type II cAMP-dependent protein kinase (Corbin et al., 1977; Rubin et al., 1979; Sommarin and Jergil, 1978).

The order of potency of binding of the cyclic nucleotides to the regulatory sites of the type I and type II cAMP-dependent protein kinase isozymes in placental cytosol and the type II isozyme in the solubilized microsomal membranes (cAMP > cGMP > $(BU)_2$ cAMP) confirms the specificity of these isozymes for cAMP. The K_Ds (shown in Table I) for cAMP binding (0.89 - 1.3 x 10^{-8}M) were very comparable to those seen in many other tissues (1.0 - 5.0 x 10^{-8}M) (Corbin and Lincoln, 1978). The K_Ds obtained cGMP and $(BU)_2$ cAMP binding are also similar to that seen in bovine adrenal cortex (Reitherman et al., 1981).

Six placental cytosol proteins demonstrated increased phosphorylation in the presence of cAMP. The identity of these proteins has not been determined nor has their possible connection with the cAMP-stimulated metabolic events summarized in the introduction: increased HCG, estrogen and lactate synthesis and decreased placental lactogen production. No cGMP-specific phosphoprotein was present in any placental fraction. Recent studies identifying guanyl cylase in placenta have failed to demonstrate increased cGMP production in response to any hormone tested (Milewich et al., 1981). The functional significance of cGMP as an intracellular messenger in the placenta becomes more questionable considering both the lack of specific stimulating hormones for its synthesis and the lack of specific phosphoproteins. Calcium increases phosphorylation of a protein of approximately 97,000 daltons in placental cytosol. The calmodulin inhibitor trifluoperazine (10-4M) inhibits this action of calcium. These results are consistent with Ca^{++} calmodulin stimulated phosphorylation. Phosphorylation of the 97,000 dalton protein is not stimulated by cAMP.

Placental microsomal membranes demonstrated a single protein of 66,000 daltons which exhibited increased phosphorylation in the presence of both cAMP and calcium. A single phosphorylated protein in human placenta microvillous membranes which contaminated placental plasma membranes of approximately this weight has been previously identified as alkaline phosphatase (Sussman et al., 1968). Although alkaline phosphatase is a major component of microvillous brush border membranes, its specific function is unknown. The effect of phosphorylation of this enzyme is also unknown.

SUMMARY

The effects of many hormones are felt to be mediated by the intracellular second messengers cAMP, cGMP and Ca^{++}-calmodulin. These in turn are known to interact in many tissues with specific protein kinases resulting in phosphorylation of specific cell proteins. Numerous effects of cAMP on placental metabolism have been described. Although the effects of cGMP and Ca^{++} calmodulin on placental function are unknown, guanyl cylase and calmodulin have both recently been described in placenta. Protein kinases and their phosphorylation substrates have not been studied in placenta. In this study, cAMP-dependent protein kinase was characterized in placental cytosol and microsomal membranes both by [^{3}H] cAMP binding and by its ability to incorporate ^{32}P from [^{32}P]ATP into histone protein. DEAE-cellulose chromatography of placental cytosol demonstrated two peaks of coincident [^{3}H]cAMP binding and cAMP-dependent kinase activity corresponding to the Type I and Type II isozymes seen in other tissue. Placental membranes, when solubilized with Triton X-100, demonstrated a single peak of cAMP-dependent protein kinase activity which chromatographed similarly to the Type II isozyme. SDS polyacrylamide gel electrophoresis and autoradiograhy of the placental fractions following exposure to [^{32}P]ATP under phosphorylation conditions revealed that cAMP stimulates increased phosphorylation of distinct proteins in cytosol, and microsomal membranes. cGMP stimulates phosphorylation of the same proteins as cAMP. Ca^{++} enhances the phosphorylation of other distinct proteins in both placental fractions.

ACKNOWLEDGMENTS

This research was supported in part by NICHD Grant No. 11725; NICHD Grant No. 07700; Maternal and Child Health Training Grant No. 000174 for JJM; RCDA-HL01024 for JAW.

REFERENCES

Cedard, L., Alsat, E. and Varangot, J. (1970) Studies on the mode of action of LH and HCG on estrogenic biosynthesis and glycogenolysis by human placenta perfused in vitro. *Steroids* 16, 361-370.

Cheng, Y. and Prusoff, P. (1973) Relationship between the inhibition constant (Ki) and the concentration of inhibitor which causes 50 percent inhibition (I50) of an enzymatic reaction. *Biochem. Pharmacol.* 22, 3099-3108.

Cho-Chung, Y.S., Archibald, D., and Clair, T. (1979) Cyclic AMP receptor triggers nuclear protein phosphorylation in a hormone-dependent mammary tumor cell-free system. *Science.* 205:1390- 1392.

Corbin, J. and Lincoln, T., (1978) Comparison of cAMP and cGMP-dependent protein kinases. *Adv. Cyc. Nuc. Res.* 9, 159-170.

Corbin,J.D., Sugden,P.H., Lincoln,T.M. and Keely,S.L. (1977) Compartmentalization of adenosine 3',5'-monophosphate and adenosine 3',5'-monophosphate-dependent protein kinase in heart tissue. *J. Biol. Chem.* 252, 3854-3861.

Coritis, S.N., Zeleznik, A.J. (1980) Effect of adrenergic agonists on progesterone production by human placental cells in culture. *Am. J. Obstet. Gynecol.* 138, 677.

Costa, M., Gerner, E.W., and Russel, D.M. (1976) Cell cycle-specific activity of type I and type II cyclic adenosine 3',5'-monophosphate-dependent protein kinases in Chinese hamster ovarian cells. *J. Biol. Chem.* 251, 3313-3319.

Demers, L., Gabbe, S., Villee, C. and Grup, R. (1973) Human choronic gonadotropin-mediated glycogenolysis in human placental villi: A role of prostaglandins. *Biochem. Biophys. Acta* 313, 202-210.

Dosdeland, S. and Ogried, D. (1981) Binding proteins of cyclic AMP in mammalian tissues. *Int. J. Biochem.* 13, 1-19, 1981.

Eppenberger, U., Roos, W., Fabbro, D., Sury, A., Weber, J., Bechtel, E., Huber, P. and Jungman, R.A. (1979) Ontogeny of the adenosine-3',5'-phosphate-dependent protein kinase system during early uterine development. Inverse relationship with the estrogen receptors. *Eur. J. Biochem.* 98, 253-259.

Fossberg, T.M., Doskeland, S.O. and Ueland, P.M., (1978) Protein kinases in human renal cell carcinoma and renal cortex. A comparison of isozyme distribution and of responsiveness to adenosine 3',5'-cyclic monophosphate. *Arch. Biochem. Biophys.* 189, 372-381.

Gharrett, A.J., Malkinson, A.M., and Sheppard, J.R. (1976) Cyclic AMP-dependent protein kinases from normal and SV40-transformed 3T3 cells. *Nature, Lond.* 264, 673-675.

Gill, G. and Walton, G. (1979) Assay of cyclic nucleotide-dependent protein kinases. Adv. Cyc. Nuc. Res. 10, 93-106.

Gilman, A. (1970) A protein binding assay for adenosine 3',5'-cyclic monophosphate. *Pro. Natl. Acad. Sci.* 67, 305-312.

Ginsburg, J. and Jeacock, M. (1964) Effect of adrenaline on human placental lactate production in vitro. *Amer. J. Obstet. Gynecol.* 90, 794-799.

Ginsburg, J. and Jeacock, M. (1968) Effect of epinephrine on placental carbohydrate metabolism. *Amer. J. Obstet. Gynecol.* 100, 357-365.

Handschin, J.G. & Eppenberger U. (1979) Altered cellular ratio of type I and type II cyclic AMP-dependent protein kinase in human mammary tumors. FEBS Let. 106, 301-304.

Krebs, E. and Beavo, T. (1979) Phosphorylation-dephosphorylation of enzymes. *Ann. Rev. Biochem.* 48, 923-959.

Laemmli, U. (1970) Cleavage of structural proteins during the assembly of the head of bacteriophage T4. *Nature (Lond)* 227, 680-685.

Lee, P.C., Radloff, D., Schweppe, J.S. and Jungmann, R.A. (1976) Testicular protein kinases. Characterization of multiple forms and ontogeny. *J. Biol. Chem.* 251, 914-921.

Lowry, O., Rosebrough, W., Fair, A., and Randall, R. (1951) Protein measurement with the Folin phenol reagent. *J. Biol. Chem.* 192, 265.

Malkinson, A.M., Gharret, A.J., and Hogg, L. (1978) Microheterogeneity of adenosine cyclic monophosphate-dependent protein kinases from mouse brain and heart. *Biochem. J.* 176, 367- 375.

Milewich, L., Hendricks, T., Gant, N., Schwartz, B., and MacDonald, P. (1981) Partial characterization of guanylate cyclase activity of the human placenta. *Placenta,* 2, 343-354.

Moore, J. and Whitsett, J. (1981) The β-adrenergic receptor in human placenta: receptor subtype analysis (β_1 and β_2) and partial characterization of the solubilized receptor. *Placenta* supple. 3, 103-113.

Moore, J., Baker, J. and Whitsett, J. (1983) 3',5'-cyclic adenosine monophosphate (cAMP) binding protein and cAMP-dependent protein kinase in human placenta. *J. Clin. Endocrinol. Metab.* 56, 1035-1041.

Moore, J., Workman, L. and Whitsett, J. (1982) Trophoblast cells of the hydatidiform mole contain a β_1 subtype adrenergic receptor. *J Clin Endocrinol Metab* 55, 341-346.

Nishizuka, Y., Takai, Y. , Hashimoto, E., Kishimoto, A., Kurda, Y., Sakai, K., Yamamura, H., (1979) Regulatory and functional compartment of three multifunctional protein kinase systems. *Mol. and Cell. Biochem.* 23, 153-165.

Reitherman, R., Chen, L., Wen, S. and Harding, B. (1981) Adenosine 3',5'-monophosphate (cAMP)-binding proteins and cAMP-dependent protein kinases in bovine adrenal cortical cell plasma membrane. *Endocrinology* 109, 301-306.

Rubin, C.J., Rangel-Aldao, R., Sarkar, D., Erlichman, J. and Fleischer, N. (1979) Characterization and comparison of membrane- associated and cytosolic cAMP-dependent protein kinases. Physiochemical and immunological studies on bovine cerebral cortex protein kinases. *J. Biol. Chem.* 254, 3797-3805.

Russel, D.H. (1978) Type I cyclic AMP-dependent protein kinase as a positive effector of growth. *Adv. Cyclic Nucl. Res.* 9, 493-506.

Satoh, K. and Ryan, J. K. (1971) Adenylate cyclase in the human placenta. *Biochem. Biophys. Acta* 244, 618-624.

Sillen, L. and Martell, A. (1964) in *Stability Constants of Metal-Ion Complexes* 2nd ed. Ser. Pub. No. 17, The Chemical Society, Burlington House, London, WIV OBN.

Sommarin, M. and Jergil, B. (1978) Protein kinases of rat liver endoplasmic reticulum. Solubilization. Partial characterization and comparison with protein kinases of rat liver cytosol. *Eur. J. Biochem.* 88, 49-60.

Sussman, H., Small P. and Cotlone, E. (1968) Human alkaline phosphatase: Immunochemical identification of organ specific enzymes. *J. Biol. Chem.* 243, 160-166.

Whitsett, J., Johnson, C., Nogouchi, A., Darovec-Beckerman, C. and Costello, M. (1980) β-adrenergic receptors and catecholamine sensitive adenylate cyclase of the human placenta. *J. Clin. Endocrinol. Metab.* 50, 27-32.

Trophoblast Research 1:197-208, 1983

INTERACTION BETWEEN MEMBRANE FUNCTION AND PROTEIN SYNTHESIS IN THE HUMAN PLACENTA IN VITRO

Olga Genbačev, Bojana Čemerikić and Milos Cvetković

INEP - Department of Endocrinology, Immunology and Nutrition, Zemun, Yugoslavia

INTRODUCTION

Membrane transport is important for all living cells. Nutrients must be taken up, waste products removed, water and ion content of the cell must be regulated. Ion gradients across the cell membrane are required to maintain membrane potentials, which play a crucial role in excitation processes, and to drive other transport processes. More recently attention has been focused on the possible primary role of the plasma membrane and inorganic cations in the regulation of cell metabolism. (Knox and Pasternak, 1977; Sanui and Rubin, 1979; Mummery et al., 1981).

In the present study we have examined the effects of changes in extracellular osmolarity and potassium (K^+) concentration on in vitro protein synthesis and release by first trimester human placenta and decidua. As we assumed that the link between membrane mediated events and the pattern of protein synthesis might be different in different tissues, porcine and rat anterior pituitary and liver have been included in the experiments as well.

MATERIALS AND METHODS

Material

Fresh human placental and decidual tissue (8-10 weeks of gestation) were obtained from legal abortions by currettage and immediately transported to the laboratory under ice in a thermal flask. For each experiment, the pool of placental and decidual tissue fragments from 10 abortions has been used.

Rat livers and pituitaries were collected from 50 adult male rats, age 2-5 months. Rat anterior pituitaries were hemisected, pooled and 4 hemipituitaries incubated per incubation flask.

Porcine pituitary glands from males of unspecified age were obtained at a slaughter house about 30-60 min after the death of the animals, and were immediately transported to the laboratory under ice. The pool of 10 adenohypophysis was used in each experiment.

Methods

Incubation of tissue slices was performed as previously described (Genbacev et al., 1977). ^{14}C-leucine (specific activity 348 mCi/mmol) used in the experiments was purchased from New England Nuclear (Boston). The control medium was minimal essential Eagle medium (MEM) prepared in our laboratory in order to modify cation concentration.

In selected experiments, the osmolarity of the medium was increased by the addition of KCl to the control medium, up to 90 mM.

In the experiments where the concentration of K^+ was altered, the osmolarity of the medium was maintained at the control level by appropriate changes in NaCl concentration. K^+ deficient medium was made by omitting KCl from the medium. Experimental medium used to examine the effects of ouabain was MEM with 0.5-1 mM ouabain added. Ouabain (ouabain octahydrate) was obtained from the Sigma Chemical Co (St. Louis).

The ^{14}C-protein determination in the tissue extracts and incubation medium was performed as previously described (Genbacev et al., 1977). Protein concentration in tissue extracts and incubation media was determined by the method of Lowry et al. (1951). Lactate production was routinely measured in the incubation media using a Behringwerke enzyme kit (W. Germany). Analysis of significant differences between control and experimental values was performed by means of the Student's-t-test. The levels of significance chosen were $p < 0.05$ and $p < 0.01$.

RESULTS

Effects of increased medium osmolarity

The effects of increased extracellular osmolarity on ^{14}C- leucine uptake and protein synthesis by first trimester placental tissue explants are shown in Figure 1. The increase of extracellular osmolarity by raising KCl concentration to 90 mM resulted in a gradual reduction of protein synthesis and a decrease of leucine uptake. This inhibition could be completely reversed by transferring the tissue explants into isotonic medium (Figure 2).

In order to test the sensitivity of different tissues to alterations of medium osmolarity, human placenta, decidua, rat anterior pituitary and liver have been investigated. The ^{14}C-leucine uptake and protein synthesis were much more affected by the hypertonic medium in the human placenta and decidua than in the rat pituitary and were not altered in rat liver tissue slices (Figure 3).

Effects of extracellular K^+ ion concentration

The effects of high K^+ concentration in isotonic medium and K^+ free incubation medium on protein synthesis by human placental, decidual, and pig pituitary tissue explants were investigated.

Incubation of tissue explants in K^+ free medium significantly ($p < 0.05$) depressed protein synthesis by human decidual explants and human placenta and was

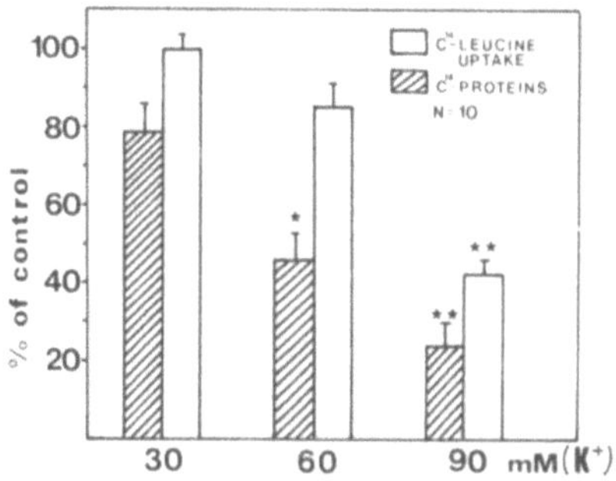

Figure 1. Effect of changes in medium osmolarity on protein synthesis and 14C-leucine uptake by human placental tissue explants. Tissue slices from the pool of 10 placentae (8-10 weeks of gestation) were randomly distributed in 40 incubation vials and incubated for 3 h in control medium and in medium with altered osmolarity. Osmolarity was increased with KCl. Each group consisted of 10 incubation flasks and the results represent the mean ± S.E.M. of the 14C-proteins/mg proteins synthesized during 3 h of incubation expressed as a percentage of control flasks. Significant differences are indicated with two asterisks for $p < 0.01$ and with one for $p < 0.05$.

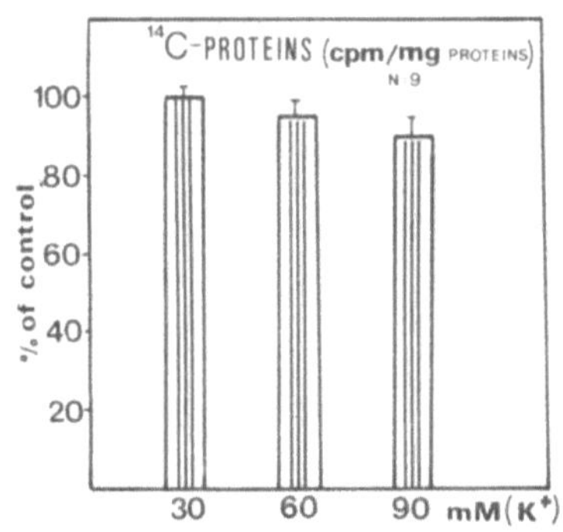

Figure 2. Protein synthesis by human placental explants incubated in hypertonic medium followed by incubation in isotonic medium. Placental explants were incubated for the next 3 h. The control group was incubated for 6 h in the isotonic medium. 14C-leucine was added to the fresh medium and tissues from both control and experimental groups were transferred and 14C-proteins were determined at the end of the experiment. Each bar represents the mean ± S.E.M. from 9 incubation flasks from the pool of ten placentae. The results are expressed as a percentage of control explants.

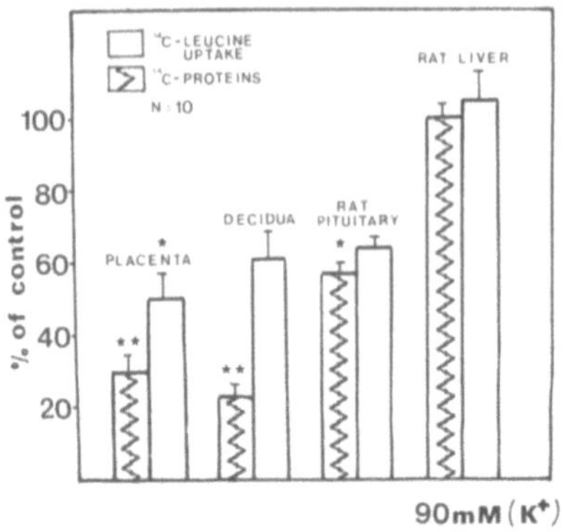

Figure 3. Protein synthesis by different tissues incubated in hypertonic medium. Human decidal, placental and rat pituitary and liver tissue explants were incubated in the medium made hypertonic with 90 mM K^+. The ^{14}C-leucine uptake and incorporation into proteins were determined after 3 h of incubation each bar is the mean of 10 incubation flasks ± S.E.M. Placental and decidual tissue slices were randomly distributed from the pool of 10 abortions, rat pituitaries were obtained from 40 male rats, dissected, pooled and 4 hemipituitaries incubated per incubation flask. The pool of rat liver tissue slices was made from 10 male rat livers. The results are expressed as a percentage of controls. Significant differences are indicated with two asteriks for $p < 0.01$ and with one for $p < 0.05$

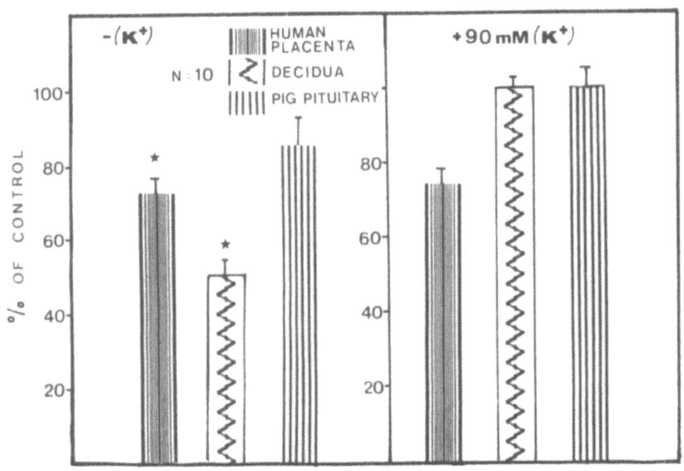

Figure 4. The effect of incubation medium K^+ concentration on protein synthesis by human placental, decidual and porcine pituitary tissue explants. Protein synthesis was determined after 3 h of incubation and the results are expressed as a percentage of the control. Placental and decidual tissue slices were obtained from the pool of the abortive material from 10 curettages, and porcine pituitary slices were obtained from the pool of 10 adenohypophysis. Each bar represents the mean of 10 incubation flasks ± S.E.M. Significant differences for $p < 0.05$ are indicated with an asterisk. Left (A): Effect of K^+ free medium Right (B): Effect of high K^+ in isotonic medium.

without effect on rat and porcine anterior pituitary (Figure 4A). The uptake of ^{14}C-leucine was only slightly reduced in both decidual and placental tissue slices. The increase of K^+ in the medium affected protein synthesis in the placenta only at extremely high concentrations (90 mM) and was without effect in all other tissues studied (Figure 4B).

The effect of K^+ deprivation on protein synthesis was tested after incubation of tissue explants in a medium containinig 0.5-1 mM ouabain, a cardiac glycoside which blocks Na^+, K^+-ATP-ase activity. Ouabain treatment significantly inhibited ^{14}C-leucine uptake (data are not presented) and protein synthesis in all examined tissues (Figure 5A). This inhibition of protein synthesis was prevented if the incubation medium was supplemented with 90 mM K^+ (Figure 5B).

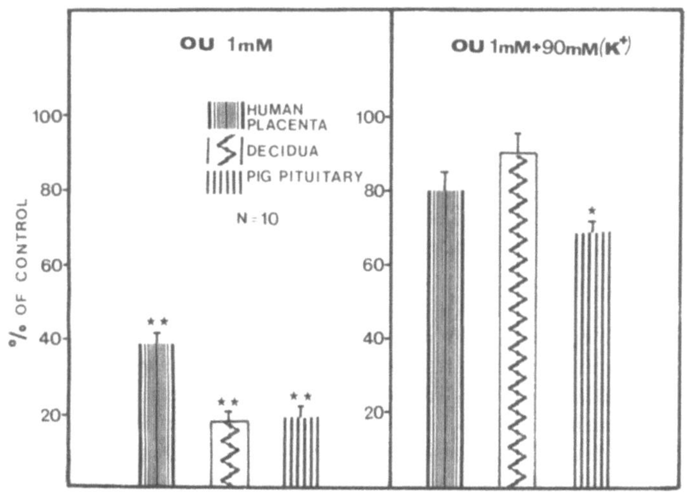

Figure 5. Ouabain effect on protein synthesis by human placental, decidual and porcine pituitary tissue explants. Tissue explants pools as under Figure 4 were incubated for 3 h and the results are expressed as a percentage of the control. Each bar is the mean of 3 experiments (9 incubation flasks) ± S.E.M. Significant differences are indicated with two asterisks for $p < 0.01$ and one for $p < 0.05$. Left (A): Effect of ouabain (1 mM); Right (B): Effect of ouabain and 90 mM K^+.

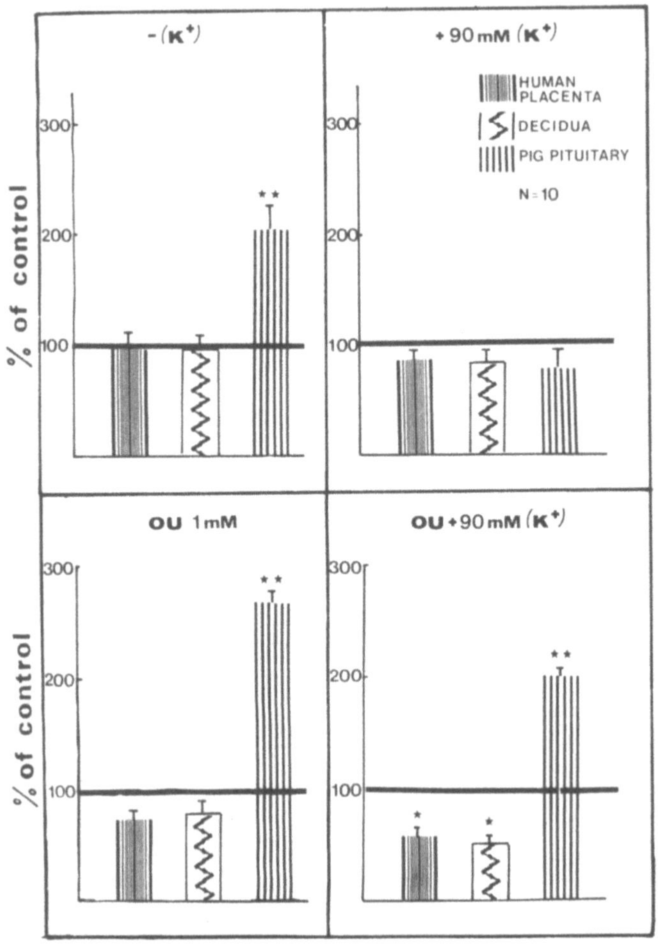

Figure 6. The effect of K+ concentration and ouabain in the medium on lactate production by human placental, decidual and porcine anterior pituitary tissue slices. Lactate concentration was measured in the incubation medium collected at the end of 3 hours of incubation. Tissue slices were obtained from the pool as described for Figure 4. Each bar is the mean of 10 incubation flasks ± S.E.M. Significant differences are indicated with two asterisks for $p < 0.01$ and one for $p < 0.05$. Placental control explants secreted 196.56 ± 26.44 µg/ml, decidual explants 261.39 ± 18.56, and porcine pituitary explants 53 ± 11.26 µg/ml.

In order to test whether K^+ inhibition of protein synthesis is direct or mediated through some other metabolic effect, glucose consumption and lactate production were also measured. Glucose consumption was not significantly affected by changes of K^+ concentrations and by the presence of ouabain in the medium. However, lactate production (Figure 6) was significantly increased in the pituitary incubated in K^+ free, ouabain and ouabain plus 90 mM K^+ containing medium. A decrease in lactate production was observed in the placenta and decidua of ouabain, and ouabain plus 90 mM K^+ containing medium.

DISCUSSION

The incubation of placental and decidual tissue slices in MEM made hypertonic by increasing KCl (30-90 mM) results in a salt concentration dependent inhibition of total protein synthesis. The ^{14}C-leucine uptake was affected only by the highest salt concentration. This effect is reversible as protein synthesis is completely restored after subsequent incubation in an isotonic medium.

It has been previously reported (Saborio et al., 1974) that the inhibition of protein synthesis could be selectively and reversibly inhibited in HeLa cells by increasing the osmolarity of the growth medium. This inhibition of peptide chain initiation is independent of the solute used (NaCl, KCl) to increase the osmolarity of the medium. It follows that the inhibition of protein synthesis by excess NaCl or KCl acts at the level of peptide chain initiation (Saborio et al., 1974; Liebowitz and Penman, 1971) leaving protein synthesizing machinery functional.

Protein synthesis by rat and porcine anterior pituitary was less affected by the increase of incubation medium osmolarity, and the rat liver was not affected at all. It may be assumed that placental cells are more sensitive to changes in the osmolarity of the incubation medium because they are involved in the active and passive transport of nutrients, electrolyte and water between mother and fetus and/or that the regulation of their protein synthesis is more dependent upon membrane mediated events (Pong et al., 1975; Herzberg et al., 1974). Decidual cells seem to be involved in the regulation of osmolarity of the amniotic fluid so that the direct feedback of osmolarity on protein synthesis could be expected.

The effect of extracellular K^+ concentration on protein synthesis has been studied in the human placenta and decidua, rat and porcine anterior pituitary and rat liver. It was anticipated that the difference in membrane architecture, distribution and number of receptor sites, in enzyme concentration between cells of different origin, may lead, in spite of the similarity of the mechanism that maintains the cation gradient across the membrane, to quantitatively and even qualitatively different responses.

The elevation of external K^+ concentration reduced protein synthesis only in the placenta and was ineffective in decidua, anterior pituitary and liver. As it has been reported that the excess of K^+ depolarizes the cell membrane, inhibits Na^+, K^+-ATP-ase activity (Skou, 1957) and inhibits K^+ influx, the observed differences might be attributed to the differences in K^+ requirements for protein synthesis by the examined tissues. To test this hypothesis, effects of K^+ deficient or K^+ free medium on protein synthesis have been investigated. Protein synthesis was strongly depressed in placental and decidual tissue explants incubated in K^+ free medium and was not affected in the pituitary. As it is known that K^+ is involved in peptide bound formation (Ledbetter and Lubin, 1977; Lehninger, 1975) and preservation of ribosomal integrity (Shank and Smith, 1976), the inhibition of protein synthesis after incubation in K^+ free medium can be expected. However, the lack of any effect on the anterior pituitary remains to be explained.

As ouabain treatment is supposed to be equivalent to K^+ deprivation, placental, decidual and pituitary tissue slices were incubated in the medium containing 1 mM ouabain. This dose has been reported to completely inhibit the ouabain sensitive flux of K^+ with no change in ouabain-insensitive flux within 60 min after addition (Johnson and Weber, 1979). This treatment lead to the strong inhibition of ^{14}C-leucine uptake and protein synthesis by all the tissues studied. However, the observed inhibition of protein synthesis cannot be attributed to the reduction of ^{14}C-leucine uptake only, as protein synthesis was lowered by 80percent while amino acid uptake was decreased for 40-50percent. However, this ouabain induced inhibition was prevented in the presence of high K^+ concentration in the medium. Because of the much more pronounced effect of ouabain containing than K^+ deficient medium on protein synthesis, some other metabolic effects of ouabain had to be considered. As it has been reported that ouabain diminishes lactate production by some cell lines (Racker and Spector, 1981), lactate concentration was systematically measured in the incubation media. A significant increase of lactate production was observed after incubation of the anterior pituitary in K^+ free and ouabain containing medium indicating that the glucose metabolism in the pituitary is primarily affected by K^+ deficiency. On the other hand, lactate production by placental and decidual tissue was reduced after incubation in the medium containing both ouabain and high K^+.

In this work, an attempt was made to couple cell membrane events with the protein biosynthesis taking place in the cytoplasm. Quantitative and qualitative differences in the role of the cell membrane in the regulation of protein synthesis in different tissues has been anticipated. These results have shown that protein synthesis by human placental and decidual cells is more influenced by membrane mediated events than for the anterior pituitary or liver. The further study of the role of the cell membrane in the regulation of cell function using human placenta and decidua may lead to the better understanding of the regulation of protein synthesis on the transcriptional level.

SUMMARY

The effect of extracellular osmolarity and K^+ concentration on protein synthesis and ^{14}C-leucine uptake were examined in human placental and decidual tissue explants incubated for 3 h in modified minimal essential Eagle's medium. Porcine and rat anterior pituitaries and rat liver were included in the experiments to test the sensitivity of different organs to alterations of incubation medium osmolarity and ion content.

Protein synthesis was strongly inhibited in placental and decidual tissue explants incubated in hypertonic medium. This inhibition was reversible if the medium osmolarity was reduced to the control level. Anterior pituitary tissue slices were less sensitive and the rat liver insensitive to changes of the incubation medium osmolarity.

Incubation in K^+ free or ouabain containing medium lead to the strong inhibition of protein synthesis in all studied tissues. Incubation in the medium containing ouabain and high K^+ prevented the reduction of protein synthesis. High K^+ concentration in the medium slightly reduced protein synthesis by placental tissue explants and was without effect on the decidua and pituitary. Potassium concentration and ouabain affected lactate production by the examined tissues to various degrees, indicating ouabain action on different metabolic patterns.

These results indicate that membrane mediated regulation of protein synthesis is more important in the placenta and decidua than in the other examined tissues.

REFERENCES

Genbačev, O., Ratković, M., Krainčanić, M. & Šulović, V. (1977) Effect of prostaglandin PGF 2 alpha on the synthesis of placental proteins and human placental lactogen (HPL). *Prostaglandins* 13, 723-733.

Herzberg, M., Breitbart, H. & Altman, H. (1974) Interactions between membrane functions and protein synthesis in reticulocytes. Effects of valinomycin and dicyclohexyl-18-crown-6. *Eur. J. Biochem.* 45, 161-170.

Johnson, M.A. & Weber, M.J. (1979) Potassium fluxes and ouabain binding in growing, Density-inhibited and Rous sarcoma virus-transformed chicken embryo cells. *J. Cell. Physiol.* 101, 89-100.

Knox, P., & Pasternak, C.A. (1977) The cell surface and growth in vitro. In: *Mammalian Cell Membranes, Responses of Plasma Membranes.* G.A. Jamieson and D.M. Robinson, (eds.), pp. 196-219, Boston: Butterworths, Vol. 5.

Ledbetter, M.L.S. & Lubin, M. (1977) Control of protein synthesis in human fibroblasts by intracellular potassium. *Exper. Cell Res.* 105, 223-236.

Lehninger, A.L. (1975) *Biochemistry.* Part III, Chapter 28, p. 790, New York: Worth Publishers.

Liebowitz, R. & Penman, S. (1971) Regulation of protein synthesis in HeLa cells. III. Inihibition during polio-virus infection. *J. Virol.* 8, 661-668.

Lowry, O.H., Rosebrough, N.J., Farr, A.L. & Randall, R.J. (1951) Protein measurement with the folin phenol reagent. *J. Biol. Chem.* 193, 265-275.

Mummery, C.L., Boonstra, J., Van Der Saag, P.T. & De Laat, S.W. (1981) Modulation of functional and optimal (Na^+ - K^+) ATPase activity during the cell cycle of neuroblastoma cells. *J. Cell. Physiol.* 107, 1-9.

Pong, S.-S., Nuss, D.L. & Koch, G. (1975) Inhibition of protein synthesis in mammalian tissue culture cells by L-1-tosylamido-2-phenylethyl chlormethyl ketone. *J. Biol. Chem.* 250, 240-245.

Racker, E. & Spector, M. (1981) Warburg effect revisited: Merger of biochemistry and molecular biology. *Science* 213, 303- 307.

Saborio, J.L., Pong, S.-S. & Koch, G. (1974) Selective and reversible inhibition of initiation of protein synthesis in mammalian cells. *J. Mol. Biol.* 85, 195-211.

Sanui, H., & Rubin, A.H. (1979) Measurement of total, intracellular and surface bound cations in animal cells grown in culture. *J. Cell. Physiol.* 100, 215-226.
Shank, B.B. & Smith, N.E. (1976) Regulation of cellular growth by sodium pump activity. *J. Cell. Physiol.* 87, 377- 388.
Skou, J.C. (1957) The influence of some cations on an adenosine triphosphatase from peripheral nerves. *Biochim. Biophys. Acta,* 23, 394-401.

DISCUSSION

KLEIN (Storrs): Have you corrected your leucine incorporation into proteins by the specific activity of the precursor pools? It is insufficient usually just to measure leucine uptake.

GENBACEV (Zemun): Yes, you are absolutely right. These corrections have been done for the placental studies. We have determined the intracellular pool of leucine and used these values to express our results in terms of total leucine.

PANIGEL (Paris): This is just a technical question about the validity of the tissue slice method for this type of an investigation. We often expect, when we make varying concentrations of electrolytes bathing the microvillar surface of the trophoblast, that variations and permeability of the membranes do occur as well as changes in its electrical activities. I wonder if your individual variations are not due to the heterogeneous material you are calling placental cells?

GENBACEV (Zemun): We have been working on the placenta for more than 10 years; we have performed numerous control studies including electron microscopic evaluation. For three to four hours, the tissue and especially the microvilli appear like controls. After that time, some alterations occur including lysosomes appearing and fluttering of the endoplasmic reticulum. So our studies have been limited to no longer than four hours.

MILLER (Rochester): In your ouabain studies you indicated that one millimolar concentrations were effective. Have you performed a dose response relationship to determine how sensitive these cells are to ouabain?

GENBACEV (Zemun): Our dose response curve includes values from 0.2 to 1.5 millimolar concentrations of ouabain. A varied dose response and sensitivity has been noted for different tissues. The most sensitive tissue was the decidua then the placenta and then the fetal organs.

MILLER (Rochester): We have observed that 10-6 M concentrations of ouabain were quite effective in inhibiting AIB uptake into human placenta slices. Did you examine concentrations in this range?

GENBACEV (Zemun): No, because the lowest concentration that we used (0.2 millimolar) did not inhibit protein synthesis to a large degree in fetal tissues. It was only inhibited 80percent in the decidua and the placenta.

BISCHOF (Geneva): I am trying to speculate about this particular sensitivity of decidua to changing osmolarity. Is the decidua in your preparation producing prolactin? There is certainly considerable speculation about the osmotic role of prolactin. Have you measured prolactin during these osmotic changes?

GENBACEV (Zemun): We have been investigating decidua prolactin for three years, and we expected that there would be tremendous changes when osmolarity, potassium, and ouabain modifications were introduced. However, there was no effect on prolactin with these treatments. Other control studies using the placental slices have demonstrated the synthesis of SP-1, hPL, and hCG during the three hour incubations.

NG (Rochester): In your system, are there changes in ATP concentration when the osmolarity in your medium is modified? Do these alterations change your intracellular water spaces?

GENBACEV (Zemun): The ADP-ATP ratio was not dramatically changed except when ouabain was used. These studies have been pursued in both the placenta and decidua. High potassium concentrations in the extracellular medium were less effective than ouabain. There was a 50 percent increase in the ratio when ouabain was present.

Trophoblast Research 1:209-222, 1983

METABOLIC CHANGES IN HUMAN PLACENTAL TISSUE IN DIABETES MELLITUS

Yoram Z. Diamant and Rita Kissilevitz

Department of Obstetrics and Gynecology, Bikur Cholim Hospital, Jerusalem, and Hebrew University Medical School, Jerusalem, Israel

INTRODUCTION

The primary responsibility of the placenta is the adequate transport of maternal fuels to the fetal circulation. The placenta, however, is not a passive channel; a proportion of glucose and lipids entering the placenta is retained and metabolized actively for its own use. The metabolic pathways of carbohydrates and lipids in the human placenta have been hitherto studied mainly by assessing the rates of the overall channeling of ^{14}C-labeled substrates through the pathways in incubated placental slices. According to these experiments, glucose can be either converted to glycogen, or degraded by glycolysis or by the pentose shunt pathway (Villee, 1953; Sakurai et al., 1969; Sybulski and Tremblay, 1969). The human placenta has been demonstrated to have an ability to assimilate fatty acids from incubation medium (Freinkel, 1965). Placental triglycerides and phospholipids appear to be formed from esterification of fatty acids or by uptake of performed lipids from the maternal blood (Szabo et al., 1973). The possibility of de novo placental fatty acids synthesis has been also suggested (Hosoya et al., 1960; Kleine, 1967; Diamant et al., 1975). Moreover, the placenta is responsive to alterations in the maternal pool of glucose and lipids with which it is in permanent contact. For example, in a perfusion study of human placentae, with increasing levels of glucose in the maternal circulation, both the transfer rate of glucose and the utilization rate rise concommitently (Nesbitt et al., 1973). Formation of glyceride-glycerol from glucose in viable human placenta slices is increased in the presence of albumin-complexed free fatty acids (Hagerman, 1962). Exogenous free fatty acids are esterified by an in vitro placental preparation in a concentration-dependent fashion, (Yoshioka and Roux, 1972; Diamant et al., 1980) and the hyperlipacidemia of starvation is attended by increased placental lipids accumulation in vivo (Herrara and Freinkel, 1975). Increases in placental glycogen have been reported to accompany the hyperglycemia of diabetes mellitus (Heijkenskjold and Gemzell, 1957; Hagerman, 1962; Fisher and Horky, 1966; Gabbe et al., 1972) and evidence in support of increased passage of lipids across the placenta in diabetes has been advanced recently (Hull and Elphick, 1979).

For its intermediary metabolism, the placenta is well-endowed with all of the necessary enzymes. During gestation, the activities of most enzymes change in order to support the metabolic needs of the vigorous, rapidly growing tissue from the primary villi stage to maturity and even senescence (Diamant and Shafrir, 1972; Diamant et al., 1975). Extensive studies in our laboratory indicate that, generally, placental enzymes are not susceptible to endocrine regulation, and imply that placental metabolism is largely independent of the physiopathological alterations affecting the maternal organism. The gradual activity decrease during gestation suggests that the enzyme complement of the placenta, once developed, is designed to last through its limited lifespan without continuous replenishment. The age of the placenta appears to be the primary factor determining its enzyme activities and metabolic performance (Shafrir and Diamant, 1979). However, in diabetic rats significant increase in the activity of placental pyruvate kinase and significant decrease in phosphoenolpyruvate carboxylase has been observed (Diamant and Shafrir, 1978). The response of these two enzymes in the placenta is the inverse of their responses in the liver, although not as extensive, and this response is considered to be incompatible with the circumstances for enhanced gluconeogenesis. The fact that the activities of these two enzymes are not altered in the placenta of starving pregnant rats indicates that these changes may be related to the direct effect of hyperglycemia rather than to adaptation to insulin deficiency (Diamant and Shafrir, 1978).

Diabetes is known to be accompanied by pronounced changes in the maternal plasma levels of glucose, lipids and amino acids as well as in the hormone levels. Since all of these alterations may profoundly influence the intermediary metabolism of the placental tissue, we have decided to examine the content of DNA, glycogen and lipids as well as the activities of rate-limiting enzymes of glycolysis, gluconeogenesis and lipogenesis in human placental tissue from diabetic pregnancies.

MATERIALS AND METHODS

Twenty three placentae from women with gestational diabetes mellitus (GDM), 12 placentae from insulin-treated patients with pregestational diabetes, and 50 placentae from women with normal carbohydrate metabolism were examined. GDM was diagnosed according to the glucose tolerance criteria of O'Sullivan and Mahan (1964). In the insulin-treated diabetic group, five patients belonged to Class B, three to class C, three to Class D, and one to Class F, according to White's classification (White, 1949). Placentae from women with GDM or normal carbohydrate metabolism were obtained following uncomplicated vaginal deliveries. Eight of the placentae from the Class B-F diabetics were obtained following elective Cesarean section under epidural anesthesia.

The gestational age as calculated from the first day of the last menstrual cycle, was matched between 38 and 40 weeks in all of the study groups. All subjects had received intravenous glucose (and insulin as necessary) to maintain the plasma glucose levels between 80-120 mg/dl throughout labor.

All placentae were obtained immediately upon delivery. They were weighed, placed in plastic bags for storage at -20°C and examined within a week. Storage of placentae at this temperature for one week, and even longer, does not change the enzyme activity and metabolic content (Diamant et al., 1975). No change in placental metabolism was observed that could be ascribed to parity, maternal age, use of oxytocin (Pitocin) or mode of delivery (Diamant et al., 1975). On the day of investigation, samples were removed from all quadrants of the placentae, defrosted and cut into slices, which were pooled and thoroughly washed in an ice-cold 0.9

percent NaCl. No decidua or chorionic plate were included in the investigated material.

Tissue lipids were extracted with chloroform:methanol (2:1, v/v). Extracts were analyzed for triglycerides and cholesterol according to the Autoanalyzer Methods (1973), and for phospholipids by the method of Fiske and Subbarow (1925). The glycogen concentration was measured by the enzymatic method described by Johnson et al. (1963). Lowry's method (1951) was used to measure protein content. Tissue DNA content was measured by the diphenylamine reaction (Richards, 1974). For enzyme activity assays, the placental slices were homogenized (1:3, v/v) in a 0.2 M sucrose solution containing triethanolamine (2 mM, pH 7.4), disodium EDTA (1 mM) and dithioerythreitol (1 mM). The homogenates were centrifuged at 100,000xg at 4^{0}C for 30 min. The supernatant fluids were used for enzyme assays. The following enzyme activities were determined by methods adapted for placental tissue as described in previous publications (Diamant and Shafrir, 1972; Diamant et al., 1975): pyruvate kinase (EC 2.7.1.40), aspartate aminotransferase (glutamate-oxaloacetate transaminase, EC 2.6.1.1), glucose-6-phosphate dehyrogenase (EC 1.1.1.49), 6-phosphogluconic dehydrogenase (EC 1.1.1.43), malate-NADP oxidoreductase dehydro-genase ("malic enzyme", EC 1.1.1.40), and phosphoenolpyruvate carboxylase (EC 4.1.1.32). All enzyme activities were determined at 37^{0}C and expressed as nmol of the substrate metabolized per min per mg protein.

The Student's t test was used for statistical evaluations of all calculations. Data were expressed as mean $\pm$ SEM.

RESULTS

The maternal values for fasting plasma glucose level during late gestation did not differ significantly in the 50 normal and 23 gestational diabetics and averaged 82 $\pm$ 6 and 101 $\pm$ 7 mg/dl respectively. Values in the 12 insulin-treated White Class B-F pregnant diabetics were significantly greater than both normal and GDM groups and averaged 132 $\pm$ 10 mg/dl ($p < 0.01$).

The effects of GDM and White Class B-F diabetes upon some of the compositional characteristics of the human term placenta were summarized in Figures 1 and 2. Placental weight tended to increase, although not to a significant extent. The DNA content of the total placenta significantly exceeded normal values in the GDM and insulin-treated groups ($p < 0.05$), although significant changes per g placenta could not be demonstrated (Figure 1). The placental content of glycogen was also significantly increased when expressed per g of placental wet weight and per unit of DNA (Figure 2).

Most placental lipid components were increased in the placentae from the diabetic women (Figure 2). The triglyceride content was significantly increased in GDM only when expressed as per g of placental wet weight or on the basis of total placental mass. The increased triglylceride was significant with all modes of expression in the insulin-treated diabetics. Significant increments in placental phospholipid content were present with all modes of expression in both GDM and in the insulin-treated White Class B-F groups. However, neither type of diabetes was associated with any demonstrable change in the placental content of cholesterol.

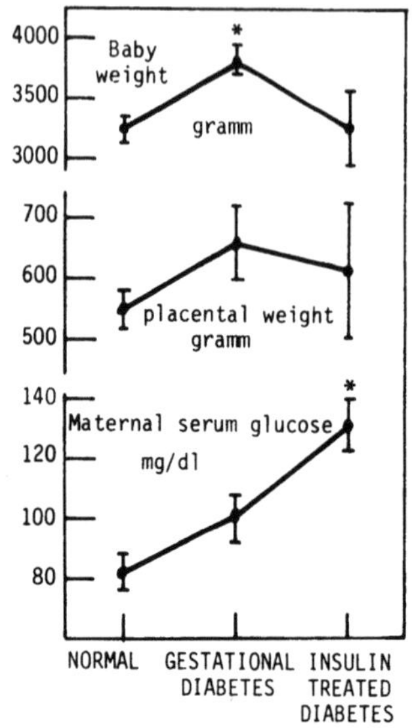

Figure 1. Maternal serum glucose level, placental weight and neonatal weight in study and control groups. The glucose values are mean ± SEM of at least 3 determination groups as compared to normal controls obtained before delivery from each patient in every group. *denotes significantly higher baby body weight in gestational diabetes.

The activities of placental enzymes were summarized in Figures 3 and 4. Pyruvate kinase activity was significantly increased in the gestational diabetic group and significantly decreased in the insulin-dependent group when compared to the normal control. The activities of glucose-6-phosphate and 6-phosphogluconate dehydrogenase were significantly elevated in both diabetic groups. The activities of the enzymes related to gluconeogenesis; phosphoenolpyruvate carboxylase and aspartate aminotransferase, were virtually unchanged. The activity of NADP-malate dehydrogenase, which is involved in lipogenesis, was significantly increased in both diabetic groups. All these changes were evident when calculated per whole placenta, per DNA or per intracellular protein content.

DISCUSSION

The present studies indicate that maternal diabetes in late pregnancy is accompanied by metabolic changes in placental tissue.

In confirmation of the results of Winick and Noble (1967) we have shown that placental weight tends to increase in diabetes and that the number of placental cells is augmented, as judged by the significant increments in total placental DNA. We have also confirmed that placental glycogen is increased in women with idiopathic diabetes (Heijkenskjold and Gemzell, 1957; Fisher and Horky, 1966; Ginsburg and Jeacock, 1966). Moreover, our studies provide the first evidence that the phenomenon of increased placental glycogen content may parallel the magnitude of the disturbance in the maternal fuel economy. Thus, our White Class B-F pregnant

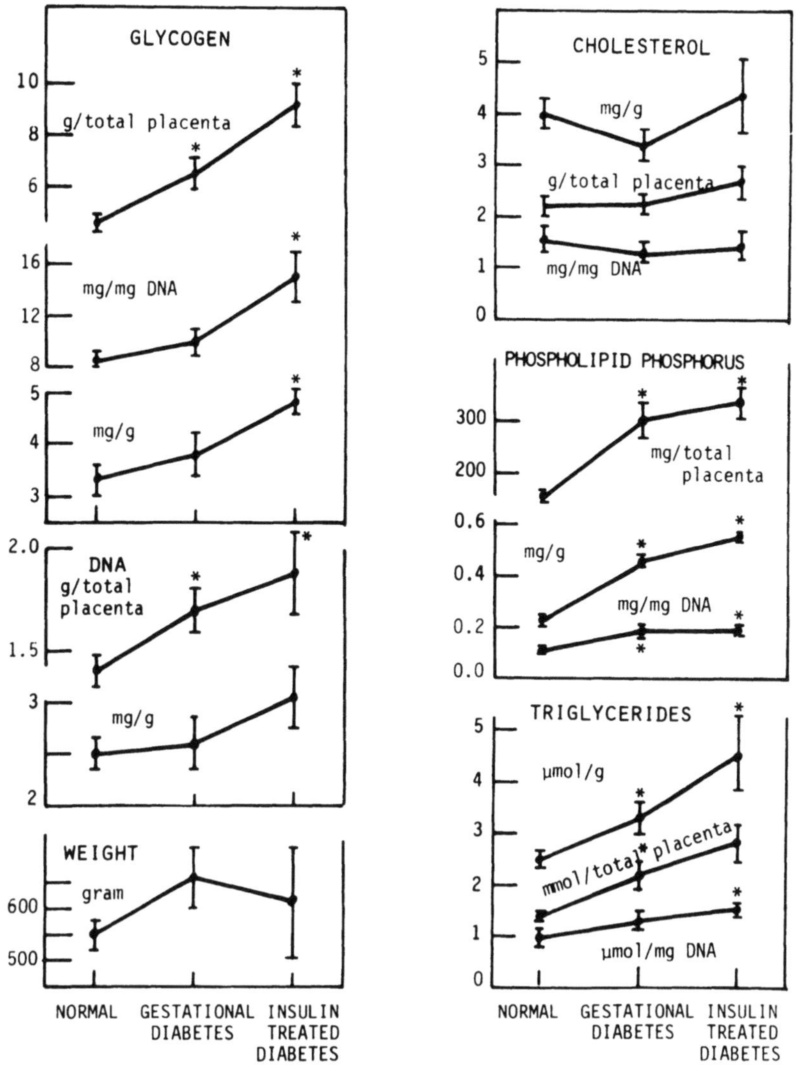

Figure 2. Content of DNA, glycogen and lipids and placental weight in study and control groups.

diabetics who had been significantly more hyperglycemic than our women with GDM, also had greater amounts of placental glycogen at delivery.

We have also shown, for the first time to our knowledge, that the placental content of lipids is also increased in diabetes. The relative increase in lipids, like that of placental glycogen, may exceed the simultaneous changes in placental mass and/or total DNA so that individual placental cells may contain more fat as well as more glycogen. The increments were not significantly greater in the White Class B-F diabetics than in the less hyperglycemic women with GDM. Thus, the correlations

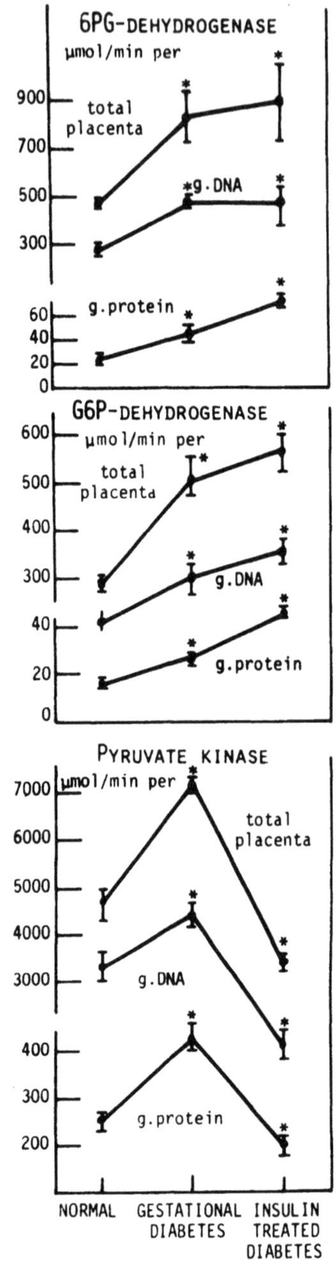

Figure 3. The results for DNA are expressed on basis of gram tissue and whole placental weight. The results of glycogen and lipids are expressed on basis of gram tissue, milligram DNA and whole placental weight. *denotes significant differences between the results in study and control groups at the level of $p < 0.05$.

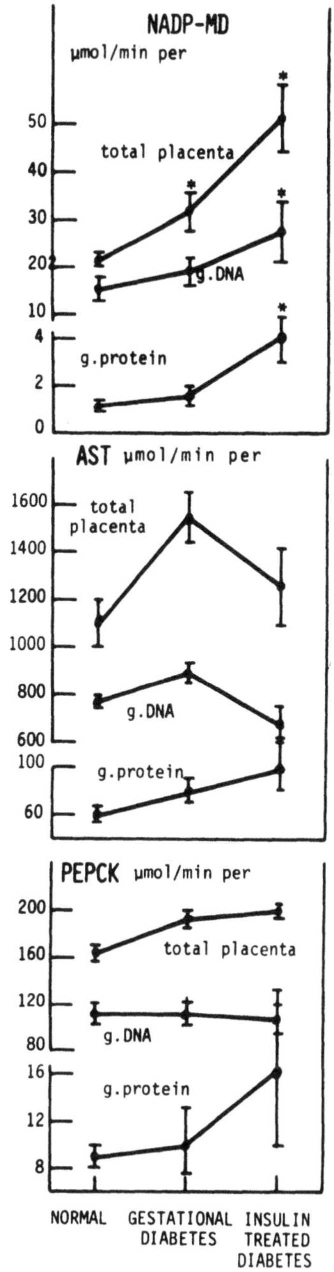

Figure 4. The activity of placental enzymes pyruvate kinase (PK), glucose- 6-phosphate dehydrogenase (G6PD) 6-phosphogluconate dehydrogenase (6PGD), NADP-malate dehydrogenase (NADP-MD), aspartate aminotransferase (AST), phosphoenolpyruvate carboxylase (PEPCK) in normal and diabetic pregnancies. The results were expressed as nmoles per min per mg protein, mg DNA and total placental weight. *denotes significant differences from normal control group on the level of $p < 0.05$.

with maternal blood sugar appear to be more equivocal for placental lipids than for placental glycogen. This observation need not exclude a relationship to the circulating fuels. Some index of maternal metabolic control other than plasma glucose could be the critical variable. For example, all forms of diabetes can exaggerate the hyperlipoproteinemic effects of pregnancy (Knopp et al., 1978). Since plasma lipids were not measured routinely in the pregnant women in this study, we do not know whether the White Class B- F pregnant diabetics and the patients with GDM differed in this regard.

Final clarification of the mechanisms underlying the increase in placental glycogen and lipids in diabetes must await further investigation. Some preliminary inferences may be justified from the available data. Direct accretion of lipids and glycogen in response to the altered ambient fuel mixtures seems likely. In the case of lipids, the placenta in diabetic pregnancies is perfused with increased quantities of albumin-complexed-free fatty acids and triglyceride-rich, very low density lipoproteins (VLDL) (Knopp et al., 1978). Earlier in vitro studies have indicated that the incorporation of free fatty acids into the triglycerides and phospholipids of viable slices of human (Yoshioka and Roux, 1972) and rat (Diamant et al., 1980) placenta is directly proportional to the fatty acid concentration in the incubation medium. Moreover, less glucose carbons are channeled into CO_2 and more to glyceride-glycol whenever preparations of human placenta are exposed to increased amounts of albumin- complexed fatty acids (Freinkel, 1965). Hence, the increased glucose in maternal blood would be conductive to esterification of fatty acids. The presence of lipoprotein lipase in rat and human placenta (Mallov and Alousi, 1965) could abet the generation of fatty acids for such esterification in-situ by acting upon the increasingly available VLDL. Finally, the direct uptake of lipoproteins by the placenta without preliminary hydrolysis could also be operative. The lack of increase in placental cholesterol that we encountered could be related to the fact that the cholesterol-rich low density lipoproteins (LDL), in contrast to VLDL, are only minimally elevated in pregnancies complicated by diabetes (Knopp et al., 1978).

The increased glycogen content may be explained by glycogen-sparing and glycogen-promoting actions that are seen in the perfused heart (Neely and Morgan, 1974) or skeletal muscle (Rennie and Holloszy, 1977) whenever fatty acids are made available. In these systems, heightened fatty acid oxidation and the accumulation of the products of fat metabolism impair glycolysis and pyruvic acid oxidation, and effect a disparate diversion of glucose-6-phosphate to glycogen. Ginsburg and Jeacock (1966) have already postulated that impairment of pyruvate oxidation may explain the heightened evolution of lactate that they observed despite normal rates of glycogen breakdown during incubation of diabetic human placentae in vitro. Moreover, a greater proportion of assimilated glucose accumulates as lactic acid when albumin-complexed-free fatty acids are added to surviving slices of normal human placenta (Freinkel, 1965). Finally, ongoing studies indicate that glucose is preferentially directed toward glycogen synthesis rather than glycolysis in the placentae of diabetic rats (Barash et al., 1983). Thus, as a working hypothesis, we would suggest that the heightened glycogen content in the placentae of diabetic mothers is linked to the increased availability and utilization of lipids by the placenta. It also reaffirms the suggestion that the placenta, like other portions of the conceptus, may be exquisitely sensitive to the fuels in the ambient substrate mixtures (Freinkel, 1965).

The increase in the activity of pentose shunt enzymes in the placentae from both gestational and insulin-dependent diabetes groups may be construed to be caused by hyperinsulinemia (maternal and/or fetal), since these enzymes are known to be insulin-dependent in the liver or adipose tissue. Our previous results in severely diabetic rats (Diamant and Shafrir, 1978) have indicated, however, that changes of placental enzyme activities are not affected by insulin deficiency in the maternal circulation. Although the diabetes was of short duration and the extrapolation to human placenta may be tenuous, there is evidence to suggest that the alterations in enzyme activities in the placenta and in some other tissues may be evoked by prolonged hyperglycemia or changes in substrates rather than by hormonal induction. Increased activity of enzymes of the pentose shunt and of glycolysis have been found in the kidneys of diabetic rats (Sochor et al., 1979) and this was explained by an increased availability of glucose to insulin-dependent tissues (Spiro, 1976).

A similar metabolic pattern was observed by us in human placental tissue from pregnancies complicated by fetal distress, due to prolonged cord compression, where local overexposure to high glucose concentrations may be expected (Diamant and Kissilevitz, 1980).

The observation of significantly decreased pyruvate kinase activity in the insulin-dependent group of placentae, when compared to the normal or gestational diabetic groups is of importance since it suggests a low functioning of the glycolytic pathway. This phenomenon may be explained by an inhibition of pyruvate kinase by increased free fatty acid and/or amino acid levels, reaching the placental tissue from the maternal circulation or produced in the placenta itself as a result of a decreased blood flow and hypoxia due to diabetes induced placental vascular abnormalities (Driscoll, 1964). Hypoxia is known to induce increased free fatty acid production and utilization which inhibits the glycolytic pathway as has been shown in other tissues (Rovetto et al., 1975; Whitmer et al., 1978). Another factor that may contribute to a reduction of glycolysis in the diabetic placenta is the accumulation of lactate also related to circulatory abnormalities. Lactate is the major product of placental glycolysis and was actually reported previously to accumulate in certain conditions (Ginsburg and Jeacock, 1966).

In view of our results of increased activity of the enzymes involved in the pentose shunt and the increased glycogen content, it may be assumed that in placentae from insulin-dependent patients with presumable hypoxia glucose-6-phosphate accumulates since its metabolism along the glycoclytic pathway is obstructed. Apart from the pyruvate kinase step, this may occur at the phosphofructokinase or pyruvate dehydrogenase stages, which may be inhibited by products of increased fatty acid oxidation or even at the glyceraldehyde-3-dehydrogenase stage as in the ischemic heart (Rovetto et al., 1975). Thus glucose-6-phosphate may be preferentially directed towards pentose shunt and/or glycogen formation.

A severe reduction in the placental energy-forming capability due to low glycolysis may cause a reduction of the energy-dependent transport of metabolites such as amino acids, and enhance the metabolism of fatty acids. This hypothesis is supported by Pedersen's observation that the decreased baby birth weight throughout the White classes B-F, is accompanied by a decrease in the amino acid content in fetal circulation (Pederson, 1976). In the present study, the mean baby weight in the gestational diabetic groups is significantly higher than in the control and insulin-dependent groups (which included White B-F group patients). No cases of intrauterine or intrapartum fetal death were observed in the present series, but as mentioned, the one-minute Agpar score was significantly lower in the insulin-dependent group of pregnancies. Since the major purpose of this study was to show some of the biochemical changes in placental tissue in human diabetes mellitus, we did not correlate all the changes with the neonatal outcome. Only the body weights and apgar scores were mentioned in this paper.

As yet, there is no direct evidence that these changes in the placental composition and enzymatic activity can be equated with changes in the placental function or neonatal outcome. If such evidence could be obtained, it would strengthen the advocacy of even more aggressive attempts to normalize maternal fuels during diabetic pregnancies. Indeed it would also mean that the success of such antepartum efforts could be gauged by the placental content of glycogen and/or lipids at delivery.

SUMMARY

The purpose of this study was to assess whether the changes in the maternal fuels in pregnancy complicated by diabetes mellitus affect the placental DNA, glycogen and lipids content, and the activities of rate- limiting enzymes in the pathways of glycolysis, gluconeogenesis and NADP generation. Plasma glucose values during late pregnancy were higher in patients with class B-F diabetes than in patients with gestational diabetes mellitus, so that they were judged to have more severe metabolic disturbances. Diabetes tended to increase placental mass, and content DNA, glycogen and lipids. However, the relative changes in glycogen and fat exceeded the alteration in mass and DNA, so that a true increase in glycogen and fat per placental cell may have occurred. Thus, placental glycogen/DNA and triglycerides/DNA significantly exceeded control values in patients with class B-F diabetes but not with gestational diabetes mellitus which suggests that these alterations in placental composition in diabetes parallel the severity of diabetes mellitus.

In placentae from the gestational diabetic group the activities of glycolytic, pentose shunt and NADP-generating enzymes were elevated and the activities of enzymes connected to glucogenesis were unchanged. This alteration of placental intermediary metabolism was explained by the oversupply of glucose to morphologically normal and well-oxygenated placental tissue. In the placentae from the insulin-dependent group, the glycolytic pathway appeared to be inhibited, the pentose shunt and NADP- generation pathway enhanced and the gluconeogenesis pathway unchanged. It was suggested that metabolic changes in these placentae occurred as a result of the exaggerated fatty acid utilization and/or lactate accumulation due to anoxia. This may be caused by obstructed placental circulation as a result of vascular changes in the placental bed in cases of insulin-dependent diabetes.

REFERENCES

Autoanalyzer Methodology - Manual N-24 and N-78 (1973) Technicon Co., Chauncey, New York.

Barash, V., Lilling, S., Gutman, A. and Shafrir, E. (1983) Mechanism of placental glucose deposition in diabetes. *Diabetologia* 24, 63-68.

Diamant, Y.Z. and Shafrir, E. (1972) Enzymes of carbohydrate and lipid metabolism in the placenta and liver of pregnant rats. *Biochim. Biophys. Acta* 279, 424-430.

Diamant, Y.Z. and Shafrir, E. (1978) Placental enzymes of glycolysis, gluconeogenesis and lipogenesis in diabetic rats and in starvation. *Diabetologia* 15, 481-485.

Diamant, Y.Z. and Kissilevitz, R. (1980) Placenta in intrauterine fetal deprivation. II. Biochemical profile of placentae from deliveries associated with fetal distress. *Israel J. Med. Sci.* 16, 7-14.

Diamant, Y.Z., Diamant, S. and Freinkel, N. (1980) Lipid deposition and metabolism in rat placenta during gestation. *Placenta* 1, 319-325.

Diamant, Y.Z., Mayorek, N., Neuman, S. and Shafrir, E. (1975) Enzymes of glucose and fatty acids metabolism in early and term human placenta. *Amer. J. Obstet. Gynecol.* 121, 58-61.

Driscoll, S. (1964) The pathology of pregnancy complicated by diabetes mellitus. *Med. Clin. N. Amer.* 49,1053-1061.

Fisher, U. and Horky, Z. (1966) Vorlalufige Untersuchungen zum Glykogengehalt sowie Sauerstoff - und Glukoseverbrauch der Plazenta in vitro bei Diabetes mellitus. *Zentralbl. Gynak.* 88, 1427-1435.

Fiske, C.H. and Subbarow, Y. (1925) Columetric determination of phosphorous. *J. Biol. Chem.* 66, 375-400.

Freinkel, N. (1965) Effects of the conceptus on maternal metabolism during pregnancy, In: *On the Nature and Treatment of Diabetes*, (eds.), Leibel, B.S. and Wrenshall, G.A., Excerpta Medica, Amsterdam, 1965, pp. 679-691.

Gabbe, S.G., Demers, L.M., Greep, R.O., Villee, C.A. (1972) Placental glycogen metabolism in diabetes mellitus. *Diabetes* 21, 1185-1191.

Ginsburg, T. and Jeacock, M.K. (1966) Some aspects of placental carbohydrate metabolism in human diabetes. *J. Obstet. Gynaecol. Brit. Cwlth.* 73, 452-455.

Hagerman, D.D. (1962) Metabolism of tissue from pregnant diabetic rats in vitro. *Endocrinology* 70, 88-89.

Heijkenskjold, F. and Gemzell, C.A. (1957) Glycogen content in the placenta of diabetic mothers. *Acta Paediat. Scand.* 46, 74-80.

Herrera, E. and Freinkel, N. (1975) Metabolism in the liver, brain and placenta of fed and fasted fetal rats. *Horm. Metab. Res.* 7, 247-249.

Hosoya, N., Hagerman, R.H., and Rosensweig (1960) Stimulation of fatty acids synthesis by estradiol in vitro. *Biochem. J.* 76, 297-301.

Hull, D. and Elphick, M.C. (1979) Evidence for fatty acids transfer across the human placenta. In: *Pregnancy, Metabolism Diabetes and Fetus*, (ed.), Beard, W.B., Ciba Foundation series 63, pp 75-86.

Johnson, J.A., Nash, J.A. and Fusaro, R.M. (1963) An enzymatic method for the quantitative determination of glycogen. *Ann. Biochem.* 5, 379-384.

Kleine, U. (1967) Studies on the lipid metabolism of villi of mature human placenta. *Clin. Chim. Acta* 17, 95-98.

Knopp, R.H., Montes, A. and Warth, M.R. (1978) Carbohydrate and Lipid Metabolism. In: *Laboratory Indices of Nutritional Status in Pregnancy*, Washington, D.C., National Academy of Sciences, pp. 35-42.

Lowry, O.H., Rosenbrough, N.J., Farr, A.Z. and Randall, R.J. (1951) Protein measurement with the Folin phenol reagent. *J. Biol. Chem.* 193, 265-271.
Mallov, S. and Alousi, A.A. (1965) Lipoproteins lipase activity of rat and human placenta, Proc. Soc. Exper. Biol. Med. 119, 301-306.
Neely, J.R. and Morgan, H.E. (1974) Relationship between carbohydrate and lipid metabolism and the energy balance of heart muscle. *Ann. Rev. Physiol.* 36, 413-419.
Nesbitt, R.E.L., Rice, P.A., Rourke, J.E. (1973) In vitro perfusion studies of the human placenta. III. The relationships between glucose utilization rates and concentration. *Gynecol. Invest.* 4, 243-253.
O'Sullivan, J.B. and Mahan, C.M. (1964) Criteria for the glucose tolerance test in pregnancy. *Diabetes* 13, 278-285.
Pedersen, J. (1976) Birth weight of newborn infants of diabetic women. In: *Diabetes. Proc. IX Congress Internat. Diabet.*, (ed.), Bajij, J.S., New Delhi 1976, pp. 353-360.
Rennie, M.J. and Holloszy, J.O. (1977) Inhibition of glucose uptake and glycogenolysis by availability of oleate in well-oxygenated perfused skeletal muscle. *Biochem. J.* 168, 161-167.
Richards, G.M. (1974) Modification of the diphenylamine reaction giving increased sensitivity and simplicity in the examination of DNA. *Anal. Biochem.* 57, 369-374.
Rovetto, M.J., Lamberton, W.F. and Neely, J.R. (1975) Mechanisms of glycolytic inhibition in ischemic hearts. *Circ. Res.* 37, 742-749.
Sakurai, T., Takagi, H., and Hosoya N. (1969) Metabolic pathways of glucose in human placenta: Changes with gestation and with added l7B-estradiol, *Amer. J. Obstet. Gynecol.* 105, 1044-1054.
Shafrir, E. and Diamant, Y.Z. (1979) Regulation of placental enzymes of the carbohydrate and lipid metabolic pathways. In: *Pregnancy, metabolism Diabetes and the Fetus*, (ed.), W.B. Beard, Ciba Foundation series 63, pp. 161-179.
Sochor, M., Baguer, N.Z. and McLean, P. (1979) Glucose overutilization in diabetes: Evidence from studies in the changes in hexokinase, the pentose phosphate pathway and glucuronate pathway in rat kidney cortex in diabetes. *Biochem. Biophys. Res.* Comm. 86, 32-39.
Spiro, R.G. (1976) Search for a biochemical basis of diabetic microangiopathy. *Diabetologia* 12, 1-14.
Sybulski, S. and Tremblay P.C. (1969) Pathways of glucose metabolism in human placentae from normal pregnancies and from pregnancies associated with intrauterine fetal malnutrition. *Amer. J. Obstet. and Gynecol.* 103, 1148-1153.
Szabo, A.J., Lellis, R. and Grimaldi, R.D. (1973) Triglyceride synthesis in human placenta. I. Incorporation of labeled palmitate into placental triglycerides. *Amer. J. Obstet. Gynecol.* 115, 257-262.
Villee, C.A. (1953) The metabolism of human placenta in vitro. *J. Biol. Chem.* 205, 113-123.
White, P. (1949) Pregnancy complicating diabetes. Amer. J. Med. 7, 609- 616.
Whitmer, J.T., Idell-Wenger, J.A., Rovetto, M.J. and Neely, J.R. (1978) Control of fatty acid metabolism in ischemic and hypoxic hearts. *J. Biol. Chem.* 253, 4305-4311.

Winick, M. and Noble, A. (1967) Cellular growth of human placenta. II. Diabetes mellitus. *J. Pediat.* 71, 216-222.
Yoshioka, T. and Roux, J.F. (1972) In vitro metabolism of palmitic acid in human fetal tissue. *Pediat. Res.* 6, 675-681.

Trophoblast Research 1:223-236, 1983

STEROID AND PROTEIN METABOLISM BY THE TROPHOBLAST

- A Review-

Arnold Klopper

Department of Obstetrics and Gynecology
Royal Infirmary
Aberdeen, AB9 2ZB, Scotland

We have been concerned with steroid metabolism in the placenta for long enough for some questions to have been settled and for others to have assumed the aspect of irksome mysteries which obstruct the advance of understanding. We know how the placenta makes steroids and a little of why; we know almost nothing of what determines the rate at which it makes them. The present investigation began as an attempt to elucidate the control of placental steroidogenesis. It cast very little light on that but raises some interesting speculations as to the targets toward which some steroids are directed. Evidence will only be offered in respect of progesterone. We have reason to believe that much the same applies to estradiol and to think that our observations bear upon generalizations concerning placental steroid metabolism rather than upon progesterone alone. By way of control we have also measured a placental protein, human placental lactogen (hPL), in the same subjects whom the progesterone measurements were made.

The study is from a cross-section of the antenatal population at the Aberdeen Maternity Hospital. Venous blood was taken at 30-34 weeks gestation from 976 women. Eighty-five percent of the women were between 31 and 33 weeks gestation and there is no reason to suppose that the material is biased by undue concentration of women at earlier or later gestation. When their records were examined 21 patients were discarded because they were found to have a twin pregnancy, or did not deliver in Aberdeen where we had access to their records or because of mistaken or uncertain dates. All of the patients were apparently healthy when the blood was drawn but no attempt was made to exclude any who subsequently showed evidence of pathology, antepartum hemorrhage, pre-eclamptic toxemia, fetal growth retardation, etc. Progesterone was measured by radioimmunoassay using an antiserum prepared against progesterone linked to bovine serum albumin at C_{11}. The hPL was also estimated by radioimmunoassay using a kit supplied by Serono.

The frequency distribution of the plasma progesterone concentration is shown in Figure 1. It is evident that the distribution is skewed by the occurrence of occasional high wild values. This finding is not peculiar to progesterone. It is seen also in Figure 2 which shows the corresponding data for hPL. None of the placental proteins or steroids display the usual Gaussian distribution curve. This may mean no more than that it is the consequence of measurements where the lowest point is fixed (zero) but there is no limit on the highest point. Measurements which show such a skewed distribution are not appropriately analyzed by determining mean and standard deviations, but require some non-parametric method of analysis. All of the results were therefore ranked, and the median and percentiles determined.

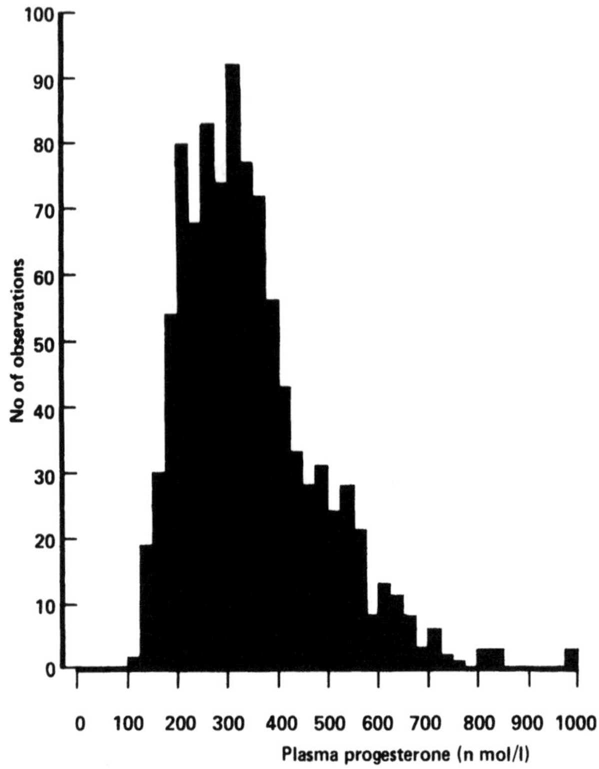

Figure 1. Frequency distribution of plasma progesterone concentration in 965 women (From Klopper, 1983a; with permission).

The subjects having a plasma progesterone concentration above the 90th percentile or below the 10th percentile were identified, and their records were scanned for any features of pregnancy associated with a low or a high plasma progesterone. If progesterone is produced at approximately the same rate by all women, it is to be expected that big women with their larger plasma volume would dilute the progesterone more and thus have a lower concentration. In Figure 3, women with a plasma progesterone concentration above the 90th percentile had the same mean height as those with a plasma progesterone concentration below the 10th percentile. There is no evidence of a dilution effect associated with taller women. A proportion of the progesterone secreted by the placenta enters the body fat, and it might be possible that in fat women a dilution effect on plasma concentration could operate by virtue of the loss of progesterone to body fat. Heavier women do not have a lower plasma progesterone concentration (Figure 4). There is thus no evidence of the physical characteristics of the women having any effect on their plasma progesterone concentration. Either the dilution effect is too small and inconsistent to show in this analysis, or there is some feedback of information from the mother to the placenta, which gives information on the dilution effect. Thus the placenta is able to compensate for the dilution. More likely, big women have big placentae which produce more progesterone and mask the dilution effect.

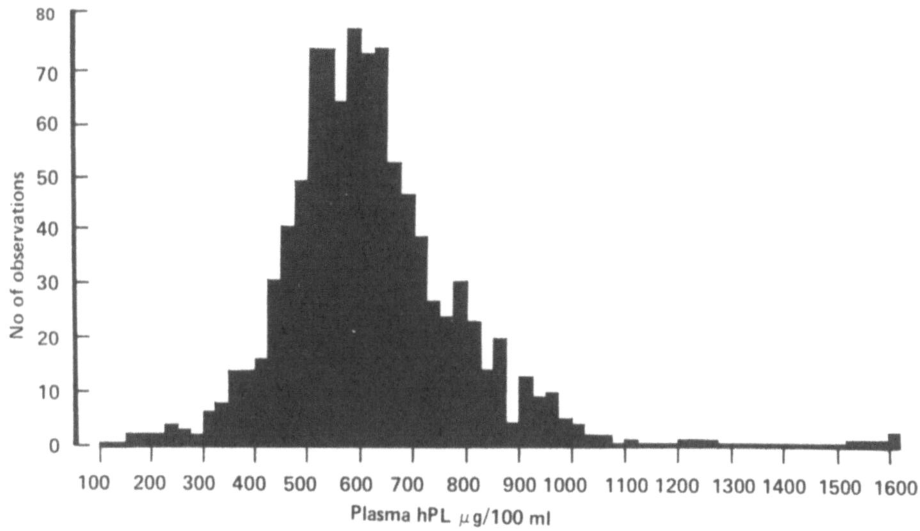

Figure 2. Frequency distribution of plasma hPL concentration in 965 women. (From Klopper, 1983a; with permission).

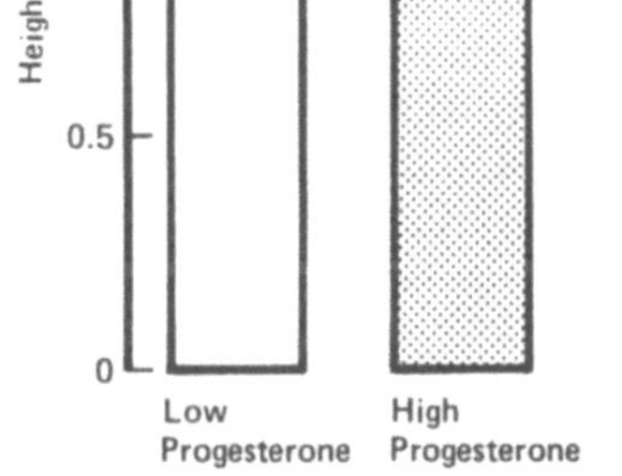

Figure 3. Average heights of women at the extremes of progesterone concentration distribution. (From Klopper, 1983a; with permission).

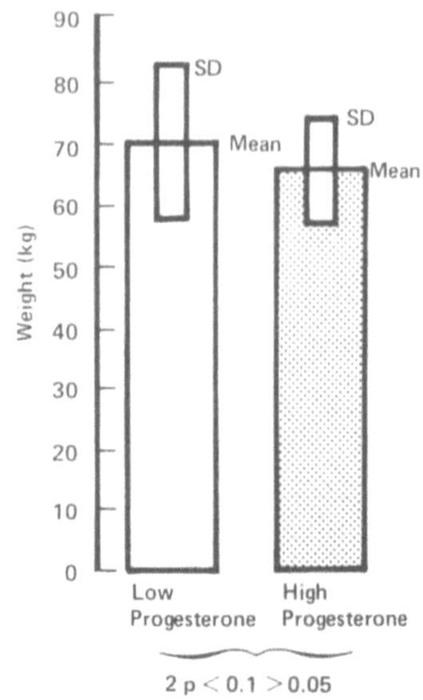

Figure 4. Average weights of women at the extremes of progesterone concentration distribution. (From Klopper, 1983a; with permission).

The question narrows down to placental size. Is the functional trophoblast mass the critical factor which determines the placental production rate and hence the plasma concentration? The findings about placental weight are shown in Figure 5. It is evident that the mean placental weight is significantly higher in the high progesterone group than in the low progesterone group. From Figure 6 it can be seen that the difference is much less marked in the case of fetal weights. Although the mean fetal weight in the high progesterone group is not significantly different from that of the low progesterone group, what difference there is, goes the expected way, i.e., higher fetal weights tend to occur in the high progesterone group. Fetal weight and placental weight are related, and it is likely that the association between fetal weight and progesterone concentration is secondary to this. The primary association is between placental weight and progesterone.

These findings raise the question, whether the results are peculiar to progesterone, or are shared by other placental products. For comparison, the same type of analysis was done for hPL, using the distribution data shown in Figure 2. The mean hPL values in the high and in the low progesterone groups are shown in Figure 7. There is a strong tendency for hPL also to be low, when progesterone is low. It is likely that the production of these two is related, either directly, or via a common factor operating on the plasma concentration of both. The only positive factor identified in the case of progesterone concentration was placental weight. The relationship between placental weight and hPL concentration was examined in the same manner as for progesterone. It was found that, like progesterone, high values of hPL tend to occur with big placentae. Some investigators have found a relationship between plasma hPL concentration and placental weight (Lindberg et al., 1973; Seppälä and Ruoslahti, 1970), others have not (Samaan et al., 1971). Perhaps the explanation is, as has been stated by Vermeulen et al. (1982), that placental weight

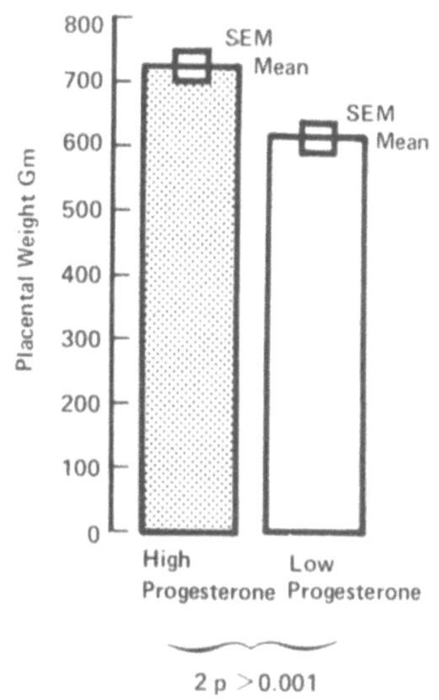

Figure 5. Average placental weights in women at the extremes of progesterone concentration distribution. (From Klopper, 1983a; with permission).

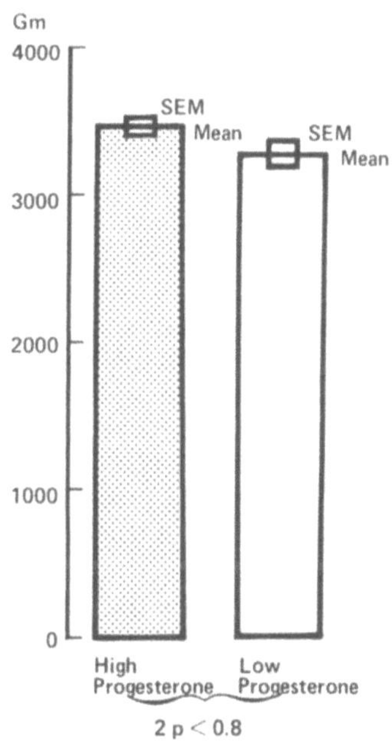

Figure 6. Average fetal weights in women at the extremes of progesterone concentration distribution. (From Klopper, 1983a; with permission).

contains an element of stromal tissue and fetal vessels which is not concerned with the synthesis of either progesterone or hPL. They found a much closer association with trophoblast surface which is composed of syncytium only. Had it been possible to measure trophoblast surface in all of these placentae, a closer association with progesterone and hPL concentration might have been found.

The analysis thus far has been directed at the maternal compartment. There is progesterone in the fetal circulation, and the question arises whether there is any equilibrium between the two compartments. This was tested by obtaining blood samples from 56 women at delivery and cannulating the umbilical vein and artery after delivery of the placenta. In neither the umbilical artery nor the vein did the progesterone concentration bear any relationship to that obtained in the mother.

A further interesting finding in this study is reflected in Figure 8. The concentration in the umbilical artery is significantly less than in the vein, i.e., there is abstraction of progesterone by the fetus. This point has been more extensively explored (Maynard et al., 1980), and there is little doubt about it. Furthermore the degree of abstraction is related to the placental production as reflected in the umbilical venous concentration (Figure 9).

All of the evidence points to the placenta being a free running system as far as maternal progesterone and hPL are concerned; an astonishing conclusion if either has any function in the mother. There is no hPL in the fetus but perhaps we are looking in the wrong place for the function of progesterone. Perhaps it is a fetal hormone and the placental production rate is controlled by fetal abstraction.

The number of newly isolated placental proteins have multiplied like well fed rabbits in recent years. There is not time for a comprehensive overview and I propose only to make some observations about two of them: Schwangerschaftsprotein 1 (SP_1) and pregnancy-associated plasma protein A (PAPP-A).

The chemical characteristics of SP_1 have been described by Bohn (1972). It proved easy to make antisera to the protein. As it is present in high concentration in late pregnancy, easy, relatively insensitive techniques, such as radial immunodiffusion and rocket immunoelectrophoresis, were adequate for its measurements. When attention turned to assays in early pregnancy, radioimmunoassay techniques were evolved. The initial findings have been reviewed (Klopper, 1983b) and will not be examined again. As it was a placental product, attention was naturally directed towards use of the assays as a measure of placental function. The picture which emerged was very similar to that of hPL, a protein whose plasma concentration is largely determined by the mass of functioning trophoblast, without overt function.

The waters have now been muddied by the discovery that there is not one, but at least two, separate proteins with SP_1 determinants (Teisner et al., 1978). It is evident that we have all been measuring a variable mixture of two substances as though there were one. It is perhaps time to call a moratorium on clinical application studies until we can sort out the methods and examine each protein separately. One observation is not likely to be substantially changed by improvements in methods. This is summarized by Figure 10 which shows some measurements of SP_1 in very early pregnancy. SP_1 can be detected as early as 6 days after ovulation, at a stage

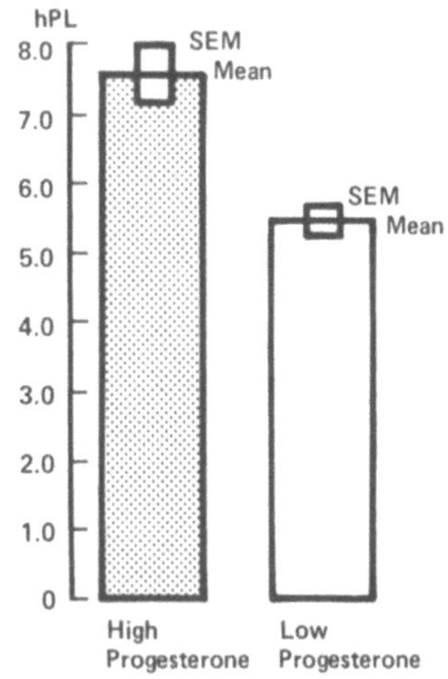

Figure 7. Average hPL (in μg/ml) in women at the extremes of progesterone concentration distribution. (From Klopper, 1983a; with permission).

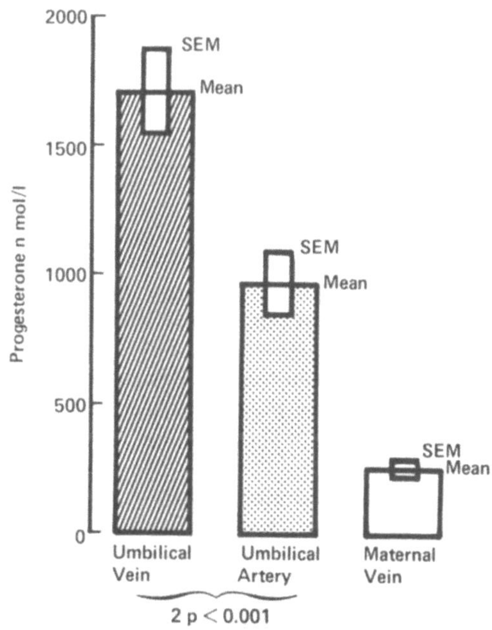

Figure 8. Average plasma progesterone concentration in umbilical vein, umbilical artery and maternal vein. (From Klopper, 1983a; with permission).

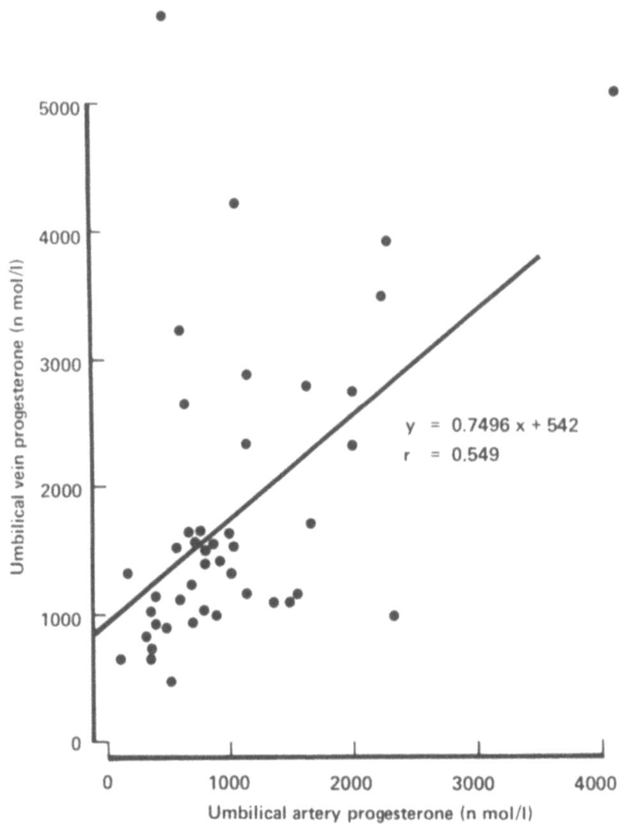

Figure 9. Relationship of umbilical arterial and venous plasma progesterone concentration. (From Klopper, 1983a; with permission).

when the blastocyst may still be lying free in the uterine cavity. All 22 pregnant women shown in Figure 10 had measurable SP_1 in their circulation before the time of the first missed period. This value suggests that SP_1 is one of the earliest and possibly most vital signals exchanged between the conceptus and the mother. There is good evidence that it may be a sensitive pregnancy test and that its assay may be a valuable aid in the study of early pregnancy wastage.

For the remaining placental protein, PAPP-A, there is a somewhat different theme to be developed. It is a maverick which fits very poorly in the tidy scheme of placental proteins. For one thing, the mean concentration curve during pregnancy does not have the shape of a placental growth curve as does hPL and SP_1. It does not flatten off in late pregnancy but instead continues to rise steeply, right up to term (Smith et al., 1979).

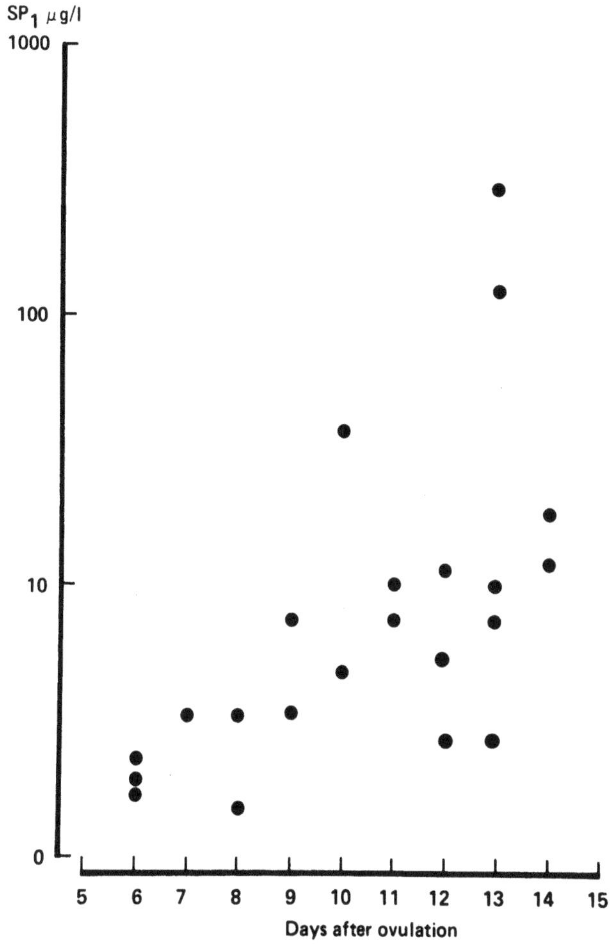

Figure 10. SP_1 concentration in pregnant women in the luteal phase before the first missed period. (From Ahmed and Klopper, 1983; with permission).

As with other placental proteins the frequency distribution in late pregnancy is skewed by some high values (Figure 11). The data in Figure 11 were used to determine the l0th and 90th percentiles as was done with progesterone, hPL and SP_1. There is no tendency for high placental or fetal weights to go with high PAPP- A (Figure 12).

The more one looks at PAPP-A, the less well does it fit the established model of a placental protein, whose production is controlled by placental mass and uterine blood flow. The greater the parity the less the PAPP-A concentration (Figure 13). How can the placenta know the mother has been pregnant before? Clearly it cannot; it must be informed by a signal from the mother. What kind of a signal? Possibly immunological: that is the obvious means by which previous pregnancies will leave their traces in the mother.

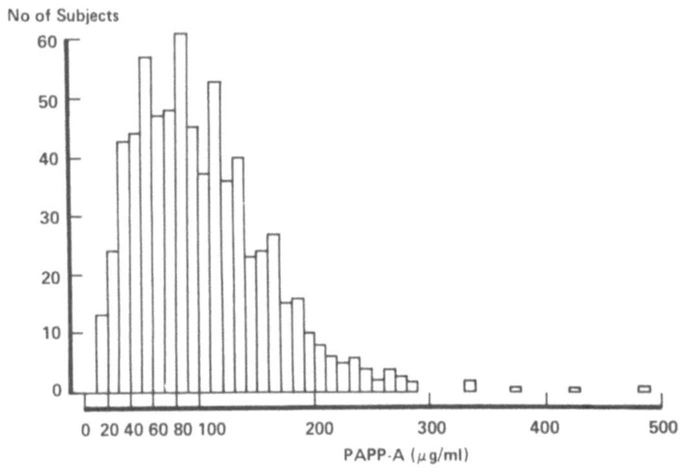

Figure 11. Frequency distribution of plasma PAPP-A concentration. (From Klopper, 1982b; with permission).

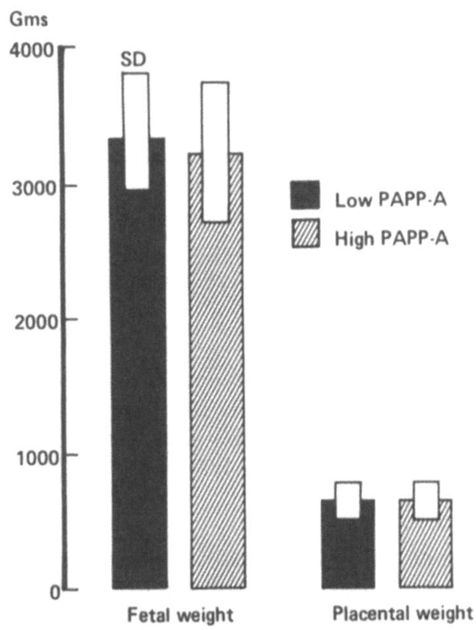

Figure 12. Average fetal and placental weights in women at the extremes of plasma PAPP-A concentration distribution. (From Klopper, 1982a; with permission).

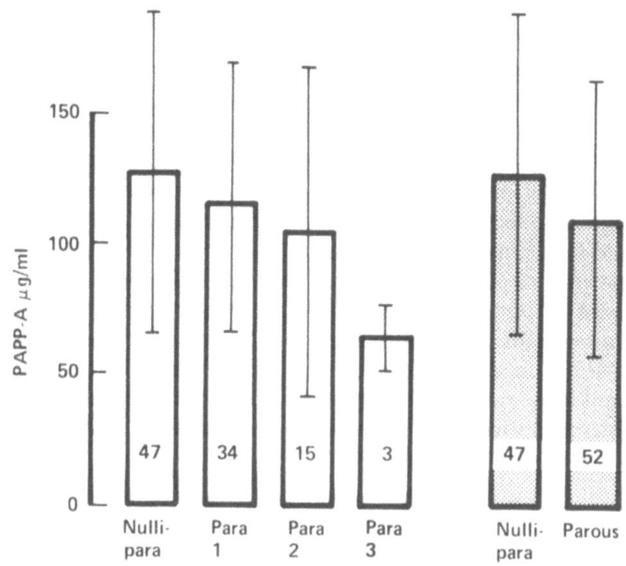

Figure 13. The effect of parity on PAPP-A concentration at 34 weeks (mean ± SD).

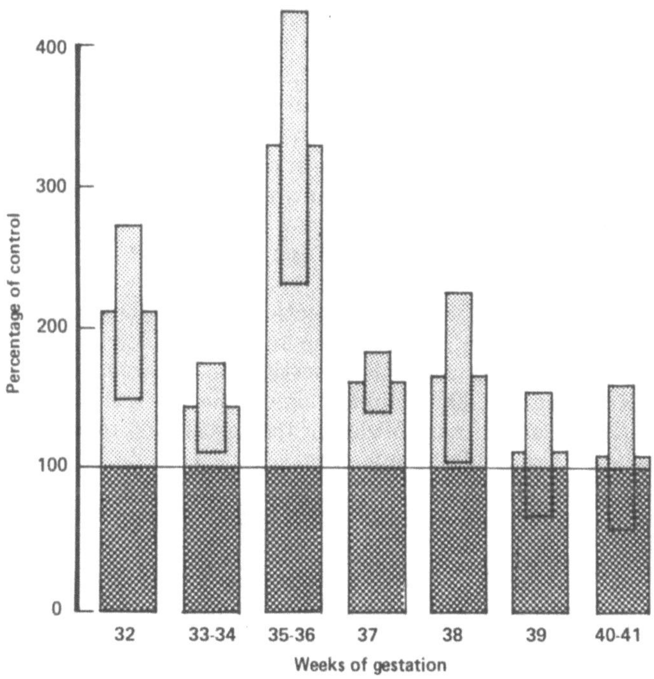

Figure 14. PAPP-A in albuminuric pre-eclampsia expressed as a percentage of control value (mean ± SD).

All through the PAPP-A story runs an immunological thread. Another observation which might have an immunological basis is the change of PAPP-A concentration which occurs in pre-eclamptic toxemia. The burden of many experiments is that PAPP-A is raised in pre-eclampsia (Klopper et al., 1979; Hughes et al., 1980; Toop and Klopper, 1981). The findings are summarized in Figure 14 which show mean PAPP-A values as a percentage of the concentration in control subjects matched for age, parity and stage of gestation. The puzzle is why PAPP-A should be raised. It is logical to expect that a process which damages the placenta like pre-eclampsia, would lower, not raise, the plasma concentration of one of its products. A challenging new view of pre-eclampsia is that it results from a failure to provoke an adequate response of protective antibodies in early pregnancy. PAPP-A is raised early in pre-eclamptic toxemia before overt manifestation of the disease. It might be argued that PAPP-A is a placental antigen which provokes a protective antibody response. When it is overproduced in women who will later develop pre-eclampsia the maternal enhancing antibody response is overwhelmed, leaving her vulnerable to more lethal antigens in later pregnancy.

It is too early to define the function of PAPP-A despite some speculations about it (Klopper, 1982a). It has been suggested by Gordon and Chard (1979) that placental proteins such as hPL and SP_1 do not have a function. The syncytiotrophoblast is simply coded to produce them and does so without biological purpose, or feedback control of their rate of synthesis. Pregnancy proceeds undisturbed in the rare patients who do not produce them. It has already been emphasized that the secretory pattern of PAPP-A is different. Whatever the truth about the function of hPL and SP_1 may be, it does not follow that the same applies to PAPP-A. Two threads run through the story of PAPP-A. The first concerns immunological interaction between trophoblast and mother. Bischof et al. (1982) have put forward evidence that PAPP-A is an immunomodulator during pregnancy. The other thread concerns a role in coagulation. PAPP-A complexes with heparin (Sinosich et al., 1981); it inhibits plasmin (Bischof, 1980) and immunofluorescent staining has shown it is bound to perivillous fibrin in the placenta (McIntyre et al., 1981). The two threads are woven together about the complement system. It only remains to unravel them.

ACKNOWLEDGMENTS

The assays demonstrating the distribution of progesterone and hPL were done on blood samples collected by a study group on carbohydrate metabolism led by Dr. Hamish Sutherland and form part of an investigation on carbohydrate metabolism in pregnancy. I am grateful to Miss Elaine Dalgarno for her secretarial assistance and to Drs. Henry Thiede and Richard Miller for the opportunity to present this material at the 9th Rochester Trophoblast Conference.

REFERENCES

Ahmed A.G. and Klopper, A. (1983) Diagnosis of early pregnancy by the assay of placental proteins. *Brit. J. Obstet. Gynaecol.* 90, (In press).

Bischof, P. (1980) Biochemical and biological characterization of pregnancy associated plasma protein A. *Experientia*, 36,717-721.

Bischof, P., DuBerg, S. and Schindler, A.M. (1982) Is pregnancy- associated plasma protein A an immunomodulator during human pregnancy. In: *Immunology of Human Placental Proteins*. Klopper, A. (ed.), Praeger, New York, 93-102.
Bohn, H. (1972) Isolation and characterisation of pregnancy specific β_1 glycoprotein. *Blut*, 24,292-302.
Gordon, Y. and Chard T. (1979) The specific proteins of the human placenta: Some new Hypotheses. In: *Placental Proteins*. Klopper, A. and Chard, T. (eds.), Springer Verlag, Heidelberg, 1-21.
Hughes, G., Bischof, P., Wilson, G. and Klopper, A. (1980) Assay of a placental protein to determine fetal risk. *Brit. Med. J.* 1:671-675.
Klopper, A. (1982a) Observations on the function of pregnancy-associated plasma protein A. In: *Immunology of Human Placental Proteins*. Klopper A. (ed.), Praeger, New York. 83- 92.
Klopper, A. (1982b) Biological and clinical aspects of PAPP-A In: *Pregnancy Proteins* Grudzinskas J.G., Teisner, B. and Seppäla, M. (eds.), Academic Press Sydney, 333-344.
Klopper, A. (1983a). Progesterone synthesis in the feto-placental unit. In: *Progestogens in Therapy*. Benagiano G., Zulli, D. and Diczfalusy, E. (eds.), Raven Press, New York, 97-108.
Klopper, A. (1983b) Specific pregnancy proteins. In: *Current Topics in Endocrinology*. Vol. 4, Martini, L. and James, V. H. T. (eds.), Academic Press, London, 127-165.
Klopper, A., Smith, R. and Davidson, I. (1979) The measurement of trophoblastic proteins as a test of placental function. In: *Placental Proteins*. Klopper, A. and Chard, T. (eds.), Springer Verlag, Heidelberg, 23-41.
Lindberg, B.S., Martinsson, K., Lindberg, P., Nilsson, B.A. and Johansson, E.D.B. (1973) Plasma levels of hCG, progesterone, oestrone, oestradiol, and oestriol during pregnancy. *Acta. Endocrinol.* 177, 231.
McIntyre, J.A., Hsi, B., Faulk, W.P., Klopper, A. and Thomson, R. (1981) Immunological studies of the human placenta: functional and morphological analysis of pregnancy associated plasma protein A (PAPP-A). *Immunology* 44, 577-584.
Maynard, P.V., Stein, P.E., and Symonds, E.M.(1980) Umbilical cord plasma progesterone at term in relation to mode of delivery. *Brit. J. Obstet. Gynaecol.* 87, 864.
Samaan, N.A., Gallager, H.S., McRoberts, W.A. and Faris, A.M. (1971) Serial estimations of hPL, estriol and pregnanediol in pregnancy correlated with whole organ section of the placenta. *Am. J. Obstet. Gynecol.* 109, 63.
Seppäla, M. and Ruoslahti, E. (1970) Serum concentrations of human placental lactogen (hPL) in pregnancy complications. *Acta. Obstet. Gynecol. Scand.* 49, 143.
Sinosich, M.J., Teisner, B., Davey, M. and Grudzinskas, J.G. (1981) Pregnancy associated plasma protein A: interaction with heparin in crossed affinity immunoelectrophoresis. *Aust. N.Z.J. Med.* 11, 429.
Smith, R., Bischof, P., Hughes, G. and Klopper, A. (1979) Studies on pregnancy associated plasma protein A in the third trimester of pregnancy. *Brit. J. Obstet. Gynaecol.* 96, 882-887.
Teisner, B., Westergaard, J.G., Folkerson, J., Husby, S. and Svehag, L. (1978) Two pregnancy-associated serum proteins with pregnancy-specific glycoprotein determinants. *Am. J. Obstet. Gynecol.* 131, 262-266.

Toop, K. and Klopper, A. (1981) Concentration of PAPP-A in patients with pre-eclamptic toxemia. In: *Placenta: Receptors, Pathology and Toxicology*. Miller, R. K. and Thiede, H.A. (eds.), Saunders, London, 167-171.

Vermeulen, R.C., Kurver, P.H., Arts, N.F., van Kessel, H., Wilson, G.R., and Klopper, A. (1982) The relationship between the surface area of the trophoblast and some placental products. *Placenta* 3, 359-366.

Trophoblast Research 1: 237-248, 1983

IN VIVO AND IN VITRO STUDIES OF THE DEHYDROEPIANDOSTERONE SULFATE METABOLISM IN CASES OF IMPAIRED ESTROGEN SECRETION

Eliane Alsat, Monique Bedin, Gisèle Tanguy, Henri Thoumsin[1] and Lise Cedard

U.166 INSERM, Maternité de Port-Royal
123, Bld de Port-Royal, 75014 Paris, France

INTRODUCTION

The estrogen production assessed in maternal fluids, formerly in 24 h urines and more recently in plasma, is considered to be a reliable method for monitoring feto-placental function. The human placenta is an incomplete steroidogenic organ and the maternal and fetal adrenals provide steroidal precursors such as dehydroepiandrosterone sulfate (DHA-S) and its derivative 16α-hydroxydehydroepiandrosterone (16α-OH-DHA-S). The placenta contains high levels of sulfatase activity (sterol sulfate sulfo-hydrolase EC 3.1.6.2) (Pulkkinen, 1961; Warren and Timberlake, 1962) so that steroid sulfates coming from the fetus or the mother are extensively hydrolyzed and made available for estrogen biosynthesis. Since the capacity of the placenta to convert androgens to estrogens in vivo is large, it is generally assumed that the regulation of estrogen synthesis depends on the substrate availability (Crystle et al., 1973).

Placental factors could also influence estrogen biosynthesis. Such factors include changes in placental blood flow and alterations in enzymatic activities (Tanguy et al., 1981).

Among the four enzyme catalyzed steps which are involved in the conversion of DHA-S to estrone (E_1) and estradiol (E_2) or 16α-OH-DHA-S to estriol (E_3), it is difficult to know which is the true rate limiting factor because the enzymes have been studied in different experimental models giving discordant results (Siiteri and Seron Ferré, 1981). It was first considered from in vivo and in vitro studies that sulfatase catalyzed the rate limiting step which could be inhibited by placental and cord blood steroids (Townsley et al., 1970). However, the aromatase (estrogen synthetase) complex is in fact operating at or near maximum velocity and cannot assume the total transformation of the androgen formed after a 50 mg DHA-S bolus injection (Klopper et al., 1976). Indeed DHA-S loading test (DLT) has been used largely as an indicator of placental dysfunction (Lauritzen, 1969; Strecker et al., 1978). The placental clearance of maternal plasma DHA-S to E_2 in normal and abnormal pregnancies is dependent upon different factors, maternal intervillous blood flow, uptake by the trophoblast, and the capacities of the enzymes to hydrolyze and convert the C19 steroids to estrogens.

[1]Present address: Clinique Gynécologique et Obstétricale, Liege, Belgium

The aim of this work is to identify, by in vivo and in vitro studies, the abnormalities of DHA-S metabolism under different pathological conditions in which the estrogen biosynthesis is impaired.

MATERIALS AND METHODS

In vivo studies

Dehydroepiandrosterone sulfate (50 mg) was given as a single bolus intravenous injection at 8 am. Antecubital venous blood samples were obtained immediately before the intravenous injection. Subsequent samples were obtained at 15, 30, 45 and 60 min. The patients were ambulatory, and blood sampling was continued at 2, 3, 4, 6, 8 h after the injection (Tanguy et al., 1980). Plasma levels of DHA-S, DHA, androstenedione (Δ^4A), testosterone (T), E_1 and E_2 were determined by radioimmunoassay. Unconjugated E_1 and E_2 were assayed after ether extraction without chromatography using specific antibodies (Institut Pasteur, Paris). The DHA-S assay was directly performed on diluted plasma using anti-DHA-S from BioMérieux (Lyon). Its cross-reactivity with DHA as assessed following Abraham (1969) is 78 percent and practically nil for the other steroids, except Δ^4A (3.3 percent). This antibody was also used for the measurement of unconjugated DHA extracted by ether. The Δ^4A and T were separated by chromatography on a column of chromatolithe (BioMérieux) using elutions with isooctane and ethyl acetate. The subsequent radioimmunoassay used specific antibodies from Institut Pasteur (Paris) (Tanguy et al., 1981). The half-life of DHA-S (DHA-S $t_{\frac{1}{2}}$) was calculated after a least square analysis performed on the plot of log DHA-S concentration versus time (Cohen and Cohen, 1977).

In vitro studies

The following experiments were performed on full-term placentae collected immediately after delivery.

Placental Perfusion. The method of perfusion of the whole organ has been described previously (Varangot et al., 1965, Cedard, 1972). In brief, the two umbilical arteries were catheterized by means of perfusion needles. The umbilical vein remained free. The perfusion fluid (Krebs-Ringer pH 7.4 + 10 percent human plasma) was set into motion by a hand pump that ensures a pulsative movement, and was maintained at 37°C by a thermostatic pump (maximal pressure: 75 to 175 mm Hg, flow rate: 50-100 ml/min).

Radioimmunoassays of DHA-S, DHA, Δ^4A, T, E_1 and E_2 were performed on 5 ml of venous fluid sampled at 15, 30, 45, 60, 90 and 120 min after the arterial injection of 10 mg of DHA-S (Thoumsin et al., 1980).

Steroid sulfatase activity

Random pieces of placenta, freed of vessels and connective tissue, were homogenized in sucrose 0.25 M and Tris HCl 0.002 M buffer, at pH 7.4. The homogenates were kept frozen at -80°C until the day of experiment.

The enzymatic activity was measured according to the method of Burstein and Dorfman (1963) at 37°C in the presence of ^{3}H-DHA- S (New England Nuclear) (Bedin et al., 1980). The incubations were stopped by addition of 1 N NaOH and the yield of liberated unconjugated steroid was measured after direct extraction by the scintillation mixture (Toluene, POPOP, PPO). The results were corrected for radioactivity loss due to extractions and sampling. For control kinetic studies, the reaction mixture contained variable concentrations (10^{-7} M to 5 x 10^{-6} M) of ^{3}H DHA-S, and the reaction rates were linear within the incubation time and the protein concentration range employed. For the inhibition studies, variable concentrations (0 to 1 x 10^{-4} M) of chlormadinone acetate were added to the reaction mixture at different substrate concentrations (3 to 5 x 10^{-6}M) (Bedin et al., 1983).

RESULTS AND DISCUSSION

Intrauterine growth retardation (IUGR)

One hundred and two DHA-S loading tests (DLT) were performed in consenting pregnant women between 30 and 41 weeks of amenorrhoea (mean 35) who were classified in different groups: 1) a control group which consisted of pregnant women hospitalized for pathology unrelated to IUGR and delivered a normal baby, and 2) a group suspected of IUGR clinically and/or by ultrasound echotomography. This latter group was subsequently divided into two subgroups depending on the baby's birthweight: appropriate for gestational age (AGA) and small for gestational age (SGA) with a birthweight under the 10th percentile as defined by Lubchenco et al. (1966). Results summarized in Table 1 indicate that the difference between the $t_{\frac{1}{2}}$ of DHA-S for the babies born with a birthweight appropriate for gestational age (either belonging to the control group or to the suspected IUGR group) and for the SGA babies is statistically significant ($p < 0.001$). For all of the SGA babies, the $t_{\frac{1}{2}}$ is greater than 4.29 h, and most of the normal ones are under this value. Rabe et al. (1982) have obtained similar results and they could detect retarded fetal growth in all cases (10/10) by a prolonged half-life (> 4.7 h). The diagnostic efficiency is reported in Table 1B.

The results obtained by this method appear to be better than those obtained by the measurement of estrogen increase in urine and in plasma (Lauritzen et al., 1976; Strecker et al., 1978; Tulchinsky et al., 1976).

Measurements of metabolic clearance rate of DHA-S (Gant et al., 1971) suggest that a decreased utero-placental blood flow is the main factor contributing to reduce estrogen production and to prolong DHA-S half-life. The in vivo placental clearance of DHA-S to E_2 is particularly blood flow dependent (Everett et al., 1980).

We have compared, in 18 cases, the results of DLT performed in vivo during pregnancy with the response obtained in vitro in the perfused placenta (Thoumsin et al., 1980). We observed a correlation between the $t_{\frac{1}{2}}$ of DHA-S assayed in vivo and in vitro when the birthweight was normal ($n = 9, r = 0.74, p < 0.005$) but a shorter half-life in vitro than in vivo in case of IUGR. Wolf et al. (1980) also observed a normal aromatization in vitro in spite of a grossly deficient DLT in a case of IUGR and

Table 1 A. DHA-S half-life in 3 groups of pregnancies

	Control	Adequate for Gestational age Infant (AGA)	Small for Gestational age Infant (SGA)
Number of cases	43	39	20
Mean Birthweight, g	3,066 ± 65	2,730 ± 68	1,881 ± 89
DHA-S half-life, h	2.90 ± 0.12	3.24 ± 0.22	5.05 ± 0.20
			$p < 0.001$*

*comparison between SGA and AGA was done with the Student's t test.

Table 1 B. Diagnostic efficiency of DHA-S half-life measurements in pregnancy

Group	Number of Cases	DHA-S half-life, h		
		≤ 3.75	3.75-4.29	≥ 4.29
Control	43	36	5	2
AGA	39	27	8	4
SGA	20	0	1	19
Total	102	63	14	25

concluded, like us, that placental perfusion experiments seem to be an interesting tool in elucidating the placental functions.

The discrepancy between the results obtained in vivo and in vitro confirms that a decreased utero-placental blood flow is the main factor contributing to the reduced estrogen production. We have not tried to confirm the effect of reducing blood flow during in vitro perfusion of normal or IUGR placentae. It is possible that hemodynamic alterations result in enzymatic changes in the placentae that could also modify the transformation of DHA-S to E_2.

In order to test this hypothesis, we have measured the maternal plasma levels of the steroids involved in metabolic processes after DLT in 17 cases of suspected IUGR.

Following DLT, the disappearance rate of injected DHA-S is slower in pregnancies with SGA infants (n = 8) than in AGA (n = 9) with $t_{\frac{1}{2}}$ of DHA-S 4.34 ± 0.83 h versus 2.94 ± 0.48 h ($p < 0.001$). The concentration changes of unconjugated DHA is similar in both groups. After an increase of about 3 to 10-fold the mean values return to the baseline within 3 to 4 h.

Blood levels of Δ^4A are higher in pregnant women with SGA fetuses than those with AGA ones. Statistical differences are observed at 30 min and 45 min, 2 h and 3 h. Following DLT, T levels do not change significantly in pregnancies with normal babies, but in the women with hypotrophic fetuses T levels rise about 2 fold over the basal values. The T levels reach values to 2000 pg/ml. The increases of unconjugated E_1 and E_2 are evident in normal pregnancies and less marked in those with small-for-age children, but the statistical analysis does not discriminate one group from another. Figure 1 shows, as a function of time, the ratio of the mean levels of the different steroids measured in both groups after DLT. This representation evaluates the activity of the following enzymes: sulfatase, Δ^5-3β hydroxysteroid dehydrogenase (HSDH), and aromatase.

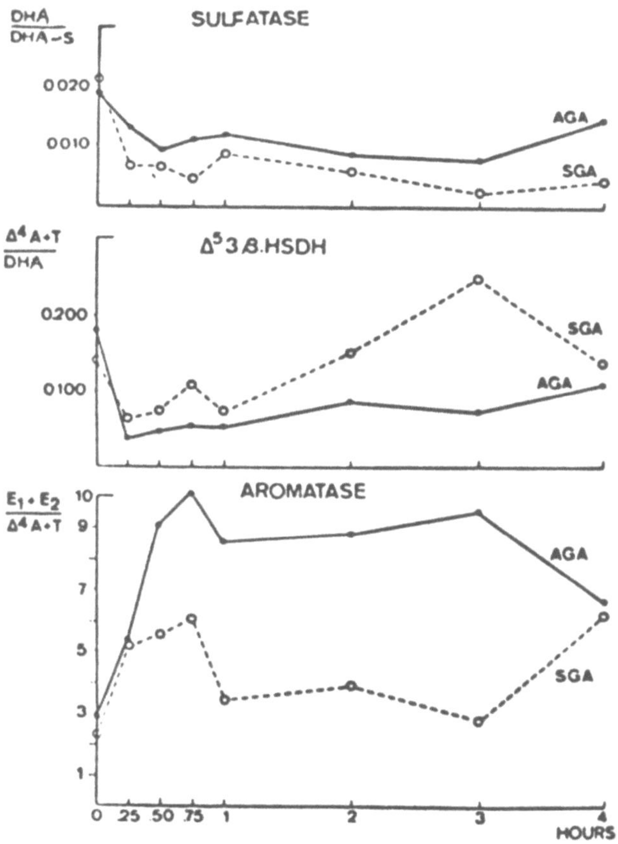

Figure 1. The ratios of plasma steroid levels following DLT in the mothers with AGA and with SGA infants.

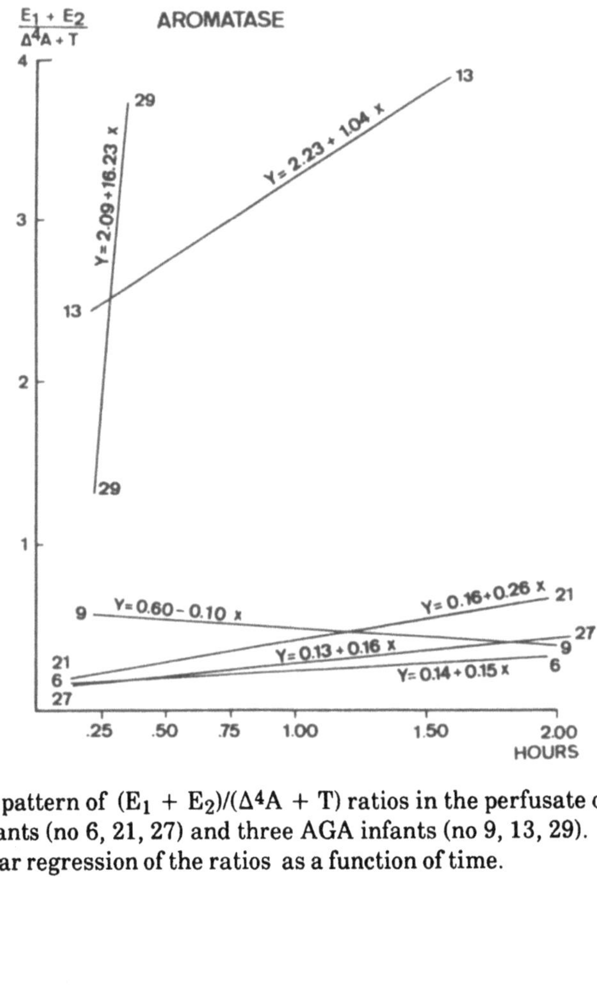

Figure 2. The pattern of $(E_1 + E_2)/(\Delta^4A + T)$ ratios in the perfusate of six placentae; three SGA infants (no 6, 21, 27) and three AGA infants (no 9, 13, 29). The results are given as a linear regression of the ratios as a function of time.

During the in vivo DLT, the sulfatase activity is rate limiting as indicated by the low DHA/DHA-S ratios (from 0 020 to 0.010) as compared to the $\Delta^4A + T$/DHA ratios (from 0.200 to 0.100) and the $(E_1 + E_2)/(\Delta^4A + T)$ ratios (from 10 to 1). Δ^5-3β HSDH activity does not seem to be disturbed in the SGA group, but in this case the aromatase activity is significantly reduced.

We have randomly selected 6 cases among the 18 perfused placentae for which the in vitro $t_{\frac{1}{2}}$ of DHA-S was already known, for the study of the time course levels of DHA-S, DHA, Δ^4A, T, E_1 and E_2 in the perfusate (Thoumsin et al., 1982). It appears clearly that a low estrogen production coincides with an accumulation of neutral steroids in the perfusate. We have calculated the

$$\frac{E_1 + E_2}{\Delta^4 A + T}$$

ratio at each time interval. For each placenta, the results are expressed as a linear regression of this ratio as a function of time (Figure 2). All placentae from SGA infants (no 6, 21, 27) are in the lower range and do not exhibit any change in aromatization activity despite an obvious increase of $\Delta^4 A + T$. It is the same for no. 9 (birth weight 2.270 g at 37 weeks of pregnancy). It appears that the placental conversion of DHA-S into estrogens may be slowed down at the aromatization step in some cases of IUGR. This phenomenon is independent of the placental blood flow, since each perfusion is performed under standardized conditions of pressure and flow.

Sulfatase deficiency

The genetic sulfatase deficiency is characterized by low levels of plasma and urinary estrogens while all other criteria of fetal development are normal (France and Liggins, 1969). The diagnosis can be made in vivo and in vitro (Bedin et al., 1980).

The in vivo diagnosis is made by DLT which does not result in a significant rise of plasma estradiol or a notable urinary estrogen increase. The $t_{\frac{1}{2}}$ for DHA-S can be either normal or greatly increased, so that its measurement is of no help for the diagnosis. This result suggests an alternative pathway allowing for the normal disappearance of DHA-S.

The in vitro diagnosis can be performed by incubation of placental homogenates in the presence of 3β-yl steroid sulfates such as DHA-S. If the defect exists, there will be a lack of hydrolysis of these precursors into free steroids contrasting with a normal aromatase activity. Babies born of the affected pregnancies are all males and develop X-linked ichthyosis with no sulfatase activity in their fibroblasts (Koppe et al., 1978; Shapiro et al., 1978; Bedin et al., 1981).

Inhibition of estrogen secretion by chlormadinone acetate administration

We observed that continuous administration of chlormadinone acetate to women at risk for premature labor induces a lowering in the urinary and plasma estrogen levels of the treated patients (Cedard et al., 1978). In 92 women who received 15-25 mg of chlormadinone acetate daily from 25 to 38 weeks of pregnancy, weekly determinations showed that plasma unconjugated E_2 and total E_3 were suppressed to below the 5th percentile as compared to normal untreated control pregnancies. A similar reduction was seen in total urinary estrogens in 65 chlormadinone acetate treated pregnancies. Phenotypic abnormalities in the newborn were not observed in any of the treated pregnancies, but we performed investigation both in vivo and in vitro, in order to clarify the mechanism of action of this progestin.

Twenty-eight hospitalized pregnant women between 30 and 38 weeks of gestation were subjected to DLT in vivo. One group (n = 14) was referred to as the "control group" presenting no severe pathology or hormonal therapy. The other group with threatened premature labor and progestin treatment (15-25 mg of chlormadinone acetate daily) was referred to as the "test group".

The $t_{\frac{1}{2}}$ for DHA-S in the two groups were not significantly different: 2.89 ± 0.4 h in the control group and 3.03 ± 0.06 h in the test group.

The variations of unconjugated E_2 and DHA-S concentrations as a function of time in the two groups are shown in Figure 3. It can be seen that in the control group the plasma levels are constantly higher for E_2 and lower for DHA-S than the corresponding values in the test group.

No difference could be shown by statistical analysis, neither for the mean values nor for their variances, except for the latter at 30, 45 and 180 min, in the case of unconjugated E_2. This observation indicates that the two groups of women do not belong to the same population.

In vitro, in a control kinetic study a mean apparent Km = 1 x 10^{-5} M (range 0.72 – 1.33 x 10^{-5} M) was calculated from six double reciprocal plots according to Lineweaver and Burk representation. The mean apparent Vm = 1.08 nmoles DHA-S hydrolyzed/min/mg protein (range 0.67 - 1.67) was also determined.

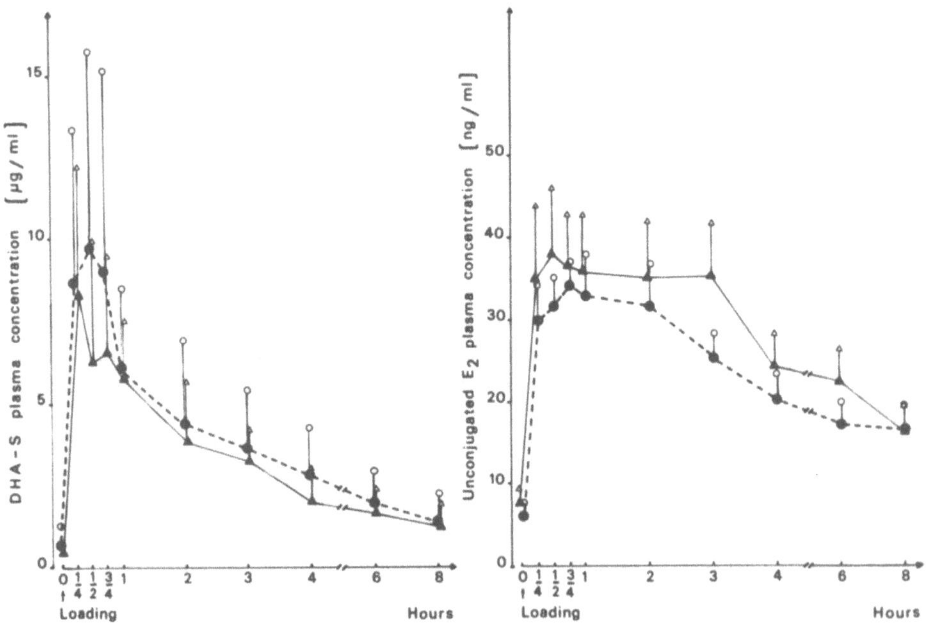

Figure 3. Mean DHA-S and unconjugated E_2 plasma concentrations following DHA-S loading test in the control and test group. Mean ± S.D. is given at each sampling time, △ control group; ○ test group

Chlormadinone acetate inhibits the sulfatase mediated DHA-S hydrolysis with a mean apparent inhibitor constant $K_i = 5.55 \times 10^{-6}M$, as calculated from the Dixon plots. These data are compatible with an inhibition of the competitive type at least in the range of substrate and inhibitor concentrations employed (Figure 4).

The results obtained in vivo and in vitro are different from those obtained in case of IUGR. The $t_{\frac{1}{2}}$ for DHA-S is not modified, which indicates that no alteration of the utero-placental blood flow occurs, but the unconjugated E_2 increase is limited. This suggests some inhibition of the placental metabolism of the substrate. The latter observation is confirmed by in vitro studies which demonstrates that chlormadinone acetate acts as a strong competitive inhibitor of DHA-S hydrolysis mediated by the placental steroid sulfatase. The aromatase activity does not seem to be modified by this progestin.

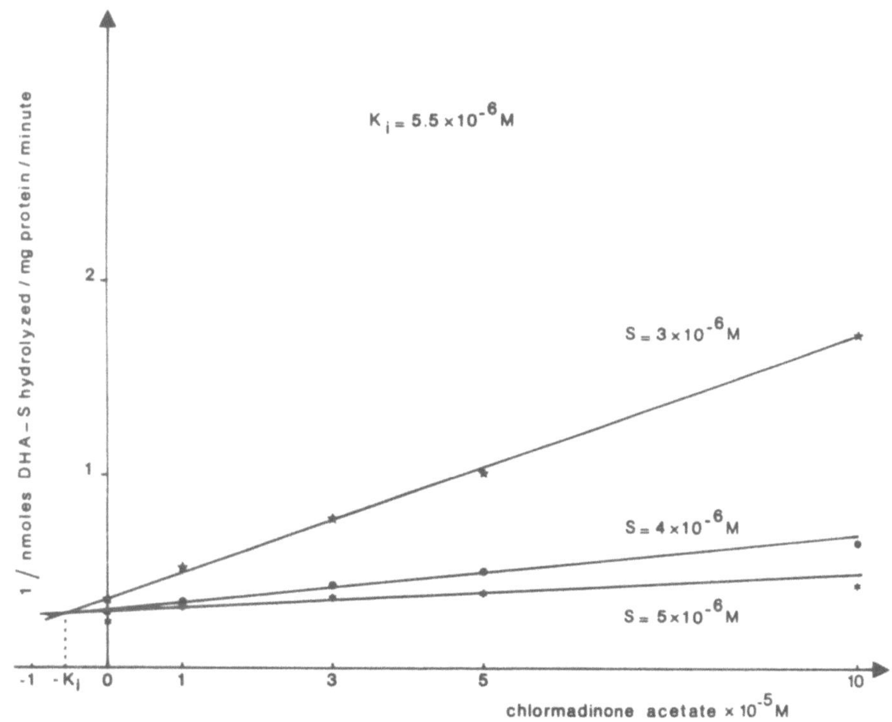

Figure 4. Typical kinetic data of the inhibitory effect of chlormadinone acetate on the placental sulfatase mediated DHA-S hydrolysis: an apparent K_i is calculated from the Dixon representation of the hydrolysis rate versus the inhibitor concentration in one experiment.

In cases of long term corticosteroid therapy for maternal diseases, where urinary and plasma estrogens are low, the DLT makes it possible to assess the fetal well-being, by showing low E_2 increase and prolonged $t_{\frac{1}{2}}$ for DHA-S in cases of fetal distress and hypotrophy, contrasting with normal results in normal pregnancies (Cedard et al., 1979).

SUMMARY

The estrogen secretion can be impaired during pregnancy for different reasons. It is often due to a lack of precursors and thus is the signal of fetal abnormalities. The DHA-S loading test has been widely used as an indicator of placental dysfunction. The placental clearance of maternal plasma DHA-S to estradiol in normal and abnormal pregnancies is dependent upon different factors: maternal intervillous blood flow, uptake by the trophoblast, and the capacity of the enzymes to hydrolyze and convert the C19 steroids to estrogens. In vitro studies of the placental metabolism of DHA-S including incubation of homogenates and perfusion of the whole organ are useful to elucidate placental function in different circumstances and to define the rate limiting factors.

In pregnancies suspected to have intrauterine growth retardation, the half-life of the DHA-S injected in vivo is significantly higher for small gestational age (SGA) babies than for newborns of adequate birthweight, but is usually normal when their placenta are perfused in vitro. This difference confirms that a decreased utero-placental blood flow is a primary contribution to the reduced estrogen production. However, in the SGA group we also observed a significant accumulation of Δ^4A and testosterone in the plasma of the mother after DHA-S administration as well as in the placental perfusion fluid. This suggests that an impairment of the aromatase activity could be superimposed on the hemodynamic alteration.

In cases of genetic deficiency of sterol sulfate sulfo-hydrolase activity, characterized by low levels of plasma and urinary estrogens in the mother during pregnancy, the $t_{\frac{1}{2}}$ for DHA-S can be either normal or increased, but the loading test does not induce a plasma estradiol increase. In vitro the aromatase activity was normal, contrasting with the absence of sulfatase activity in the placental homogenates.

Chlormadinone acetate, a synthetic progestin, produces a decrease of estrogen production in women treated for threatened premature labor. In vivo the $t_{\frac{1}{2}}$ for DHA-S is normal, and the plasma estradiol increase is reduced. In vitro, the drug acts as a strong competitive inhibitor of DHA-S hydrolysis, but does not modify the aromatase activity.

The comparison of in vivo and in vitro DHA-S metabolism makes it possible to determine the predominant abnormalities in different physiopathological conditions.

REFERENCES

Abraham, G.E. (1969) Solid phase radioimmunoassay of oestradiol-17β. *J. Clin. Endocr. Metab.* 29, 866-870.

Bedin, M., Alsat, E., Tanguy, G., and Cedard, L. (1980) Placental sulfatase deficiency: Clinical and biochemical study of 16 cases. *Eur. J. Obstet. Gynaecol. Reprod. Biol.* 10, 21-34.

Bedin, M., Weil, D., Fournier, T., Cedard, L., and Frezal, J. (1981) Biochemical evidence for the non-inactivation of the steroid sulfatase locus in human placenta and fibroblasts. *Hum. Genet.* 59, 256-258.

Bedin, M., Fournier, T, Tanguy, G., Cedard, L., Zorn, J.R., and Sureau, C. (1983) In vivo and in vitro study of the mechanism of action of a synthetic progestin in lowering unconjugated E_2 and total E_3 in plasma during normal human pregnancy. *Amer. J. Obstet. Gynecol.* 145, 373-374.

Burstein, S., and Dorfman, R.I. (1963) Determination of mammalian steroid sulfatase with 7α-^{3}H-3β-hydroxy-androst-5-en-17-one sulfate. *J. Biol. Chem.* 43, 1656-1660.

Cedard, L. (1972) Placental perfusion in vitro. 4th Karolinska Symposia on Research Methods in Reproductive Endocrinology. *Acta Endoc.*, Suppl. 158, 331-346.

Cedard, L., Breart, G., Cohen, M., Uzan, M., Prinos, C., Tanguy, G., and Sureau, C. (1978) Insuffisance des taux plasmatiques et urinaires d'oestriol liés à l'administration d'acétate de chlormadinone au cours de la grossesse. *La Nouvelle Presse Médicale* 7, 944.

Cedard, L., Bedin, M., Leblond, J., and Tanguy, G. (1979) Maternal plasma total oestriol and DHEA sulfate loading test as indicators of feto-placental function or placental sulfatase deficiency. *J. Steroid Biochem.* 11, 501-507.

Cohen, H., and Cohen, M. (1977) DHA-S half-life value in pregnancy, its prognostic value in high risk pregnancies. *J. Steroid Biochem.* 8, 381-383.

Crystle, C.D., Dubin, N.H, Grannis, G.F., Stevens, V.C., and Townsley, J.D. (1973) Investigation of precursor availability in the regulation of estrogen synthesis in normal human pregnancy. *Obstet. Gynecol.* N.Y. 42, 718-724.

Everett, R.B., Porter, J.C., Mac Donald, P.C., and Gant, N.F. (1980) Relationship of maternal placental blood flow to the placental clearance of maternal plasma dehydroisoandrosterone sulfate through placental estradiol formation. *Amer. J. Obstet. Gynecol.* 136, 435-439.

France, J.T., and Liggins, G.C. (1969) Placental sulfatase deficiency. *J. Clin. Endocrinol. Metab.* 36, 1-9.

Gant, N.F., Hutchinson, H.T., Siiteri, P.K., and MacDonald, P.C. (1971) Studies of the metabolic clearance rate of dehydroisoandrosterone sulfate in pregnancy. *Amer. J. Obstet. Gynecol.* 111, 555-561.

Klopper, A., Varela-Torres, R., and Janvial, V. (1976) Placental metabolism of dehydroepiandrosterone sulphate in normal pregnancy. *Br. J. Obstet. Gynaecol.* 83, 478-483.

Koppe, J.G., Marinkovic-Ilsen, A., Rijken, Y., De Groot, W.P., and Jobsis, A.C. (1978) X-linked ichthyosis. A sulphatase deficiency. *Arch. Dis. Child.* 53, 803-806.

Lauritzen, C. (1969) Conversion of DHEA sulfate to estrogens as a test of placental function. *Horm. Met. Res.* 1, 1-96.

Lauritzen, C., Strecker, J., and Lehmann, W.D. (1976) Dynamic tests of placental functions. In *Plasma hormone assay in evaluation of fetal wellbeing*, Klopper, A. (ed.), pp. 113-123 London: Churchill Livingstone.

Lubchenco, L.O., Hansman, C., and Boyd, E. (1966) Intra-uterine growth in length and head circumference as estimated from live birth at gestational age from 26 to 42 weeks. *Pediatrics* 37, 403- 409.

Pulkkinen, M.O. (1961) Arylsulfatase and the hydrolysis of some steroid sulfates in developing organism and placenta. *Acta Physiol. Scand. Suppl.* 180, 1-92.

Rabe, T., Runnebaum, B., Koepen, U., Widmaier, G., and Kubli, F. (1982) Diagnosis of intrauterine fetal growth retardation by prolongation of DHA-S half life after DHA-S loading. *Europ. J. Obstet. Gynaecol. Reprod. Biol.* 13, 145-158.

Shapiro, L.J., Weiss, R., Webster, D., and France, J.T. (1978) X-linked ichthyosis due to steroid-sulfatase deficiency. *Lancet, Jan.* 14, 70-72.

Siiteri, P.K., and Seron-Ferré, M. (1981) Some new thoughts on the feto-placental unit and parturition in primates. In *Fetal Endocrinology*, Novy, M.J. and Resko, J.A. (ed.), pp. 1-34, New York: Academic Press.

Strecker, J.R., Killus, C.M., Lauritzen, C., and Neumann, G.K. (1978) The clinical value of the dehydroepiandrosterone sulfate loading test in normal and pathologic pregnancies. *Amer. J. Obstet. Gynecol.* 131, 239-249.

Tanguy, G., Zorn, J.R., Sureau, C., and Cedard, L. (1980) Exogenous DHA-S half-life: A good index of intrauterine growth retardation. *Gynecol. Obstet. Invest.* 11, 170-174.

Tanguy, G., Thoumsin, H.J., Zorn, J.R., and Cedard, L. (1981) DHEA-S loading test in cases of intrauterine growth retardation: Relationship between the pattern of the maternal plasma metabolites and the fetoplacental dysfunction. *Gynecol. Obstet. Invest.* 12, 305-316.

Thoumsin, H.J., Alsat, E., Tanguy, G., Germeau, P., and Cedard, L. (1980) Test de charge au DHEA-S in vivo et in vitro: Hypotrophie et debit sanguin uteroplacentaire. *J. Gynecol. Obstet. Biol. Reprod.* 9, 205-210.

Thoumsin, H.J., Alsat, E., and Cedard, L. (1982) In vitro aromatization of androgens into estrogens in placental insufficiency. *Gynecol. Obstet. Invest.* 13, 37-42.

Townsley, J.D., Scheel, D.A., and Rubin, E. (1970) Inhibition of steroid-3-sulfatase by endogenous steroids. A possible mechanism controlling placental estrogen synthesis from conjugated precursors. *J. Clin. Endocr. Metab.* 31, 670-678.

Tulchinsky, D., Osathanondh, R., and Finn, A. (1976) Dehydroepiandrosterone sulfate loading test in the diagnosis of complicated pregnancies. *New Eng. J. Med.* 94, 517-522.

Varangot, J., Cedard, L., Yannotti, S. (1965) Perfusion of the human placenta in vitro. Study of the biosynthesis of oestrogens. *Amer. J. Obstet. Gynecol.* 92, 534-547.

Warren, J.C., and Timberlake, C.E. (1962) Steroid sulfatase in the human placenta. *J. Clin. Endocr. Metab.* 22, 1148-1151.

Wolf, A.S., Musch, K., and Lauritzen, C. (1980) Metabolism of the physiological precursor steroid dehydroepiandrosterone (DHA) in the perfused human placenta. In *The Human Placenta: Steroids and Proteins*. Klopper, A., Genazzani, A. and Crosignani, T. (eds.), New York Academic Press, pp. 215-223.

Trophoblast Research 1:249-270, 1983

THE PLACENTA AS A TARGET TISSUE FOR STEROIDS

- A Review-

Carolyn B. Coulam and
Thomas C. Spelsberg

The Mayo Clinic and Mayo Foundation
Rochester, Minnesota 55905, U.S.A.

INTRODUCTION

Although the function of the placenta as a steroid-producing organ is well known, its function as a target tissue for steroid hormones is less well documented. The physiologic actions of steroid hormones are believed to be mediated by cytoplasmic protein macromolecules, known as receptors, which are found in the cells of target tissues (Spelsberg and Toft, 1976). Each steroid binds to its specific cytoplasmic receptor, and each complex undergoes activation that results in translocation and binding of the complex to nuclear acceptor sites. By interacting with the chromatin, the activated complex alters DNA transcription, thus causing production of steroid-induced messenger RNA (Mainwaring, 1977). To be classified as a receptor, a steroid-binding protein should exhibit steroid specificity, high affinity for the steroid, low tissue concentration, and ability to translocate into the nucleus (Toft and Gorski, 1966; Jensen and DeSombre, 1972).

The presence of steroid receptors has been demonstrated in a number of tissues (Milgrom et al., 1970; Chan and O'Malley, 1976; Spelsberg and Toft, 1976; Mainwaring, 1977; Do and Leavitt, 1978; McCarty and McCarty, 1978; Baxter and Funder, 1979; Boyd and Spelsberg, 1979a; Giannopoulos and Tulchinsky, 1979) that synthesize steroids or are involved in reproduction. The placenta has long been suspected to be a target tissue for steroids, and indeed it has been reported to contain receptors for certain steroids (Diczfalusy, 1968; Schwartz et al., 1977; Kneussel et al., 1982). We have screened cytosolic and nuclear fractions from placentae at various lengths of gestation for the presence of receptors for estrogens, androgens, glucocorticoids, and progesterone.

MATERIALS AND METHODS

Chemicals

Tritiated estradiol, progesterone, R 5020 (17α promestone, or 21-dimethyl-19-nor-pregna-4,9-diene-3,20-diene), R 1881 (methyltrienolone, or 17β hydroxy-17α-methylestra-4,9,11-trien-3-one), dexamethasone, and unlabeled R 5020 and R 1881 were products of New England Nuclear (Boston, MA). All other steroids and chemicals were purchased from Sigma Chemical Co. (St. Louis, MO) and Fisher Scientific Co. (Pittsburgh, PA).

Tissue preparation

All preparations were made at 0°C to 4°C unless otherwise specified. Placentae at various weeks of gestation were separated from the fetal membranes and placed on ice immediately upon delivery. For general receptor studies the tissues were stored at -75°C. For some purposes, e.g., nuclear binding of the steroid in intact tissues--the fresh placentae were used within 2 h of surgical removal.

Cytosol preparation

Frozen or fresh placental tissue was pulverized and homogenized for approximately 15 seconds (Waring blender) at 4°C with three volumes (v/w) of buffer A, which consisted of 50 mM tris (hydroxymethyl) aminomethane hydrochloride (tris HCl), 1 mM ethylenediamine tetraacetic acid (EDTA), and 12 mM monothioglycerol, adjusted to pH 7.4. The homogenate was filtered through fine mesh organza cloth and further homogenized at 4°C (Thomas homogenizer). The final homogenate was centrifuged at 20,000 x g for 10 min and at 100,000 x g for 1 h. This supernatant was then recentrifuged at 100,000 x g for 1 h. The resultant supernatant is termed the "cytosolic" fraction. In some processes, the cytosolic fraction was then brought to 35 percent saturation with $(NH_4)_2SO_4$ at 4°C, and the precipitated protein was collected by centrifugation and stored at -75°C until needed.

Nuclear preparation

Placental tissue was homogenized as described above, but with 10 volumes (v/wt) of buffer B, which was comprised of 50 mM tris HCl, 25 mM potassium chloride, 20 mM magnesium chloride, and 2 M sucrose, adjusted to pH 7.5 The homogenate was centrifuged at 100,000 x g_{max} for 90 min, and the pellet of purified nuclei was resuspended in three volumes (relative to starting tissue weight) of buffer A with 0.3 M potassium chloride. The mixture was further homogenized (Glenco homogenizer), incubated at 0°C for 30 min, and centrifuged at 20,000 x g for 10 min. The supernatant was brought to 35 percent saturation with $(NH_4)_2SO_4$ at 4°C, and the precipitate was stored frozen as previously described.

Labeling and exchange with (^{3}H) steroid

Tritiated steroid, supplied in benzene-ethanol (9:1, v/v), was lyophilized and redissolved in an equal volume of absolute ethanol. This was diluted serially with absolute ethanol to provide a stock solution. Aliquots of this stock were added directly to the cytosolic and nuclear fractions to make the final desired concentration. Incubations continued for 4 to 22 h at 4°C until maximal binding was demonstrated.

Analysis of specific binding

Bound (^{3}H) steroid was measured by the dextran charcoal method modified from the method of Korenman (1968). All steps were performed at 4°C. The supernatants from the cytosolic and nuclear fractions were tested for specific steroid binding by incubation with (^{3}H) E_2, (^{3}H) R 5020, (^{3}H) R 1881, or (^{3}H) dexamethasone (0.05 to 20 nM) in the presence or absence of 100-fold excess of the same unlabeled substances. The incubation mixtures were sampled at various times, and bound (^{3}H) steroid was determined by treatment of the samples with 4 volumes of 1 percent (w/w) dextran coated charcoal at 0°C for 5 min to remove the free steroid. The charcoal was pelleted by centrifugation, and one half the volume was removed for liquid scintillation counting to determine the bound (^{3}H) steroid. At each time point, the bound (^{3}H) steroid from the incubation without additional unlabeled steroid represented the total bound steroid. Specifically bound steroid was determined as the difference between the total bound steroid and the nonspecifically bound steroid (obtained by the same incubation containing an excess of the known unlabeled steroid).

Determination of binding constants

A Scatchard analysis (Scatchard, 1949) was performed to determine the equilibrium dissociation constant (Kd) and concentration of binding sites in human placental cytosol and nuclei. The protein pellets were resuspended and dialyzed as previously described. The protein concentration in each of the preparations was determined by Bradford's modification (1976) of the Lowry method. Aliquots (0.25 ml) of the term and preterm placental cytosolic fractions or their nuclear fractions were incubated at 0°C for 4-22 h with different concentrations of (^{3}H) steroid (from 0.05 to 10 nM), with and without a 100-fold excess of unlabeled steroid for specific binding determinations. At the end of the incubation, 50 µl of each sample was removed, and the concentration of (^{3}H) steroid present in the sample was determined by liquid scintillation counting. The remainder of each sample (0.2 ml) was assayed for bound steroid by the charcoal assay, as previously described. The binding constants were determined by linear regression analysis of the Scatchard plots.

Steroid specificity

Competition experiments were conducted to determine the specificity of the binding protein. Aliquots of 0.5 ml of the cytosol were incubated at 0°C for 20 h with 10 nM (^{3}H) R 1881 with and without various concentrations of unlabeled R 1881, dihydrotestosterone, testosterone, progesterone, estradiol, esterone, or cortisol; and with 20 nM (^{3}H) dexamethasone, with and without various concentrations of unlabeled dexamethasone, triamcinolone, dihydrotestosterone, estradiol, and progesterone. Ammonium sulfate precipitation was performed as described above, and the protein pellets were again resuspended in 0.2 ml of buffer A and were treated with dextran-coated charcoal. The steroid specificity was estimated as the difference between total and nonspecific binding in the assays containing only the particular labeled steroid (20 nM) and that containing both the labeled steroid and unlabeled steroids (1 to 2 nM).

Sucrose density gradients

Cytosol was prepared as described above from both term and preterm placental tissues and was incubated for 20 h with 10 nM (^{3}H) R 1881, with and without 1 µM unlabeled R 1881, or with 20 µM (^{3}H) dexamethasone with and without 2 uM unlabeled dexamethasone. A 0.6 ml fraction of cytosol from each incubation was added to a charcoal pellet prepared by centrifuging 2.4 ml of the dextran-coated charcoal solution described above. The mixture was vortexed, incubated on ice for 5 min, and then centrifuged at 2,000 x g for 5 min. Aliquots (0.2 ml) of each supernatant were loaded on sucrose density gradients of 5 to 20 percent (w/w) previously prepared with a Buchler Auto Densi Flow at 11°C. Both high salt gradients (containing 0.5 ml M KCl) and low salt gradients (0.01 M KCl) were run for each incubation mixture. The gradients were centrifuged at 30,000 x g for 16 h, with low acceleration and no braking at the end of the centrifugation. Each gradient was removed with the Buchler Auto Densi Flow and was separated into sequential fractions of 8 drops each. The fractions were mixed with Spectrafluor solution, allowed to stand in the dark for 4 h, and then counted. by the liquid scintillation method.

Cell-free binding of receptor to isolated placental chromatin

Chromatin was isolated from 20 g of a 40-week placenta, as described by Pikler et al. (1976); Boyd and Spelsberg (1979b), and Thrall and Spelsberg (1980). The DNA concentration was determined by the method of Burton (1956). Binding of the glucocorticoid receptor to chromatin in a cell-free system was demonstrated by resuspending the ammonium sulfate precipitates of the (^{3}H) dexamethasone-labeled term and preterm placental cytosols in one-fourth the original volume of cytosol in buffer A and dialyzing them against 10 volumes of the same solution for 1 h. The receptor solution was then clarified by centrifugation at 20,000 x g_{max} for 10 min.

The nuclear binding assay used is a modification of that described by Boyd and Spelsberg (1979b) and was performed by adding an increasing amount of chromatin to a constant amount of receptor. The total reaction volume was 1 ml, with a final KCl concentration of 0.2 M. The sample was incubated on ice for 90 min and frequently mixed on a vortex. The chromatin was then pelleted in the assay tubes at 2,000 x g for 5 min and the pellet was washed twice, each time with 1 ml of buffer C (2 mM tris HCl, 0.1 mM EDTA, pH 7.5). Background assays consisted of (1) zero time incubations wherein chromatin was pelleted within 10 to 20 seconds after adding the receptor solution, (2) incubations containing no chromatin, or (3) those containing no receptor. After the final washing, the pellets were resuspended in 1 ml of buffer C, mixed, and filtered over numbered Millipore filters. The assay tubes were rinsed twice, the rinses were passed through the same filters, and the filters were dried under a heat lamp for 10 min and counted in 5 ml of scintillation fluid. After counting, the filters were dried again, and the DNA per filter was quantitated as described by Spelsberg and Hnilica (1971).

Studies were performed to determine the optimal time, temperature, and concentration of chromatin for receptor to DNA binding in the placental system. It was determined that optimal binding was achieved at 90 min, at 0 to 4°C, with 50 µg of chromatin (as DNA), and with varying the levels of the receptor per assay. Comparisons of the chromatin bindings of the steroid receptors from preterm (27 week) and term placentae were then conducted using these specific parameters.

Nuclear binding of receptor in intact tissue

The assay for the nuclear binding of (^{3}H)-labeled steroid receptors in whole tissue sections is the subject of another study (Razel et al., unpublished data). Briefly, fresh 40-week placental tissue was frozen on dry ice and pulverized with a modified staple gun. After the quick, transient freezing, the rate of nuclear uptake of the (^{3}H)-labeled steroid was higher than with unfrozen tissue, but the maximal levels of binding were not altered. It is surmised that transient freezing of small sections of tissue generates a greater surface area, thus enhancing the rate of steroid uptake. Most cells in the frozen tissue appear intact on microscopic examination.

In a typical experiment, four 0.5 g samples were incubated with 50 nM of (^{3}H) R 1881 or (^{3}H) dexamethasone; 5 µM of unlabeled R 1881 or dexamethasone was added to two of the samples to determine nonspecific binding. One sample with and one without unlabeled steroid was incubated at 22°C in 1 ml of 50 percent McCoy's medium for 90 min. For the zero-time control, samples were processed immediately after addition of McCoy's medium. For processing after the incubations, each sample of minced tissue was washed thoroughly and the nuclei were isolated, as described elsewhere (Boyd and Spelsberg, 1979b). The nuclear pellets were resuspended in buffer E (50 mM trisHCl, pH 7.5, and 10 percent glycerol) and filtered on nitrocellulose filters. The filters were counted by scintillation spectrometry, and the DNA per filter quantitated, as described elsewhere (Spelsberg and Hnilica, 1971).

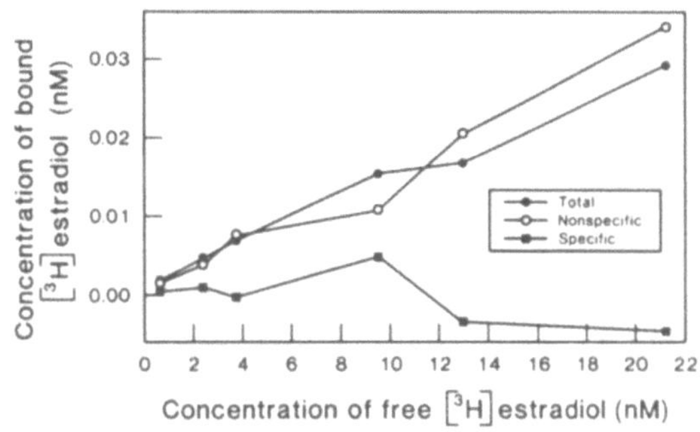

Figure 1. Binding of (^{3}H)-labeled estradiol to cytosolic fractions of term placentae. Pellets of ammonium sulfate-precipitated protein from placental cytosol were resuspended, dialysed, clarified, and incubated for 8 h at 0°C with increasing concentrations of (^{3}H) E_2. Preparations were incubated with and without 100-fold excess of unlabeled estradiol. Specifically bound (^{3}H)-labeled estradiol was determined as difference between total and non-specifically bound (^{3}H)-labeled estradiol.

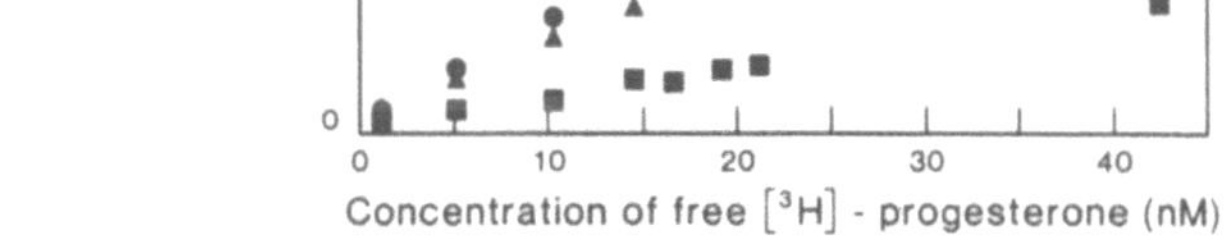

Figure 2. Binding of (^{3}H)-labeled progesterone to cytosolic fractions of term placentae. Pellets of $(NH_4)_2SO_4$-precipitated protein from placental cytosol were resuspended, dialysed, clarified, and incubated for 2 h at 0°C with increasing concentrations of (^{3}H)-labeled progesterone. Preparations were incubated with and without 200-fold excess of unlabeled progesterone. Specifically bound (^{3}H)-labeled progesterone was determined as difference between total and nonspecifically bound (^{3}H)-labeled progesterone.

Quantitation of protein and DNA

Protein concentrations in cytosols were determined by a modification of the Bradford method (Bradford, 1976). Protein standards were bovine serum albumin. DNA in the initial homogenates or on the filters was assayed according to the method of Burton (1956).

RESULTS

Characterization of estrogen binding

An apparent saturation of macromolecular binding of (^{3}H) E_2 occurred by 8 h in the timed binding assays. However, no specific binding could be demonstrated in either cytosolic or nuclear fractions from preterm or term placental tissue (Figure 1). Scatchard studies failed to reveal any high-affinity, low-capacity binding expected of a steroid receptor. Furthermore, competitive binding assays failed to demonstrate any specific steroid binding.

Characterization of progesterone binding

An apparent specific binding of (^{3}H) progesterone was detected during a 24 h incubation period. This binding was observed at approximately 2 h. However, more detailed analysis (by Scatchard method) showed no high affinity, low-capacity binding sites, nor any steroid specificity (Figure 2). Similarly, specific binding of (^{3}H) R 5020 over a 24 h incubation period at 4°C or room temperature did not reveal any specific binding in either the cytosolic or nuclear fractions of placentae from term deliveries.

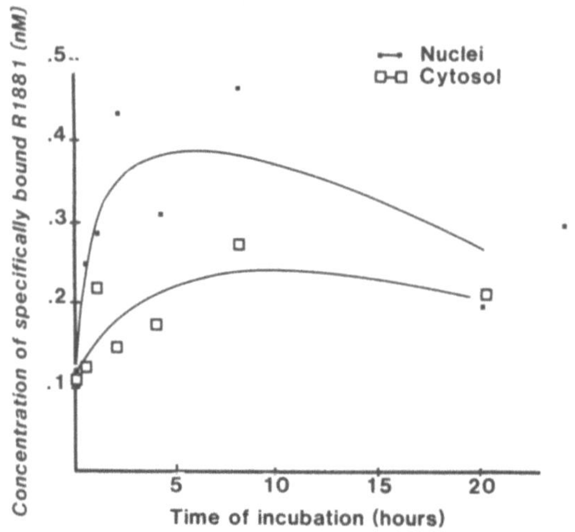

Figure 3. Kinetics of binding of (^{3}H) R 1881 to placental cytosol. Pellets of $(NH_4)_2SO_4$-precipitated protein from placental cytosol and nuclei were resuspended, dialyzed, and clarified as described in the text and were incubated at 0°C with 10 nM (^{3}H) R 1881, with and without 1 μM unlabeled R 1881. At various times, 0.2 ml of the mixtures was removed and treated with 0.8 ml of 1 percent (w/w) dextran-coated charcoal to remove free R 1881. The concentration of specifically bound (^{3}H) R 1881 in each treated sample was estimated as the difference between the (^{3}H) R 1881 bound in the absence of unlabeled R 1881 and that bound in presence of unlabeled R 1881. (From McCormick et al., 1981a; by permission)

Characterization of androgen binding

Specific binding of (^{3}H) R 1881 in term placental cytosolic and nuclear fractions was found. The latter showed a rapid increase in concentration of specifically bound ligand during the first h of incubation at 0°C (Figure 3). Maximal specific binding was reached between 4 and 8 h of incubation in both preparations. Thereafter, the specifically bound concentrations of ligand appeared to decrease in the nuclear fraction and remained relatively steady in the cytosol. By Scatchard analysis, the placental cytosol (Figure 4) showed that the specific binding had an apparent Kd of 3.8 nM and a binding site concentration of 1.2 pmoles/g tissue (10 fmoles/mg protein). Figure 5 shows that the placental nuclear fraction also had a specific binding with an apparent Kd of 8.8 nM and a concentration of binding sites of 0.17 mole/g tissue.

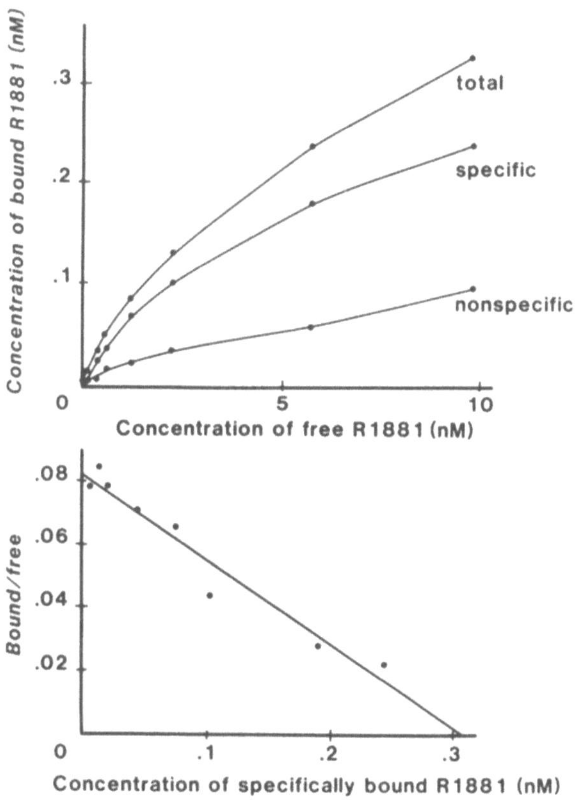

Figure 4. Scatchard analysis of (^{3}H) R 1881 binding to placental cytosol. To determine binding characteristics of R 1881, protein preparations from placental cytosol were incubated with various concentrations of (^{3}H) R 1881, with and without 100-fold excess of unlabeled R 1881, for 4 h at 0°C. Specifically bound (^{3}H) R 1881 was determined by subtracting nonspecific binding from total binding. Concentration of free (^{3}H) R 1881 was determined as difference between concentration of (^{3}H) R 1881 in an aliquot of each incubation and concentration of total bound (^{3}H) R 1881. Binding constants were determined according to method of Scatchard, by fitting a line to plotted points by linear regression. (From McCormick et al., 1981a; by permission)

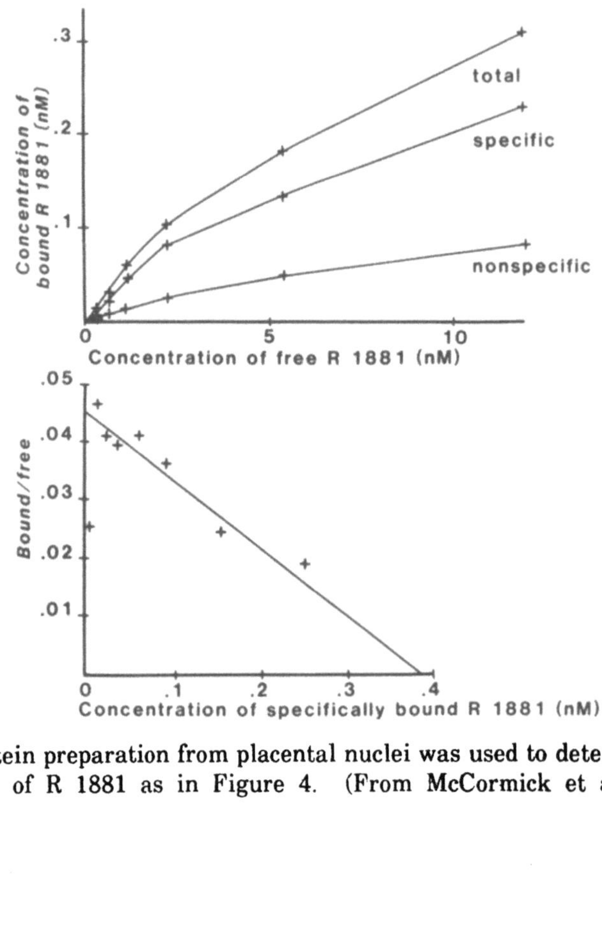

Figure 5. Protein preparation from placental nuclei was used to determine binding characteristics of R 1881 as in Figure 4. (From McCormick et al., 1981a; by permission)

Steroid specificity of the binding

The specificity of R 1881 binding to term placental cytosol protein was examined by treating the binding mixture with various concentrations of unlabeled competing steroids. As expected, the most effective competitor for R 1881 binding to term placental cytosol protein was 5 α- dihydrotestosterone (Figure 6). By comparison of the amounts of each required to reduce (^{3}H) R 1881 binding to 50 percent of the original binding values, 5 α-dihydrotestosterone appeared to bind with affinity approximately 50-fold weaker than that of R 1881. Next in competing effectiveness was testosterone, with about 700-fold weaker affinity, followed by progesterone and estradiol. Estrone and cortisol did not appear to compete, even at levels of 1,000-fold excess over (^{3}H) R 1881. These results support the existence of an androgen receptor.

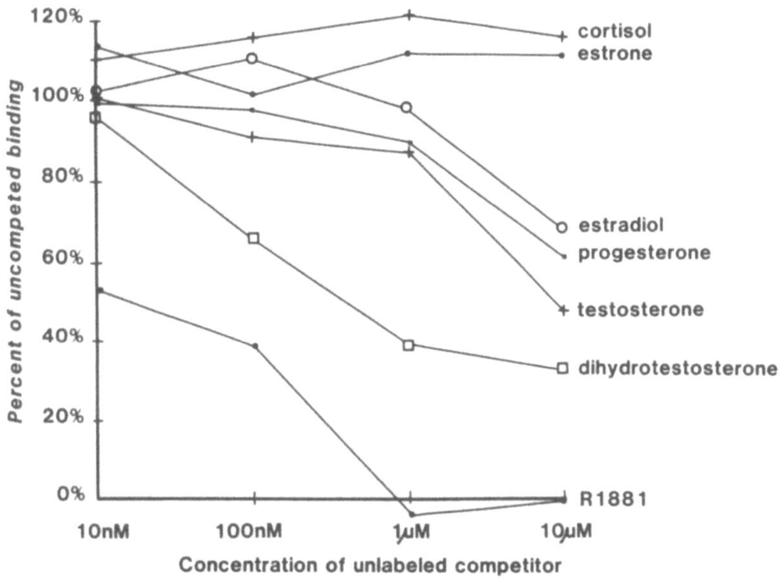

Figure 6. Steroid specificity of androgen binding in placenta. Binding to protein preparations from placental cytosol was subjected to competition of (^{3}H) R 1881, unlabeled R 1881, and other steroids. Protein preparations were incubated at 0°C for 4 h with 10 nM (^{3}H) R 1881 and various concentrations of unlabeled steroids. Specifically bound (^{3}H) R 1881 was estimated as in Figure 4 by means of replicate incubation of each with 1 µM unlabeled R 1881. Concentration of specifically bound (^{3}H) R 1881 was expressed as percentage of uncompeted (^{3}H) R 1881. (From McCormick et al., 1981a; by permission)

Sucrose density gradients

Figure 7 shows the sedimentation of the specifically bound (^{3}H) R 1881 "receptor" in sucrose gradients under low salt conditions. This action occurs with an 8S value under low salt conditions and with a 4S value under high salt conditions. The presence of molybdate appears to stabilize the 8S species. These results are characteristic of receptors in general (Jensen and DeSombre, 1972; McCarty and McCarty, 1978; Baxter and Funder, 1979).

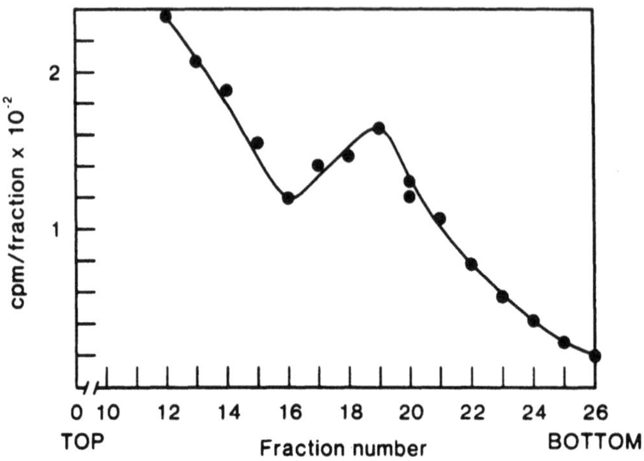

Figure 7. Sucrose gradient analysis of androgen receptor from full-term human placenta. Crude cytosol 10^5 x g supernatant from full-term human placenta was labeled with 20 nM (^{3}H) R 1881 for 4 h at 4°C. Then 0.2-ml aliquots were layered over 5 to 20 percent (w/w) sucrose gradients in SW-50.1 centrifuge tubes. In the low-salt assays a standard marker, (^{14}C) aldolase, was added alone and its sedimentation (7.2S) pattern noted. Tubes were centrifuged at 30,000 rpm for 20 h at 4°C, after which the 0.2 ml fractions were collected by Buchler Auto Densi-Flow apparatus and 5 ml Spectrofluor added. Cpm per fraction is plotted against fraction number.

Cell free and intact tissue binding of the androgen receptor to nuclear acceptor sites in placenta

Since steroid receptor complexes translocate and bind to nuclear acceptor sites in vivo, we examined this aspect with this preparation. Figure 8 shows the binding of the partially purified androgen receptor (ammonium-sulfated (^{3}H) R 1881 receptor) to isolated chromatin from full-term placenta. A saturable specific binding of the androgen receptor to the chromatin is evident. Free labeled R 1881 (i.e., without receptor) showed minimal binding, as did heat-denatured androgen receptor.

For a check of the intact cell function of this "receptor," tissue cultures using (^{3}H) R 1881 incubations were performed. Figure 9 represents a typical time-dependent incorporation of the (^{3}H) R 1881 into nuclei in intact sections of placental tissue supporting the presence of functioning receptor in this tissue.

Thus both intact cell and cell-free assays imply that a functional androgen receptor is present in full term placenta. Next, quantitative and qualitative comparisons of the androgen receptor between normal-term and preterm placentae were performed.

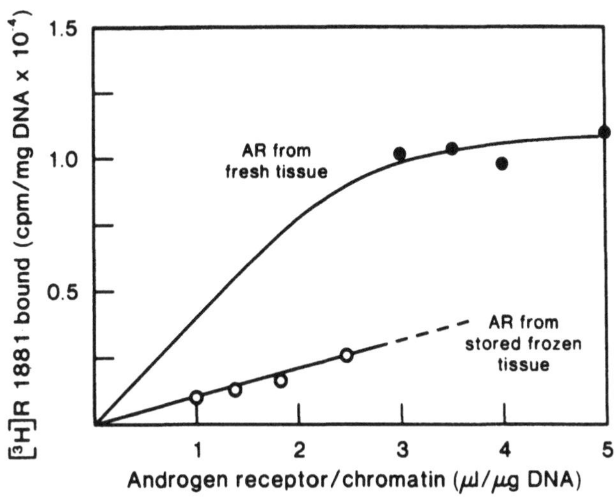

Figure 8. Cell-free binding of (^{3}H) androgen receptor (AR) to chromatin isolated from full-term human placenta. Chromatin was purified from fresh human placenta as described by Pikler et al., (1976). Androgen receptor was isolated and labeled with (^{3}H) R 1881 (ammonium sulfate precipitated and resuspended in 1/10 the original volume) as described by McCormack and Glasser (1976), except receptor was kept constant (150 μl) and chromatin varied from 50 to 300 μg per assay. Nuclei were then washed and placed on nitrocellulose filters. After counting, filters were analyzed for DNA and cpm/mg DNA was calculated. That value is plotted against the ratio of androgen receptor (μl) to chromatin (μg DNA).

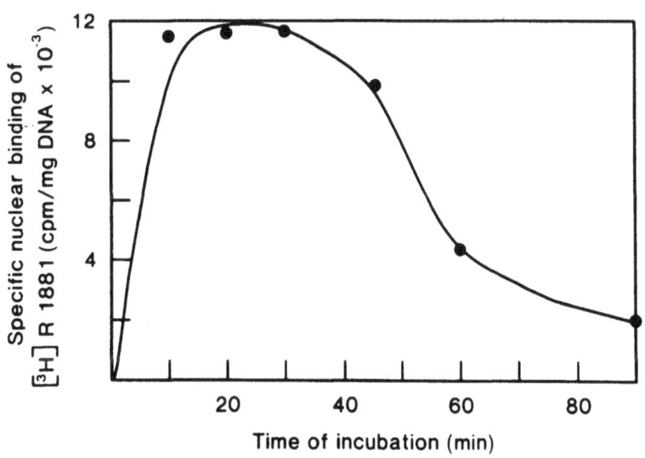

Figure 9. Intact cell nuclear binding of androgen receptor: time course of (^{3}H) R 1881 binding to nuclei of intact tissue. Concentration of specifically bound (^{3}H) R 1881 was estimated as difference between (^{3}H) R 1881 bound in the absence of unlabeled R 1881 and that bound in the presence of a 100-fold excess of unlabeled R 1881.

The binding constants of the receptors in crude cytosols from placentae at various lengthS of gestation were determined (Figure 10). Five experiments using cytosol from term placentae (different in each experiment) produced a spectrum of Kd values ranging from 1.3 to 27 nM and binding site concentrations of 1.4 to 15 fmoles/mg protein (20 to 340 fmoles/mg DNA). In the five experiments with cytosol from different preterm placentae, the Kd values ranged from 1.5 to 50 nM and the binding site concentrations from 1.2 to 21 fmoles/mg protein (19 to 335 fmoles/mg DNA). Thus, the ranges and distribution of the binding constant for term and preterm placentae were equivalent. No relationship was noted between the length of gestation and the magnitude of the binding constant or the concentration of receptor.

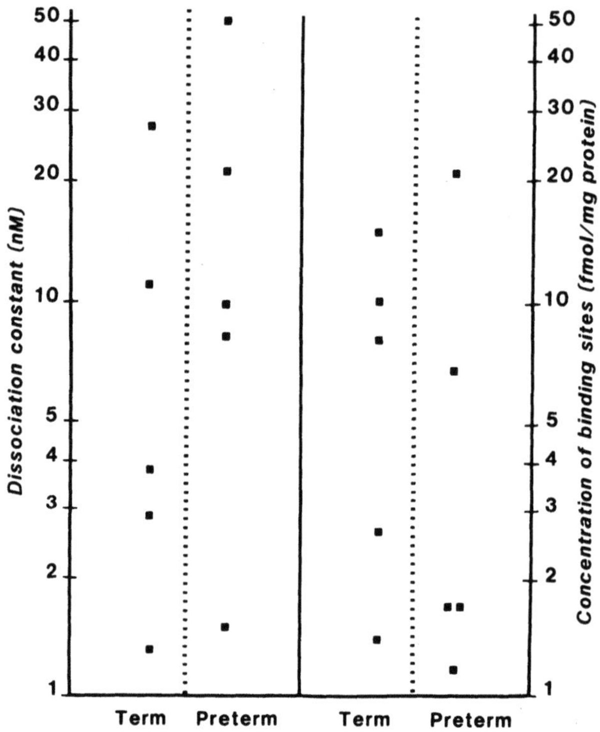

Figure 10. Equilibrium dissociation constants (Kd) and concentrations of binding sites for 10 placentae of various gestational periods, determined by Scatchard method. The columns on the left side of the figure plot the Kd values obtained from specific binding of the (^{3}H) R 1881 to the androgen receptors; those on the right side indicate the concentrations of the androgen receptor in the various specimens. (From McCormick et al., 1981a; by permission)

Characterization of glucocorticoid binding

Binding of (^{3}H) dexamethasone -- As shown in Figure 11, the amount of specifically bound (^{3}H) dexamethasone increased to a maximal level at 12 h and remained fairly constant up to 30 h of incubation. Scatchard analysis demonstrated that the placental cytosol contains a binding site concentration of 86.2 fmole/mg protein (2,763 fmole/mg DNA), with an apparent Kd of 24.7 nM (Figure 12). The placental nuclear fraction revealed a similar affinity, with a Kd of 28 nM.

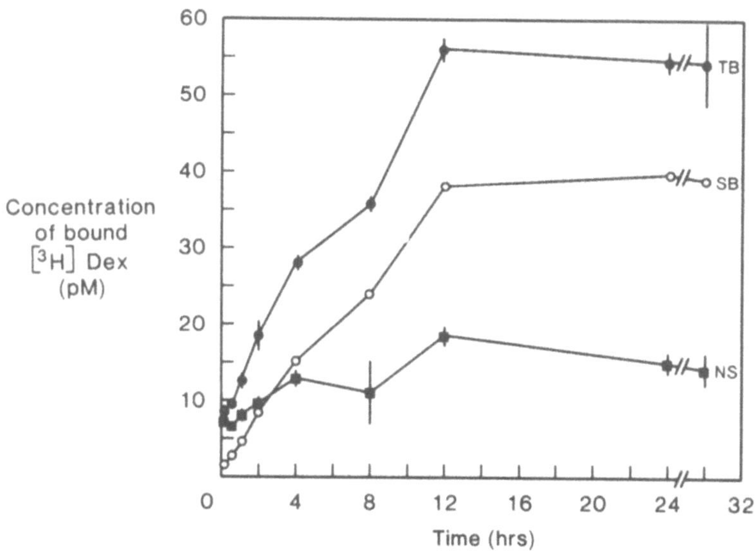

Figure 11. Kinetics of binding of (^{3}H) dexamethasone in mature placental cytosol. Placental cytosol was incubated with 20 nM (^{3}H) dexamethasone at 4°C for 30 min to 30 h. At each time point, total binding (TB) and nonspecific (NS) binding were determined by dextran-coated charcoal method, as described in the text. Specific binding (SB) was obtained by subtracting nonspecific binding from total binding. Each point represents the mean of triplicate analyses. (From Lageson et al., 1983; with permission)

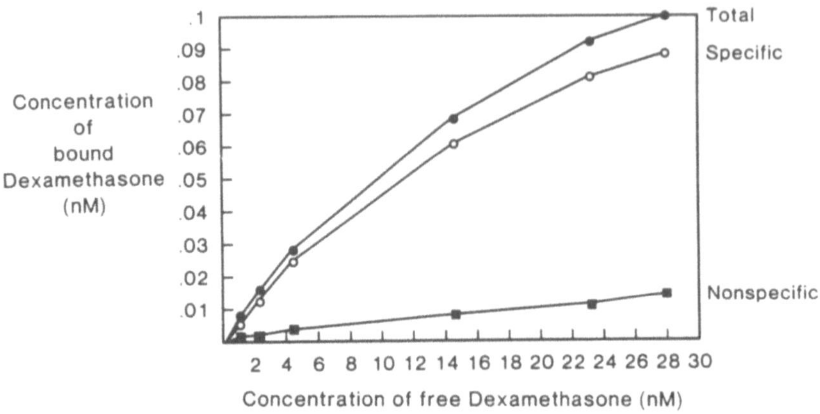

Figure 12A. Titration of specific dexamethasone binding sites in mature placental cytosol. Saturation analyses of (^{3}H) dexamethasone binding were performed by incubating aliquots of cytosol for 20 h with 11 different concentrations of (^{3}H) dexamethasone (ranging from 0.05 to 40 nM). Total, specific, and nonspecific bindings were determined by dextran-coated charcoal assay, as described in the text, and are plotted against (^{3}H) dexamethasone concentration. Each point represents the mean of triplicate analyses.

Steroid specificity of binding

The steroid specificity of the binding sites in term placentae was demonstrated by competition between (^{3}H) dexamethasone and various unlabeled steroids. As shown in Figure 13, unlabeled triamcinolone and dexamethasone readily competed with (^{3}H) dexamethasone for specific binding sites. Dihydrotestosterone and estradiol, however, demonstrated no competition for (^{3}H) dexamethasone binding in the range of 2 to 2,000 nM. Progesterone competed with specific binding only at 10-fold or higher concentrations, as it characteristically does in experiments with glucocorticoid receptors in other tissues. Thus a steroid specificity was demonstrated for the glucocorticoid binding.

Sucrose density gradients

Sedimentation analysis of the (^{3}H) dexamethasone binding in term placental cytosol demonstrated an 8S binding region under low salt conditions and a shift to a 4S binding region with a high salt treatment (Figure 14). This is also a typical characteristic of steroid receptors.

Cell-free binding of glucocorticoid receptor to isolated placental chromatin

A cell-free nuclear binding assay was performed to examine the biologic activity of the glucocorticoid receptor. Partially purified dexamethasone receptor and chromatin isolated from a 40-week placenta were used. The background assays were conducted under zero-time and chromatin-deficient conditions. Figure 15 shows the nuclear binding to be a time- and chromatin-dependent process that can lead to saturation. Previously determined optimal conditions of 90 min of incubation at 0 to 4°C and a DNA concentration of 25 μg/ml were used.

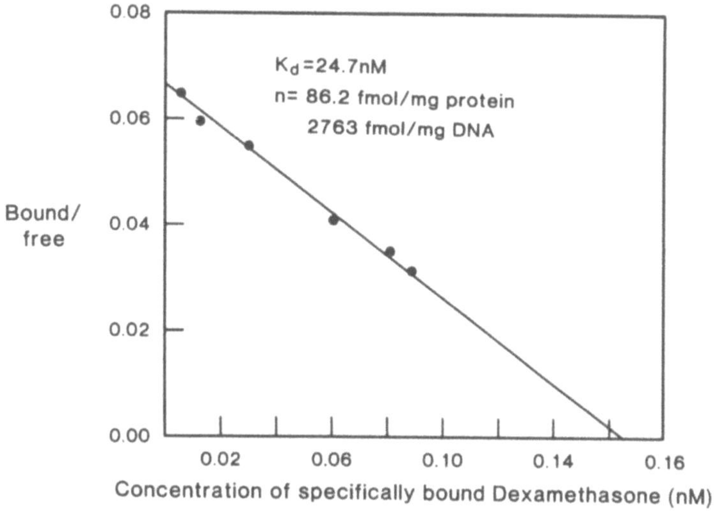

Figure 12B. Scatchard analysis of (^{3}H) dexamethasone binding in mature placental cytosol. Calculations were made with the data in Figure 3. Data are plotted according to method of Scatchard, with dissociation constant (Kd) and the number of binding sites (n) calculated. Each point represents the mean of triplicate analyses. (From Lageson et al., 1983; with permission)

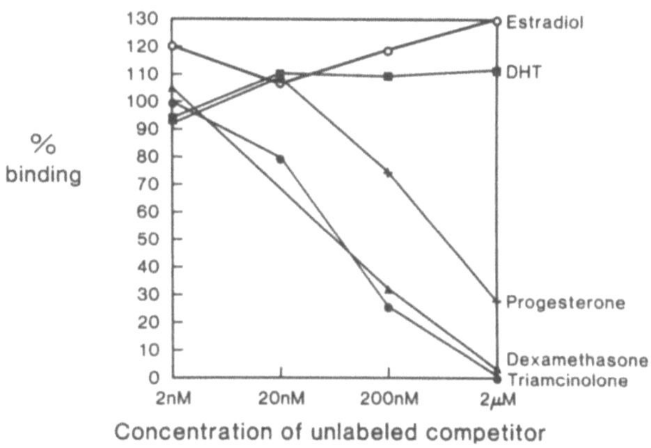

Figure 13. Competition for specific (^{3}H) dexamethasone-binding sites by unlabeled steroids. (^{3}H) dexamethasone at a concentration of 20 nM was added to aliquots of cytosol in the absence and presence of excess of unlabeled triamcinolone, dexamethasone, progesterone, dihydrotestosterone (DHT), and estradiol, and was incubated for 20 h at 4°C. Ammonium sulfate precipitation at 35 percent was performed, and specific binding of (^{3}H) dexamethasone was determined by the dextran-coated charcoal method. Each incubation was assayed in duplicate, and mean value is given. (From Lageson et al., 1983; with permission)

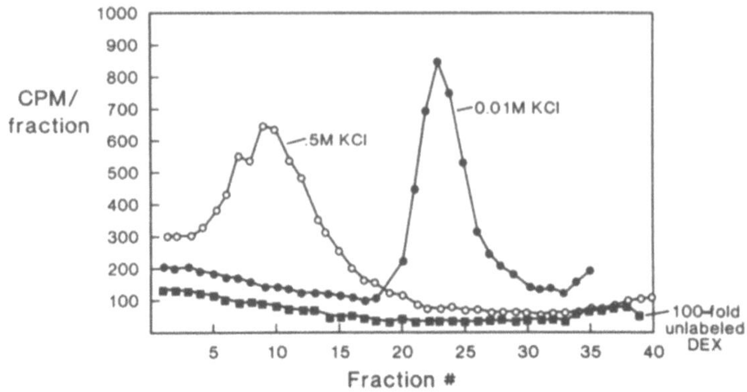

Figure 14. Sedimentation analysis of (^{3}H) dexamethasone-binding proteins in mature placental cytosol. Cytosol was incubated for 20 h with 20 nM (^{3}H) dexamethasone and then mixed with a pellet of dextran-coated charcoal and centrifuged. Aliquots from this supernatant were loaded on density gradients of 5 to 20 percent sucrose. Both high salt (0.5 M KCl) and low salt (0.01M KCl) gradients were centrifuged, as described in the text. (From Lageson et al., 1983; with permission)

Nuclear binding of glucocoroticoid receptor in intact cells

To corroborate, by tissue culture methods, the finding that placenta contains functional glucocorticoid receptor, we analyzed the translocation of (^{3}H) dexamethasone to nuclei. Incubation in culture medium at 22°C of minced pieces of term placenta with 50 nM (^{3}H) dexamethasone demonstrated time-dependent specific nuclear binding (Figure 16). Thus, functional glucocorticoid receptor appears to exist in the term placenta.

Comparison of binding between term and preterm placentae

Thirteen experiments using cytosols from third trimester placentae (28 to 40 weeks) produced dissociation constants in the range of 16.9 to 96.7 nM and concentrations of binding sites (the receptor) in the range of 16.0 to 260.0 fmole/mg protein (426 to 4,882 fmole/mg DNA). Two experiments with cytosol from second-trimester placentae (20 and 27 weeks) also disclosed a broad range of dissociation constants, 14.8 and 77.3 nM, as well as of binding-site concentrations, 66.1 and 452.0 fmole/mg protein (366 and 3,431 fmole/mg DNA). Tissue from two surgical abortions (approximately 8-week gestations) yeilded receptors with dissociation constant values of 26.1 and 33.4 nM and binding-site concentrations of 6.1 and 12.7 fmole/mg protein (295 and 267 fmole/mg DNA).

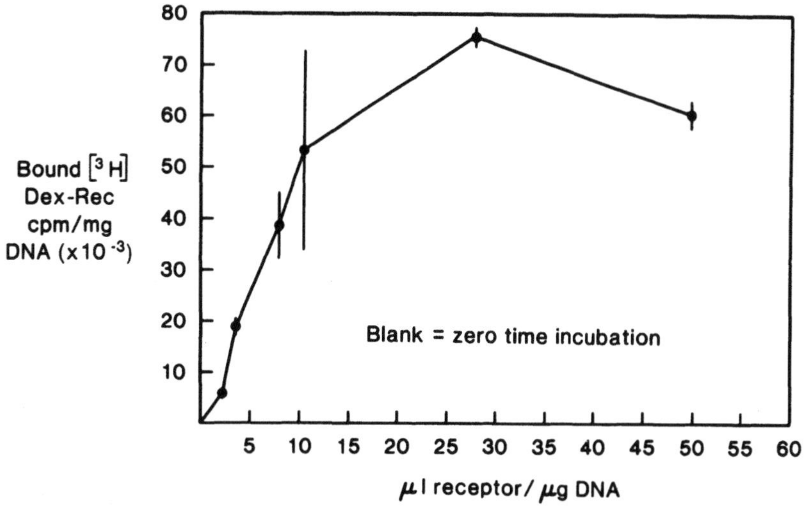

Figure 15. Cell-free binding of glucocorticoid receptor to isolated chromatin. Cell-free nuclear binding assay was performed by adding increasing amounts of isolated chromatin to a constant amount of partially purified (by 35 percent ammonium sulfate precipitation) (^3H) dexamethasone-labeled receptor (Dex-Rec). Control blanks of zero time and no chromatin were also processed. After incubation, chromatin was pelleted and binding of receptor was quantitated, as described in the text. (From Lageson et al., 1983; with permission)

Comparisons of the data from the three trimesters reveal no significant differences among the dissociation constants. These results suggest that similar receptor protein is present in the placenta at every stage of gestation. Comparisons of the mean concentrations of the receptor in the second and third trimesters on the basis of either mass of protein or mass of DNA in the tissue sample also showed no significant differences. In contrast, the receptor concentration in the first trimester was significantly lower.

Differences appeared also in the ability of cytoplasmic receptor from the three trimesters to bind to chromatin in vitro. Such binding measured from 53,000 to 56,000 cpm/mg DNA in the test with receptor from a second-trimester placenta, and 74,000 to 78,000 with term placental receptor (Figure 17). Because the preparations of receptor from these two stages of placenta had been adjusted to equivalent concentrations of bound (^3H) dexamethasone, the observed differences may reflect different capacities of the two receptors for binding to nuclear acceptor sites. Alternatively, the different levels of binding may reflect a difference in the stability of the two receptor preparations during the binding assay.

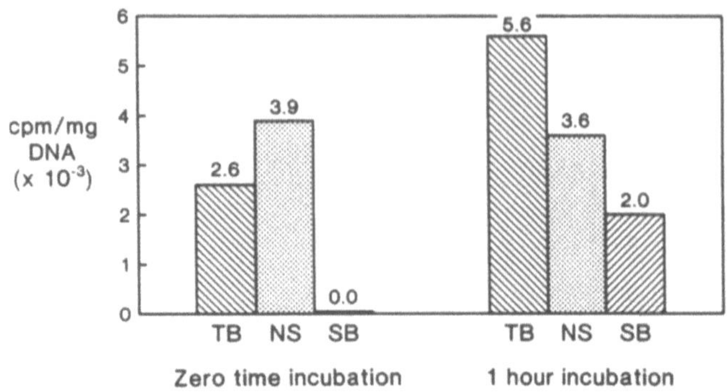

Figure 16. Intact-cell nuclear binding of glucocorticoid receptor. Fresh, pulverized mature placental tissue was incubated with 50 nM (^{3}H) dexamethasone at 22°C for 1 h in 50 percent McCoy's medium. The tissue was washed after incubation, and nuclei were isolated. Radioactivity on filters was quantitated by liquid scintillation method. Approximately 100 to 300 µg of DNA (as tissue) was collected on filters. Zero-time control was used as background. (TB = total binding; NS = nonspecific binding or that performed with an excess of unlabeled steroid; SB = specific binding.) (From Lageson et al., 1983; with permission)

DISCUSSION

Previous work has suggested that the placenta might be a target tissue for steroids as well as a source of steroid production. Estrogen, progesterone, and glucocorticoid-binding proteins ("receptors") have been investigated in rodent placentae (Wong and Burton, 1974; McCormack and Glasser, 1976; Guerne and Stutinsky, 1978; Ogle, 1980; Kneussel et al., 1982); and an androgen receptor has been identified in human placental tissue (Barile et al., 1979; McCormick et al., 1981a). Reports of the presence of estrogen and progesterone receptors in human placentae have been conflicting (Fujimori and Yamada, 1977; McCormick et al., 1981b; Younes et al., 1981).

Our study revealed no estrogen or progesterone receptor. By contrast, specific androgen and glucocorticoid binding to soluble proteins from human placentae showed the presence of high-affinity, low-capacity, and steroid-specific receptors. Similar binding proteins were identified in the nuclear fraction. In addition, a nuclear binding capacity was identified in both cell-free and intact cell assays for both steroids. These data strongly suggest that both androgen and glucocorticoid receptors are present in human placenta. R 1881 has been shown to bind specifically to receptors but not to sex hormone binding globulin, as natural androgens do (Bonne and Raynaud, 1975). R 1881 has also been shown to bind to progesterone receptors (Zava et al., 1979). However, no progesterone receptors are demonstrable in cytosol from human placenta by use of (^{3}H) progesterone or its synthetic analogue (^{3}H) R 5020. Because the placenta is exposed to high concentrations of progesterone, most of the progesterone receptor, if present, is likely to be translocated to the nucleus; yet no specific R 5020 binding was demonstrated in the nuclear fraction, even with a 22-hour exchange period.

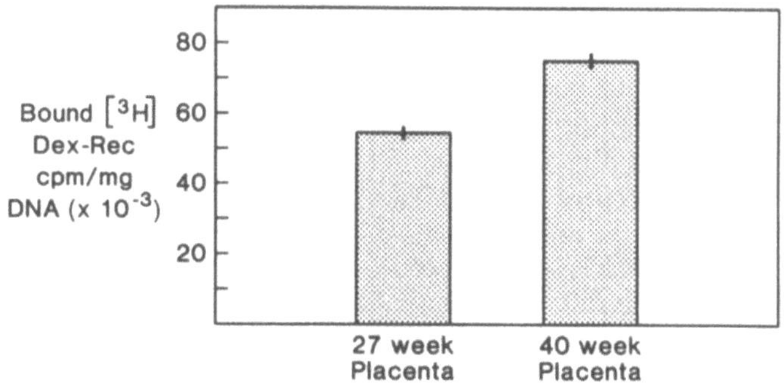

Figure 17. Comparison of cell-free binding of glucocorticoid receptors from preterm and term placentae to isolated chromatin. Ammonium sulfate precipitates of (^{3}H) dexamethasone-labeled 27-week and 40-week placental cytosols were resuspended in buffer A and used to demonstrate chromatin binding by receptors. Previously determined optimal conditions of 90 min of incubation at 0°C to 4°C and a DNA concentration of 25 µg/ml were used for binding. Both histograms represent mean of triplicate analyses; range is indicated by error bars. (From Lageson et al., 1983; with permission)

This observation disagrees with data in another report that described estradiol and progesterone binding in human term placental cytosol (Younes et al., 1981; Kneussel et al., 1982). In that study, the progesterone receptor was thermolabile at temperatures above 15°C and no R 5020 binding was found on sucrose density gradients. Additionally, no nuclear translocation was demonstrated. Several changes, including buffer compositions, failed to identify an estrogen or progesterone receptor. The reason for the discrepancies between these results and those reporting the presence of such receptors in placenta is unknown. It is possible that the present conditions cause a loss or degradation of the estrogen receptor and the progesterone receptor. Alternatively, these steroids bind to many proteins, including serum proteins. It is possible that previous reports describing the presence of estrogen receptors and progesterone receptors in placenta were measuring other binding proteins.

As mentioned earlier, current theory holds that the function of a steroid receptor, after binding the steroid and undergoing an activation process, is to translocate to the nucleus of the target cell and there change the transcription process, leading to an alteration of gene expression (Toft and Gorski, 1966; Jensen and DeSombre, 1972; Mainwaring, 1977). That the estrogen and progesterone binding proteins have not been demonstrated in the placental nuclear fraction in the previous studies (Younes et al., 1981; Kneussel et al., 1982) is evidence that binding proteins may not be steroid receptors. In contrast, the glucocorticoid and androgen binding demonstrated in our experiments are characteristic of a receptor role. Recent studies have implicated the glucocorticoid receptor in placental production of heat-stable alkaline phosphatase (Speeg and Harrison, 1979) and of human chorionic gonadotropin (Wilson and Jaward, 1982). The ability of the androgen to alter transcription in the placenta would further support the concept that the placenta is a target organ for androgen.

Although no differences in the androgen receptor concentrations were observed throughout gestation in the present study, a 7- to 12-fold increase in concentration of glucocorticoid receptor was found between samples of placental tissue from the first to the third trimesters. This difference confirms a previous report (Speeg and Harrison, 1979) of a 27-fold difference between first and third trimester placentae. The pattern of increasing glucocorticoid receptor during gestation suggests an increasing responsiveness of the placenta to the steroid. Whether the glucocorticoids are involved in premature parturition is unclear. The present data indicate that no mechanism for premature parturition can be hypothesized readily on the basis of the relative biologic activity or properties of the receptor from premature placenta, but one may be hypothesized on the basis of the concentration of the receptor.

SUMMARY

Although the function of the placenta as a steroid-producing organ is well known, its function as a target tissue for steroid hormones is less well documented. Human placentae from each trimester were studied for the presence of estrogen, progesterone, androgen, and glucocorticoid receptors. Placental tissue was homogenized in dilute Tris buffer containing thioglycerol (TESH) and centrifuged for 1 h at 10^5 x g. The cytosolic and nuclear fractions were incubated with tritiated estradiol, R 5020, R 1881, and dexamethasone in separate experiments. When (^{3}H)-E_2 and (^{3}H) R 5020 binding were studied, no specific binding was demonstrated. In contrast, (^{3}H) R 1881 and (^{3}H) dexamethasone demonstrated specific binding with saturation between 8 and 16 h. Scatchard analysis revealed high-affinity (Kd = 1.7-3.6 x 10^{-8}), low-capacity (n = 1.35-2.16 x 10^{-13} mol/g protein) binding of (^{3}H) dexamethasone and high-affinity (Kd = 1.3-50 nM), low-capacity (n = 1.2-21 fmole/mg protein) binding of (^{3}H) R 1881. Results of competitive binding assays and sucrose density gradient analyses were characteristic of steroid receptors. Similar binding proteins were identified in the nuclear fraction, suggesting that nuclear translocation occurs in vivo. Ammonium sulfate precipitation showed that the receptor bound to nuclear acceptor sites in cell-free assays. The data suggest the placenta is a target tissue for glucocorticoids and androgen, but not for estrogen and progesterone.

REFERENCES

Barile, G., Giani, S., Montemurro, A., Mango, D. and Scirpa, P. (1979) Evidence for a testosterone binding macromolecule in human placental cytosol. *J. Ster. Biochem.* 11, 1247-1252.

Baxter, J.D. and Funder, J.W. (1979) Hormone receptors. *N. Eng. J. Med.* 301, 1149-1161.

Bonne, C. and Raynaud, J.-P. (1975) Methyltrienolone, a specific ligand for cellular androgen receptors. *Steroids* 26, 227-232.

Boyd, P.A. and Spelsberg, T.C. (1979a) Analysis of the molecular species of the chick oviduct progesterone receptor using isoelectric focusing. *Biochemistry* 18, 3679-3685.

Boyd, P.A. and Spelsberg, T.C. (1979b) Seasonal changes in the molecular species and nuclear binding of the chick oviduct progesterone receptor. *Biochemistry* 18, 3685-3690.

Bradford, M.M. (1976) A rapid and sensitive method for the quantitation of microgram quantities of protein utilizing the principle of protein-dye binding. *Anal. Biochem.* 72, 248-254.

Burton, K. (1956) A study of the conditions and mechanism of the diphenylamine reaction for the colorimetric estimation of deoxyribonucleic acid. *Biochem. J.* 62, 315-323.

Chan, L. and O'Malley, B.W. (1976) Mechanism of action of the sex steroid hormones (first of three parts). *N. Eng. J. Med.* 294, 1322-1328.

Diczfalusy, E. (1968) Steroid metabolism in the foeto-placental unit. *Exerpta Medica, International Congress Series* 183, 65-109.

Do, Y.-S. and Leavitt, W.W. (1978) Characterization of a specific progesterone receptor in decidualized hamster uterus. *Endocrinology* 102, 443-451.

Fujimori, K. and Yamada, M.O. (1977) In vitro evidence of 17-β estradiol receptor in human placenta. *Cell. Mol. Biol.* 22, 357-365.

Giannopoulos, G. and Tulchinsky, D. (1979) Cytoplasmic and nuclear progestin receptors in human myometrium during the menstrual cycle and in pregnancy at term. *J. Clin. Endocrinol. Metab.* 49, 100-106.

Guerné, J.M. and Stutinsky, F. (1978) Estradiol and progesterone binding in rabbit placenta during gestation. *Horm. Metab. Res.* 10, 548-553.

Jensen, E.V. and DeSombre, E.R. (1972) Mechanism of action of the female sex hormones. *Ann. Rev. Biochem.* 41, 203-230.

Kneussel, E.S., Ances, I.G. and Albrecht, E.D. (1982) A specific cytosolic estrogen receptor in human term placenta. *Amer. J. Obstet. Gynecol.* 144, 803-809.

Korenman, S.G. (1968) Radio-ligand binding assay of specific estrogens using a soluble uterine macromolecule. *J Clin Endo Metab*, 28, 127-130.

Mainwaring, W.I.P. (1977) The mechanism of action of androgens. *Monog. Endocrinol.* 10, 1-178.

McCarty, K.S., Jr. and McCarty, K.S., Sr. (1978) Steroid hormone receptors in the regulation of differentiation: A review. *Amer. J. Path.* 86, 705-744.

McCormack, S.A. and Glasser, S.R. (1976) A high-affinity estrogen-bibnding protein in rat placental trophoblast. *Endocrinology* 99, 701-712.

McCormick, P.D., Razel, A.J., Spelsberg, T.C. and Coulam, C.B. (1981a) Evidence for an androgen receptor in the human placenta. Amer. J Obstet. Gyneco. 140, 8-13.

McCormick, P.D., Razel, A.J., Spelsberg, T.C. and Coulam, C.B. (1981b) Absence of high-affinity binding of progesterone (R 5020) in human placenta and fetal membranes. *Placenta Suppl. 3*, 123-132.

Milgrom, E., Atger, M. and Baulieu, E.E. (1970) Progesterone in uterus and plasma. IV - Progesterone receptor(s) in guinea pig uterus cytosol. *Steroids* 16,741-754.

Ogle, T.F. (1980) Characteristics of high affinity progesterone binding to rat placental cytosol. *Endocrinology* 106, 1861-1868.
Pikler, G.M., Webster, R.A. and Spelsberg, T.C. (1976) Nuclear binding of progesterone in hen oviduct: Binding to multiple sites in vitro. *Biochem. J.* 156, 399-408.
Scatchard, G. (1949) The attractions of proteins for small molecules and ions. *Ann. NY Acad. Sci.* 51, 660-672.
Schwartz, B.E., Milewich, L., Gant, N.F., Porter, J.C., Johnston, J.M. and MacDonald, P.C. (1977) Progesterone binding and metabolism in human fetal membranes. *Ann. NY Acad. Sci.* 286, 304-310.
Speeg, K.V., Jr. and Harrison, R.W. (1979) The ontogony of the human placental glucocorticoid receptor and inducibility of heat-stable alkaline phosphatase. *Endocrinology* 104, 1364-1368.
Spelsberg, T.C. and Hnilica, L.S. (1971) Proteins of chromatin in template restriction. I. RNA synthesis in vitro. *Biochem. Biophys. Acta.* 228, 202-211.
Spelsberg, T.C. and Toft, D.O. (1976) The mechanism of action of progesterone. In *Receptors and Mechanism of Action of Steroid Hormones (in two parts)* (ed.), Pasqualini, J.R., Part 1, p. 261- 309. New York: Marcel Dekker.
Thrall, C.L. and Spelsberg, T.C. (1980) Factors affecting the binding of chick oviduct progesterone receptor to deoxyribonucleic acid: Evidence that deoxyribonucleic acid alone is not the nuclear acceptor site. *Biochemistry* 19, 4130-4138.
Toft, D. and Gorski, J. (1966) A receptor molecule for estrogens: Isolation from the rat uterus and preliminary characterization. *Proc. Nat. Acad. Sci. U..Amer.* 55, 1574-1581.
Wilson, E.A. and Jaward, M.J. (1982) Stimulation of human chorionic gonadotropin secretion by glucocorticoids. *Amer. J. Obstet Gynecol.* 42, 344-349.
Wong, M.D. and Burton, A.F. (1974) Studies on corticosterone-receptor complexes from mouse placenta. *Can. J. Biochem.* 52, 190-195.
Younes, M.A., Besch, N.F. and Besch, P.K. (1981) Estradiol and progesterone binding in human term placental cytosol. *Amer. J. Obstet. Gynecol.* 141, 170-174.
Zava, D.T., Landrum, B., Horwitz, K.B. and McGuire, W.L. (1979) Androgen receptor assay with (^{3}H)methyltrienolone (1881) in the presence of progesterone receptors. *Endocrinology* 104, 1007-1012.

Trophoblast Research 1: 271-278, 1983

THE PLACENTAL SECRETION OF SP_1: A COMPARISON OF CONCENTRATIONS IN RETROPLACENTAL AND PERIPHERAL BLOOD

Abdel Ghaffar Ahmed, Dorothy Goodwin and Arnold Klopper

Department of Obstetrics and Gynaecology
University of Aberdeen
Royal Infirmary, Aberdeen, AB9 2ZB Scotland

INTRODUCTION

Schwangerschafts protein 1 (SP_1) is a placental protein. It was originally extracted from the placenta by Bohn in 1971. Its presence in the syncytiotrophoblast was subsequently demonstrated by immunofluorescent staining (Bohn and Sedlacek, 1975; Tatarinov et al., 1976; Lin and Halbert, 1976). The issue was clinched by Horne et al., (1976) who demonstrated the incorporation of radioactive amino acids into SP_1 by trophoblast explants. A secondary question arose when it was found there was not one, but two, proteins with SP_1 determinants in the blood of pregnant women (Teisner et al., 1978; Ahmed and Klopper, 1980). The original investigators made no distinction between the two, and it is not clear whether the placenta produces $SP_1\beta$, or $SP_1\alpha$ or both.

There is an odd finding about SP_1 which is difficult to reconcile with its placental origin: Several groups of investigators have found that the concentration of SP_1 is higher in the peripheral venous blood than in retroplacental blood (Klopper and Hughes, 1978; Klopper et al., 1979; Grudzinskas et al., 1979; Grudzinskas et al., 1980). This is very surprising if the retroplacental space is the place where SP_1 is released from the placenta. We have recently devised a technique for the separate measurement of $SP_1\beta$ and $SP_1\alpha$ and have applied this to examine whether it is $SP_1\beta$ and $SP_1\alpha$ or both that is secreted by the placenta.

MATERIALS AND METHODS

Blood samples were taken from 22 women who delivered in the Aberdeen Maternity Hospital. They were all uncomplicated pregnancies at term and gave birth to babies ranging in weight from 2880-4250 gm with an average birthweight of 3458 gm. The placental weight averaged 595 gm (range 400-950 gm). Five of the women were undergoing elective Caesarean section; the remainder had spontaneous vaginal deliveries. Ten of the 22 women were primiparae.

Venous blood was drawn from an antecubital vein just before delivery. When the placenta was delivered, the membranes were inverted over the placenta and the retroplacental blood collected from the maternal surface by syringe, taking care to avoid contamination with amniotic fluid, fetal blood or antiseptic solutions. At Caesarean section we found we could get retroplacental blood free from fetal fluid by sampling the blood which came up between the placenta and the uterine wall, as the placenta separated.

Human chorionic gonadotropin (hCG) was measured by radioimmunoassay using the β-hCG kit supplied by Serono Diagnostics (Hypolab S.A. Switzerland). Measurement of hPL was also by radioimmunoassay using the kit marketed by the Radiochemical Centre, Amersham. Pregnancy-associated plasma protein A (PAPP-A), another placental protein, was measured by immunoelectrophoresis (Bischof et al., 1979). SP_1, without separating the two components, was measured by the immunoelectrophoretic technique of Bruce and Klopper (1978), adding 4 percent of polyethylene glycol to the agarose used for electrophoresis to ensure adequate precipitation of $SP_1\alpha$. Both proteins are precipitated by the antiserum in the conditions of assay and the value obtained represents roughly the total of $SP_1\beta$ and $SP_1\alpha$. A further aliquot of serum was assayed for $SP_1\beta$ and $SP_1\alpha$ using the method of Ahmed and Klopper (1982a) to separate the proteins and an immunoelectrophoretic endpoint. In this technique, the separation of $SP_1\alpha$ and $SP_1\beta$ is achieved by chromatography of the serum on hydroxylapatite. The intra-assay precision for $SP_1\alpha$ is 3.7 percent on this method and for $SP_1\beta$ is 4.1 percent. The interassay precision for both proteins is 4.8 percent.

All samples were assayed in duplicate, and the average used in the analysis. The retroplacental value of each protein was compared to the peripheral value in the same patient using Student's paired-t-test.

RESULTS

Table 1 shows the mean and standard error of the values found in peripheral venous and in retroplacental blood. Figure 1 shows the mean values obtained when the concentrations of each protein in retroplacental blood were expressed as a percentage of the corresponding value in the peripheral blood. The concentrations of βhCG, hPL and of PAPP-A are significantly higher in retroplacental blood than in peripheral blood as might be expected if they are secreted into the retroplacental space in the first instance.

The concentration of $SP_1\beta$, on the other hand, is lower in the retroplacental blood than in peripheral blood. As $SP_1\beta$ is by much the major component of the mixture designated SP_1, the latter is also, not surprisingly, lower in retroplacental blood than in peripheral blood. By contrast, $SP_1\alpha$ follows the same pattern as other placental proteins and is higher in retroplacental blood.

The individual results for PAPP-A and SP_1 are contrasted in Figure 2. In the case of PAPP-A the retroplacental values were higher than the peripheral vein in 11 subjects, there was no significant difference in 9 subjects and only 2 women had peripheral blood concentrations of PAPP-A higher than the retroplacental value (Figure 2A). On the other hand, SP_1 values were higher in retroplacental blood in only 3 subjects, much the same in 11, and significantly higher in peripheral blood in 8 women (Figure 2B).

Table I

The concentrations of pregnancy-specific proteins in the peripheral venous blood and retroplacental blood in 22 women

Type of protein	Peripheral blood		Retroplacental blood		P
	Mean	Standard error	Mean	Standard error	
β-hCG	10.71 IU/ml	2.54	12.88 IU/ml	2.76	<0.025
hPL	8.85 mg/l	0.96	13.56 mg/l	0.50	<0.0005
PAPP-A	152.43 IU/ml	26.81	163.73 IU/ml	26.76	<0.01
SP_1	173.79 mg/l	13.22	166.57 mg/l	12.74	(-)<0.01
$SP_1\beta$	149.48 mg/l	11.27	141.63 mg/l	2.28	(-)<0.005
$SP_1\alpha$	28.33 mg/l	1.48	31.96 mg/l	2.28	<0.005

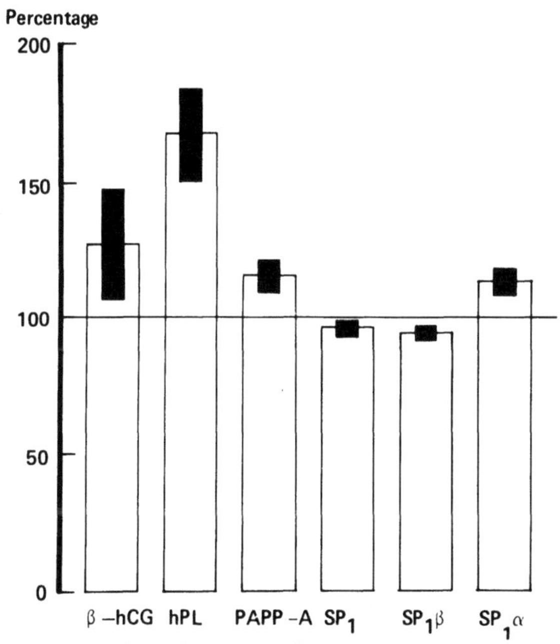

Figure 1. The concentrations (mean and standard error) of pregnancy-specific proteins in the retroplacental blood expressed as a percentage of the value in the maternal peripheral blood, taken as 100 percent.

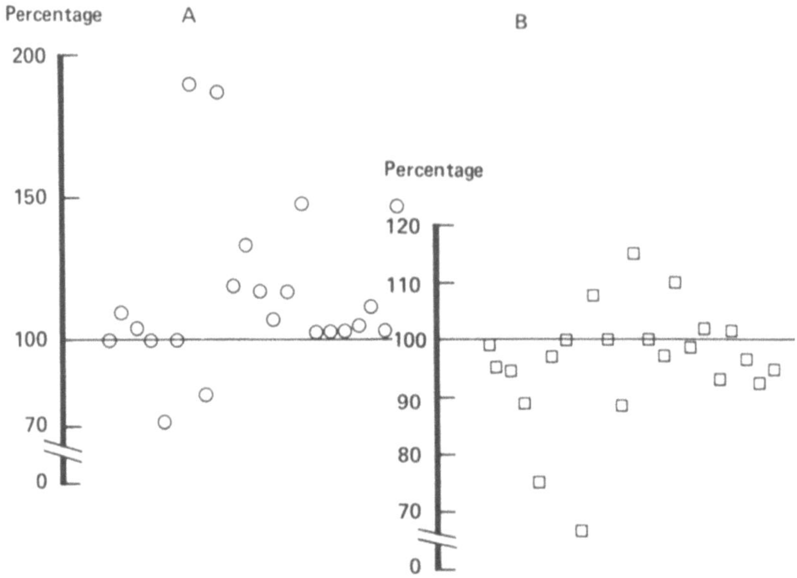

Figure 2. The concentrations of PAPP-A (2A) and of SP_1 (2B) in the retroplacental blood expressed as a percentage of the value in peripheral blood in 22 subjects.

The individual results for $SP_1\beta$ and $SP_1\alpha$ are shown in Figures 3A and 3B. In the case of $SP_1\beta$ the surprising reversal of concentration is even clearer than for SP_1. The retroplacental concentration was significantly higher in only one subject; there was no difference in 12 patients, and in 9 the peripheral value was higher. By contrast, $SP_1\alpha$ follows the same pattern as hCG, hPL and PAPP-A. Retroplacental values were higher than peripheral blood in 15 patients, there was no difference in 4 and only in 3 patients were the peripheral blood values higher.

DISCUSSION

The previous finding that SP_1 concentration is higher in peripiheral blood than in retroplacental blood has been confirmed. It appears that this reversal of what might be expected with a placental product applies to the β component of SP_1. As this is the major constituent of the SP_1 mixture, measurements of SP_1 show the same pattern in spite of the lesser component, $SP_1\alpha$, having the normal pattern of higher values in retroplacental than in peripheral blood.

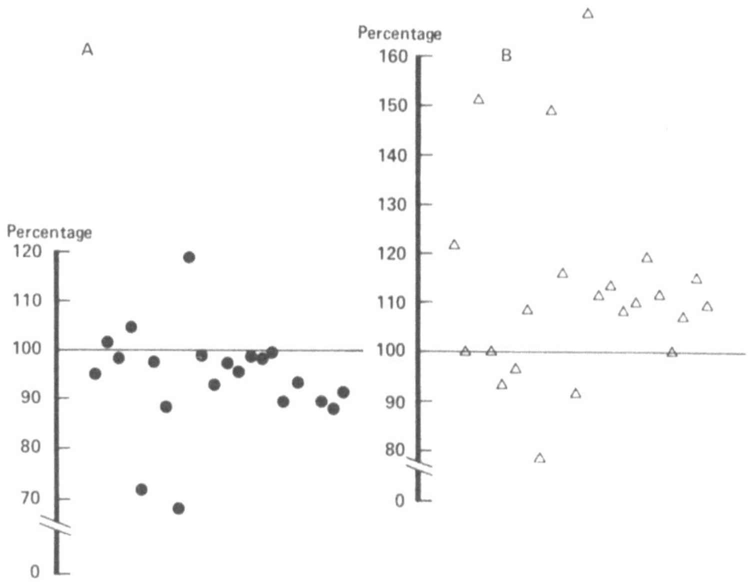

Figure 3. The concentrations of $SP_1\beta$ (3A) and $SP_1\alpha$ (3B) in the retroplacental blood expressed as a percentage of the value in peripheral blood in 21 subjects.

The finding that $SP_1\beta$ is higher in peripheral than in retroplacental blood raises the possibility that its point of entry into the maternal circulation may not be the retroplacental space. Klopper and associates et al. (1979) speculated that SP_1 might not be released by the trophoblast but make its way into the maternal circulation by dissolution of embolic or migrating trophoblast. While this remains a possibility it must be acknowledged that this suggestion does not account for the normal pattern of $SP_1\alpha$. An alternative explanation is that $SP_1\alpha$ is secreted by the placenta. It is certainly present in the placenta and can be extracted from it (Ahmed et al., 1981). The immunological studies localizing SP_1 in the trophoblast do not distinguish between $SP_1\alpha$ and $SP_1\beta$ and could equally well be demonstrating either in the placenta. $SP_1\alpha$ consists of $SP_1\beta$ combined with another protein (Bohn, 1979, Ahmed and Klopper, 1982b). This combination could take place either in the placenta or in the maternal circulation, although in the latter case one would have to postulate that $SP_1\alpha$, formed in the retroplacental blood, is then absorbed by the trophoblast to account for its presence in the placenta. The retroplacental concentration of $SP_1\beta$ would then be lowered by its incorporation into the $SP_1\alpha$ molecule. Alternatively additional amounts of $SP_1\beta$ could be generated in the maternal circulation by the dissolution of $SP_1\alpha$ outside of the retroplacental space.

SUMMARY

The concentrations of pregnancy specific β1 glycoprotein (SP_1) as well as its β and α components ($SP_1β$ and $SP_1α$), human chorionic gonadotropin (hCG), human placental lactogen (hPL) and pregnancy-associated plasma protein A (PAPP-A) were measured in peripheral venous blood and in the retroplacental blood at delivery in 22 women. The values of hCG, hPL, PAPP-A and $SP_1α$ were higher in the retroplacental than in the peripheral blood. By contrast, the concentrations of SP_1 and $SP_1β$ were lower in retroplacental than in peripheral blood.

ACKNOWLEDGMENTS

We are grateful to the Medical Illustration Department, Universtiy of Aberdeen, for preparing the figures, and to Miss Elaine Dalgarno for secretarial assistance. A.G. Ahmed is supported by the University of Assuit, Egypt.

REFERENCES

Ahmed, A.G. and Klopper, A. (1980) Separation of two pregnancy- associated plasma proteins with SP_1 determinants and the conversion of $SP_1β$ to $SP_1α$. *Arch. Gynecol.* 230, 95-108.

Ahmed, A.G., Toop, K. and Klopper, A. (1981) The demonstration of two pregnancy-associated proteins with SP_1 determinants in placental extracts. *Placenta* 2, 45-52.

Ahmed, A.G. and Klopper, A. (1982a) A method for separate measurement of the β- and -α- components of SP_1 in pregnancy serum. *Arch. Gynecol.* 231, 307-313.

Ahmed, A.G. and Klopper, A. (1982b) Immunological observations on the relationship of $SP_1α$ to $SP_1β$. *Gynecol. Obstet. Invest.* 13, 249-256.

Bischof, P., Bruce, D., Cunningham, P. and Klopper, A. (1979) Measurement of pregnancy associated plasma protein A (PAPP-A). *Clinica Chimica Acta* 95, 243-247.

Bohn, H. (1971) Nachweis und Charakterisierung von Schwangerschaftsproteinen in des menschlichen Plazenta, sowie ihre quantitative immunologische Bestimmung im Serum Schwangerer Frauen. *Archiv. für Gynäkol.* 210, 105-121.

Bohn, H. and Sedlacek, H. (1975) Eine vergleichende Untersuchung von plazentaspezifischen Proteinen bei Mensch und subhumanen Primaten. *Archiv. für Gynäkol.* 220, 105-121.

Bohn, H. (1979) Placental and pregnancy proteins. In: Lehmann, H. (Ed.) *Carcinoembryonic proteins*. Amsterdam: Elsevier-North Holland. pp. 289-299.

Bruce, D. and Klopper, A. (1978) The measurement of pregnancy- specific $β_1$ glycoprotein by electroimmunodiffusion. *Clinica Chimica Acta* 84, 107-113.

Grudzinskas, J.G., Menabey, M., Wiley, B.A., Teisner, B. and Chard, T. (1979) The relation between the concentration of placental specific proteins in retroplacental and peripheral blood. *Brit. J. Obstet. Gynaecol.* 86, 891- 893.

Grudzinkas, J.G., Teisner, B. and Chard, T. (1980) The ratio between molecular variants of pregnancy-specific $β_1$ glycoprotein (SP_1) in peripheral and retroplacental circulation during late pregnancy. *Placenta* 1, 223-226.

Horne, C.H., Towler, C.M., Pugh-Humphreys, R.G., Thomson, A.W. and Bohn, H. (1976) Pregnancy-specific $β_1$ - glycoprotein - a product of the syncytiotrophoblast. *Experientia.* 32, 1197-1199.

Klopper, A. and Hughes, G. (1978) Placental secretion of oestrogens and protein hormones. *Archiv. für Gynäkol.* 225, 171-177.
Klopper, A., Smith, R. and Davidson, I (1979) The measurement of trophoblastic proteins as a test of placental function. In: Klopper, A. and Chard, T. (Eds.) *Placental Proteins.* Heidelberg: Springer Verlag. pp. 23-41.
Lin, T.M. and Halbert, S.P. (1976) Placental localization of human pregnancy-associated plasma proteins. *Science* 193, 1249-1252.
Tatarinov, V.S., Falaleeva, D.M., Kalashniikov, V.V. and Toloknov, B.O. (1976) Immunofluorescent localization of human pregnancy-specific β-globulin in placenta and chorioepithelioma. *Nature* 260, 263.
Teisner, B., Westergaard, J.G., Folkersen, J., Husby, S. and Svehag, S.E. (1978) Two pregnancy-associated serum proteins with pregnancy specific β-glycoprotein determinants. *Amer. J. Obstet. Gynecol.* 131, 262-266.

Trophoblast Research 1: 279-288,1983

STORAGE AND RELEASE OF RENIN AND hCG IN TROPHOBLAST FROM HUMAN CHORION LAEVE

Alan M. Poisner[1], Hsien-Chen Cheng[2], Gary W. Wood[3] and Roselle Poisner[1]

Department of Pharmacology [1]
Department of Obstetrics and Gynecology [2]
Department of Pathology [3]
University of Kansas College of Health Sciences, Kansas City
Kansas 66103, U.S.A.

INTRODUCTION

We have recently demonstrated by immunocytochemical and biochemical methods that the trophoblast layer of the term chorion laeve and isolated chorionic cells contain renin (Poisner et al., 1981a). We have also shown that cultured chorionic cells continue to synthesize and release renin for periods up to six weeks (Poisner et al., 1982a). Since the principal cell in the trophoblast layer is the cytotrophoblast (Bourne, 1962), we have examined two other potential cell markers of trophoblast, hCG and progesterone. The origin of hCG in the placenta is generally considered to be the syncytiotrophoblast (Friesen, 1973), although cells with the appearance of cytotrophoblast or transitional cell types have also been reported to contain hCG (Thiede and Choate, 1963; Patillo et al., 1971). Progesterone has also been found in trophoblast, but the localization of hCG and progesterone in the chorion laeve has not been well studied.

The present study is part of an ongoing investigation into the cellular regulation of renin and other hormones in human fetal membranes. In addition to studying the cellular localization of renin, hCG and progesterone in human chorion laeve, we have also examined the release of these substances from a variety of model systems, including cultured cells and superfused membranes. Preliminary portions of this work have been reported (Poisner et al., 1982b).

MATERIALS AND METHODS

Chorion laeve were obtained from term vaginal deliveries. The amnion was stripped away and the chorion was rinsed with saline. The rinsed chorion was then used (a) to prepare isolated cells, (b) for direct extraction, or (c) for membrane perfusion. Preparation of isolated cells and cell culture were carried out as previously described, using enzymatic digestion with collagenase and separation on a Percoll density gradient (Poisner et al., 1981a; Poisner et al., 1982b). Aliquots of 5×10^5 cells were plated (renin content averaged 147 $\mu U/10^6$ cells). Tissues were extracted with 0.1% Triton X-100 after freezing and thawing. For membrane perfusion, 2 cm circular pieces of fetal membranes were clamped between the two chambers of a Ussing-type apparatus and perfused at 0.5-1.0 ml/min with modified Krebs solution without stripping away the amnion (Poisner et al., 1982a). The two sides of the membrane were perfused independently, and perfusates from the two sides were collected separately in a fraction collector.

Immunofluorescence techniques

For immunofluorescence studies, standard techniques previously reported were carried out using rabbit antiserum to hCG and FITC-labeled goat anti-rabbit antiserum (Poisner et al., 1981a). Controls were performed with non-immune rabbit serum.

Renin assays

Renin in chorionic extracts and cultured chorionic cells has previously been shown to be almost exclusively in the form of inactive renin (trypsin-activated) (Poisner et al., 1981a,b; Poisner et al., 1982a). It was assayed using 2 µg/ml trypsin for activation, nephrectomized sheep serum for substrate, and radioimmunoassay of the generated angiotensin 1 (Poisner et al., 1981a,b).

Radioimmunoassays

The hCG was assayed using the second antibody technique. Antiserum to the beta subunit of hCG-SB6 was provided by the NIAMD-Human Pituitary Agency. The Second International Standard for hCG was obtained from the Division of Biological Standards, Holly Hill, London. Highly purified hCG for iodination was purchased from Calbiochem-Behring Corp. and goat anti-rabbit Immunobeads second antibody was purchased from Bio-Rad Laboratories. The limit of sensitivity was 1.0 mIU/ml. hCG was also assayed in some samples with the immunoradiometric assay (Hybridtech-Tandem hCG assay) which employs two monoclonal antibodies and measures only the intact hormone. Progesterone was assayed as previously described for our laboratory (Johnson and Cheng, 1978).

RESULTS

hCG and progesterone in chorion and isolated cells

Immunofluorescence studies for hCG in term chorion laeve revealed positive fluorescence in the trophoblast layer (Figure 1). The pattern was identical to that previously shown for renin (Poisner et al., 1981a). Control experiments with non-immune rabbit serum were negative. These results were identical to the immunofluorescence studies on renin in the chorion laeve which indicated presence in trophoblast (Poisner et al., 1981a). In one sample of lyophilized chorion, hCG was also assayed by the TANDEM immunoradiometric assay which measures the intact hormone (Tandem hCG - Hybridtech, San Diego, CA). The concentration of hCG by the standard radioimmunoassay using the antibody to the beta subunit was 35.0 mIU/ml extract; with the TANDEM assay the value found was 35.6 mIU/ml. Therefore, the hCG assayed with the standard antiserum to the beta subunit reflected the intact hormone.

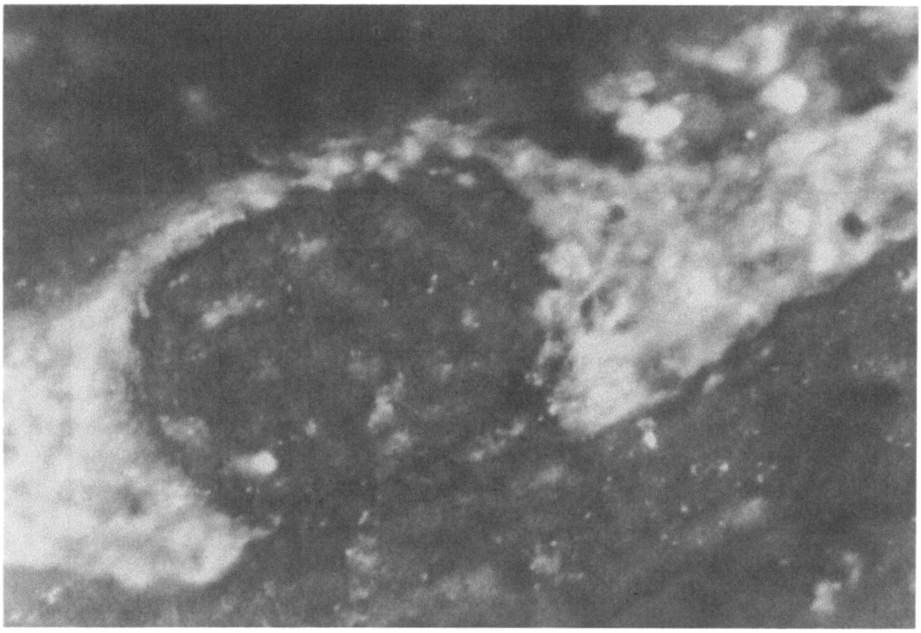

Figure 1. Immunocytochemical localization of hCG in the trophoblast layer of term chorion laeve. Standard indirect immunofluorescence technique reveals a positive fluorescence in the trophoblast layer. The dark atrophic villus does not fluoresence. The pattern is identical to that found for human renin (Poisner et al., 1981a). Control sections treated with non- immune serum are negative. (Magnification x 320)

Analysis of the isolated cells for renin and hCG showed a stoichiometric relationship between renin and hCG (Table 1). The mean ratio in 8 preparations of cells was 5.14 µU renin/mIU hCG and the correlation coefficient was 0.993. In three other preparations of cells the mean ratio of renin to progesterone was 48.0 ± 5.0 µU/ng progesterone, and the ratio of hCG to progesterone was 7.6 ± 1.5 mIU/ng.

Release of renin and hCG from cultured cells

When isolated chorionic cells were incubated for periods up to six weeks, renin was continuously released into the culture medium (Poisner et al., 1981a). More than 99% of the renin was in the form of trypsin-activated renin (inactive renin). The concentration of renin in the culture medium reached values of more than 40,000 micro Units (µU)/ml. However, measurements of hCG in these samples revealed only traces. Thus the ability to synthesize and release hCG apeared to disappear after long term culture. In short term cultures (six days), hCG was detectable in the medium bathing the cultured cells. After six days of culture, fresh medium (minus fetal calf serum) was replaced on the cells at 30 min intervals. Renin and hCG were found in the medium. The hCG levels ranged from 14-35 mIU/ml and renin from 5.5- 8.2 µU/ml. When cells were exposed to digitonin, an agent known to release substances from cells by acting on the cell membrane (Mackall et al., 1979), there was an increased release of hCG and of renin (Table 2).

Table 1
Renin and hCG in isolated chorionic cells.

Sample	Renin μU/ml	hCG mIU/ml	Ratio
1	57.5	10.7	5.38
2	47.0	11.7	4.02
3	31.5	8.3	3.79
4	1050.0	200.0	5.25
5	158.0	33.8	4.66
6	498.0	74.7	6.77
7	1298.0	211.0	6.15
8	563.0	111.0	5.07
mean			5.14 ± 0.36

Isolated chorionic cells were prepared from term chorionic laeve by digestion, filtration and density gradient centrifugation as described previously (Poisner et al., 1981a). After extraction in 0.1% Triton X-100, samples were assayed for renin and hCG.

Release of renin and hCG from superfused fetal membranes

In an initial experiment, a 2 cm diameter circular piece of chorion laeve (with amnion still attached) was clamped between two chambers of a Ussing-type membrane holder and perfused with modified Krebs solution at 0.5 ml/min. A period of 80 minutes of washout was allowed for the preparation to equilibrate and then the medium was changed to calcium-free Krebs containing 1 mM EGTA and 0.1 mM verapamil for 30 minutes. Renin and hCG were measured in the effluent appearing on the amnion side and on the chorion side (Table 3).

DISCUSSION

The present results provide several pieces of evidence which suggest that renin and hCG are in the same cells in the chorion laeve, namely trophoblast. First, immunofluorescence studies indicate that hCG-positive cells are localized in the same layer of the chorion laeve as is renin, the trophoblast layer. Secondly, biochemical analysis shows a stoichiometric relationship between renin and hCG in isolated cells, with a correlation coefficient of 0.99. Finally, superfusion of the chorion laeve produces a parallel release of renin and hCG. The presence of progesterone in the same preparations of chorionic cells which contain renin and hCG indicates the broad endocrine potential of the fetal membranes. Experiments in progress indicate that progesterone is released from the superfused fetal membranes. Further studies will

Table 2
Release of renin and hCG from cultured chorionic cells.

Experiment	Treatment	(Time)	Renin µU/ml	hCG mIU/ml
1	Control	0-30	8.2	24.6
	"	30-60	7.5	30.6
	"	60-90	6.5	32.0
2	"	0-30	5.5	15.4
	"	30-60	6.5	14.0
	Digitonin	60-90	19.4	34.2

Isolated chorionic cells were cultured for 6 days in RPMI medium + 10% fetal calf serum (FCS). A 2.0 ml fresh medium solution minus FCS was then added and replaced at 30 minute intervals. Digitonin concentration was 0.1 mg/ml.

Table 3
Release of renin and hCG from dual perfused chorio-amnion

Time	Treatment	Fetal Side		Maternal Side	
		Renin µU/ml	hCG mIU/ml	Renin µU/ml	hCG mIU/ml
75-80	Control	28.8	2.6	41.3	2.6
80-85	Ca-free	33.5	3.0	53.3	3.0
85-90	Ca-free	55.5	7.9	63.3	5.0
90-95	Ca-free	62.5	6.8	75.0	3.0
96-100	Ca-free	44.0	5.2	39.3	1.0

A 3.14 cm^2 piece of chorio-amnion was clamped between two chambers of a Ussing-type apparatus, and both chambers were perfused separately at 0.5 ml/min with Krebs solution containing 1 mg/ml BSA for 80 minutes. Then perfusion was changed to a calcium-free medium containing 2.0 mM EGTA and 0.1 mM verapamil. The concentrations of renin and hCG appearing in the medium emerging from the two chambers are shown.

be required to determine if the release of these various factors can be independently regulated.

There is now evidence for the presence in both plasma and the placenta of a number of proteins presumed to be of trophoblastic origin (Klopper, 1980). Most of these are thought to be produced by syncytiotrophoblast. The protein content of trophoblast in the chorion laeve is less well documented. As mentioned earlier, current indications are that hCG in the placenta is almost exclusively in the syncytiotrophoblast. We have found that cytotrophoblast (but not syncytiotrophoblast) in 18-20 week placentae is positive for renin by immuno-fluorescence (Wood and Poisner, unpublished observations). The increase in the concentration of inactive renin in the plasma of patients during pregnancy is consistent with a source in the placenta (and/or fetal membranes) (Hsueh et al.,1982). The time course of the rise of plasma inactive renin during pregnancy resembles to some extent the changes in hCG levels, but not that of hPL (Simpson and McDonald, 1981). It is also worth noting that plasma renin levels are often elevated in cases of molar pregnancy, a trophoblastic tumor (Mulrow, 1977).

The trophoblast of the chorion laeve include transitional elements as well as cytotrophoblast-appearing cells (Anderson and McKay, 1966). Cells isolated from amniotic fluid and grown in tissue culture contain hCG and differentiate into multinucleate cells (Priest et al., 1979; Priest and Priest, 1980). This has led to the suggestion that these cells are of trophoblastic origin (Priest and Priest, 1980). We have recently found that cells isolated from amniotic fluid also contain renin (Poisner, Wood and King, unpublished observations).

The functional significance of renin in trophoblast is unknown (as is that of most placental proteins) but it has been speculated that it could be related to local vascular control, membrane permeability or events associated with parturition (Poisner et al., 1982c). Most of the renin in the chorion laeve is inactive and its physiological activation is unknown (Poisner et al., 1981b). The association of renin with hCG brings into question whether the release of these substances may be under different physiological control. There is not yet any information on this question, but cyclic AMP has been implicated in the release of both renin and hCG in other systems (Michelakis et al., 1969; Simpson and MacDonald, 1981). The increased release of renin and hCG on calcium deprivation is of interest in terms of the mechanisms of hormone release. Calcium deprivation has been reported to cause renin release from the kidney in certain experimental conditions, but its role is still uncertain (Fray, 1980). Under certain experimental conditions, calcium has been shown to increase renin release (Chen and Poisner, 1976). EGTA inhibits hCG release from malignant trophoblast but so does the calcium ionophore A23187 (Hussa, 1977). It was suggested that there are basic differences between hormone secretory mechanisms in the malignant trophoblast and other endocrine tissues (Hussa, 1977). EGTA inhibits renin release from cultured chorionic trophoblast (Poisner et al., 1982). In most secretory systems, extracellular calcium is required for stimulus-secretion coupling. The evidence to date indicates that the release of renin from the kidney and from trophoblast and the release of hCG from trophoblast may follow a different pattern.

There are reasons to consider a role for the renin- angiotensin system in the endocrine physiology of the placenta. Angiotensin can release LH, GH and PRL from anterior pituitary glands in vitro (Steele et al., 1981), and there are high affinity receptors for angiotensin II on membranes from the anterior pituitary gland (Muhrejee et al., 1981). Renin has been detected in the LH-containing cells in the anterior pituitary of the rat, but not in the other endocrine cells of the anterior pituitary (Naruse et al.,1981). Therefore, there is evidence that the renin-angiotensin system may be a factor in regulating the release of LH and related hormones.

We have reported on the presence of renin in the epithelial cells of the amnion (Poisner et al., 1982c). However, no evidence for synthesis of renin could be demonstrated in organ culture of amnion (Symonds et al., 1968) or in cells cultured from amnion (Poisner et al., 1982a). It was suggested that one explanation for the renin in the amnion could be due to an uptake from the extracellular fluid (Poisner et al., 1982a). Uptake of hCG might also explain the reports of hCG in the amnion (delkonicoff and Cedard, 1973; Thiede and Fierer, 1966). Uptake mechanisms for various peptides, including hCG, have been described (Ahmed et al., 1981).

These studies which began with an investigation of renin in amniotic fluid (Johnson et al., 1979a,b) have more recently been concerned with the fetal membranes (Poisner et al.,1981a,b; Poisner et al., 1982a,b; Poisner, 1982). It now appears that the fetal membranes are not only of interest with respect to the renin-angiotensin system, but also as a potential source and target for a variety of hormones.

SUMMARY

Immunofluorescence studies on human chorion laeve have revealed that both hCG and renin are present in the trophoblast layer. Analysis of cells isolated from the chorion shows a correlation of renin with hCG; the ratio of renin to hCG was 5.14 μU/mIU. The isolated cells also contain progesterone. Cultured chorionic cells release renin and hCG in short term culture and their release is enhanced by treatment with digitonin, an agent known to labilize the cell membrane. When a piece of chorioamnion was superfused in a dual perfusion apparatus, both renin and hCG were released into the medium on the fetal and the maternal sides. A period of calcium deprivation (calcium omitted, EGTA = 1.0 mM, verapamil = 0.1 mM) causes a transient increase in the release of renin and hCG on both sides of the membrane. The presence in the chorion of renin (together with hCG and progesterone) and its reported identification in the LH cells of the anterior pituitary suggest that the renin-angiotensin system may be involved in reproductive physiology. The fetal membranes are considered to be a source of and a target for a variety of hormones.

ACKNOWLEDGMENTS

This work was supported by grants from the Kansas Heart Association and NIH HD-14065. We wish to acknowledge the help of Dr. Charles King in obtaining the clinical material.

REFERENCES

Ahmed, C.E., Sawyer, H.R. and Niswender, G.D. (1981) Internalization and degradation of human chorionic gonadotropin in ovine luteal cells: Kinetic studies. *Endocrinology* 109, 1380-1387.

Anderson, W.R. and McKay, D.G. (1966) Electron microscope study of the trophoblast in normal and toxemic placentas. *Amer. J. Obstet. Gynecol.* 95, 1134-1148.

Bourne, G. (1962) *The Human Amnion and Chorion.* London: Lloyd-Luke, p. 10.

Chen, D.S. and Poisner, A.M. (1976) Direct stimulation of renin release by calcium. *Proc. Soc. Exper. Biol. Med.* 152, 565-567.

delkonicoff, L.K. and Cedard, L. (1973) Localization of human chorionic gonadotropin and somatommamotropic hormone by the immunohistoenzymologic method in villi and amniotic epithelium of human placentas (from six weeks to term). *Amer. J. Obstet. Gynecol.* 116, 1124-1129.

Fray, J.C.S. (1980) Stimulus-secretion coupling of renin. *Circul. Res.* 47, 485-492.

Friesen, H. (1973) Placental protein and polypeptide hormones. In *Handbook of Physiology - Endocrinology*, Vol. II, Female Reproductive System, Part 2. (ed.), Greep, R., Washington, D.C.: American Physiological Society, pp. 295-309.

Hsueh, W.A., Luetscher, J.A., Carlson, E.J., Grislis, G., Fraze, E. and McHargue, A. (1982) Changes in active and inactive renin throughout pregnancy. *J. Clin. Endocrinol. Metabol.* 54, 1010-1016.

Hussa, R.O. (1977) Studies on human chorionic gonadotropin secretion: Effects of EGTA, lanthanum, and the ionophore A23187. *J. Clin. Endocrinol. Metabol.* 44, 520-529.

Johnson, D.C. and Cheng, H.C. (1978) Effect of stilbesterol on ovarian responses to pregnant mare's serum gonadotropin in hypophysectomized immature rats. *Endocrinology* 102, 1563-1569.

Johnson, R.L., Fleming, N.W. and Poisner, A.M. (1979a) Chromatographic and kinetic properties of acid- and pepsin-activated renin from human amniotic fluid. *Biochem. Pharm.* 28, 2597-2600.

Johnson, R.L., Poisner, A.M. and Crist, R.D. (1979b) Partial purification and chromatographic properties of inactive renin from human amniotic fluid. *Biochem. Pharm.* 28, 1791-1799.

Klopper, A. (1980) The new placental proteins. *Placenta* 1, 77- 89.

Mackall, J., Meredith, M. and Lane, M.D. (1979) A mild procedure for the rapid release of cytoplasmic enzymes from cultured animal cells. *Anal. Biochem.* 95, 270-274.

Michelakis, A.M., Caudle, J. and Liddle, G.W. (1969) In vitro stimulation of renin production by epinephrine, norepinephrine, and cyclic AMP. *Proc. Soc. Exp. Biol. Med.* 130, 748-753.

Muhrejee, A., Kulkarni, P., McCann, S.M. and Negro-Vilar, A. (1982) Evidence for the presence and characterization of angiotensin II receptors in rat anterior pituitary membranes. *Endocrinology* 110, 665-670.

Mulrow, P.J. (1977) Renin aldosterone system in pregnancy. In *Endocrinology of Pregnancy* (ed.), Fuchs, F. and Klopper, A., Hagerstown: Harper and Row p. 177.

Naruse, K., Takii, Y. and Inagami, T. (1981) Immunohistochemical localization of renin in luteinizing hormone-producing cells of rat pituitary. *Proc. Nat. Acad. Sci.* 78, 7579-7581.

Patillo, R.A., Gey, G.O., Delfs, E., Huang, W.Y., Hause, L., Garancis, J., Knoth, M.,

Amatruda, J., Bertino, J., Friesen, H.G., and Mattingly, R.F. (1971) The hormone-synthesizing trophoblastic cell in vitro: A model for cancer research and placental hormone synthesis. *Annals. NY. Acad. Sci.* 172, 288-298.

Poisner, A.M., Wood, G.W., Poisner, R. and Inagami, T. (1981a) Localization of renin in trophoblasts in human chorion laeve at term pregnancy. *Endocrinology* 109, 1150-1155.

Poisner, A.M., Johnson, R.L., Hanna, G. and Poisner, R. (1981b) Activation of renin in human amniotic fluid and placental membranes. In *Heterogeneity of Renin and Renin Substrate* (ed.), Sambhi, M., Amsterdam: Elsevier North Holland pp. 335-347.

Poisner, A.M., Wood, G.W. and Poisner, R. (1982a) Release of inactive renin from human fetal membranes and isolated trophoblasts. *Clin. Exp. Hypertension* A4,2007-2017.

Poisner, A.M., Cheng, H.C., Wood, G.W. and Poisner, R. (1982b) Simultaneous storage and release of renin and hCG from trophoblasts in human chorion laeve. *Fed. Proc.* 41, 1231.

Poisner, A.M, Wood, G.W., Poisner, R. and Inagami, T. (1982c) Renin and inactive renin in human amnion at term pregnancy. *Proc. Soc. Exp. Biol. Med.* 169, 4-6.

Priest, R.E. and Priest, J.H. (1980) Specialized functions and origins of cultured cells from human amniotic fluid. *In Vitro* 16, 243A.

Priest, R.E., Priest, J.H., Moinuddin, J.F. and Sgoutas, D.S.C. (1979) Differentiation in human amniotic fluid cell cultures: Chorionic gonadotropin production. *In Vitro* 15, 142-147.

Simpson, E.R. and MacDonald, P.C. (1981) Endocrine physiology of the placenta. *Ann. Rev. Physiol.* 43, 163-188.

Steele, M.K., Negro-Vilar, A. and McCann, S.M. (1981) Effect of angiotensin II on in vitro release of anterior pituitary hormones in the female rat. *Endocrinology* 109, 893-899.

Symonds, E.M., Stanley, M.A. and Skinner, S.L. (1968) Production of renin by in vitro cultures of human chorion and uterine muscle. *Nature* 217, 1152-1154.

Thiede, H.A. and Choate, J.W. (1963) Chorionic gonadotropin localilzation in the human placenta by immunofluorescent staining: II. Demonstration of hCG in the trophoblast and amnion epithelium of immature and mature placentas. *Obstet. Gynecol.* 2, 433-443.

Thiede, H.A. and Fierer, M.B. (1966) Detection of hCG in the amnion by biologic and immunologic assay. *Obstet. Gynecol.* 27, 363-370.

Trophoblast Research 1:289-300, 1983

THE ARACHIDONIC ACID PATHWAY AND THE SECRETION OF CHORIONIC GONADOTROPIN (hCG) AND PROGESTERONE BY THE CULTURED HUMAN CHORIOCARCINOMA JEG-3 CELL

John Ilekis and Robert Benveniste

Division of Reproductive Endocrinology and Infertility
Department of Obstetrics and Gynecology
Michael Reese Hospital and Medical Center
Pritzker School of Medicine, University of Chicago
Chicago, Illinois 60616, U.S.A.

INTRODUCTION

Approximately eight weeks after conception, the progesterone producing activity of the human corpus luteum is virtually taken over by the trophoblast, which is already contributing to peak hCG secretion. From this point until term, the production of progesterone by the trophoblast increases in contrast to the decline in hCG. Little is known about the mechanisms which control these sequential hormonal patterns during pregnancy. As an exploratory model, we used the cultured human choriocarcinoma JEG-3 cell to investigate the biochemistry underlying the control of hCG and progesterone secretion.

The JEG-3 cell retains several characteristics of the normal trophoblastic cell. In addition to hCG and progesterone, the cell secretes free hCG alpha subunit and is capable of estradiol synthesis when incubated with dehydroepiandrosterone sulfate (Kohler and Bridson, 1971; Benveniste et al., 1979). Like the normal trophoblastic cell, the JEG-3 cell has a high affinity receptor to Epidermal Growth Factor (EGF), a 6,045 daltons peptide also known in human as beta-urogastrone (Cohen and Taylor, 1974; Gregory, 1975; Benveniste et al., 1978a). At the last Trophoblast Conference, we reviewed results on the stimulatory effect of EGF on hCG secretion by the JEG-3 cell (Benveniste and Scommegna, 1981). Salomon (1981), reported that the number of EGF receptors present on a mouse carcinoma cell was reduced after exposure to phorbol myristate acetate (herein referred to as phorbol), a derivative of a plant alkaloid with tumor-promoting properties. The binding of phorbol to mammalian cells is followed by the stimulation of phospholipase which results in an increase of arachidonic acid (Levine and Ohuci, 1978). The binding of phorbol to the JEG-3 cell and its effect on EGF receptors (Ilekis and Benveniste, unpublished) has lead us to study the influence of both phorbol and the arachidonic acid pathway on the secretion of hCG and progesterone by the choriocarcinoma cell.

MATERIALS AND METHODS

JEG-3 cells, kindly provided by Dr. Peter Kohler (Department of Medicine, University of Arkansas) were grown in 25 cm^2 culture plastic flasks in Dulbecco's modified Eagles medium (DMEM) enriched with 10 percent heat- inactivated fetal calf serum (FCS) at 37°C, in a 90 percent air-10 percent CO_2 atmosphere. FCS and DMEM were purchased from GIBCO laboratories, Grand Island, NY. For each experiment, cells were collected by scraping, aliquoted to replicate flasks and were fed with DMEM supplemented with 10 percent FCS. At 30-50 percent confluency, media were changed to FCS-free DMEM. After 2 days in that medium, cultures were refed with DMEM alone (control) or DMEM plus various experimental agents. Unless otherwise stated, culture media were collected 24 hours later and after addition of bovine serum albumin (1 mg per ml) were stored frozen until measured by radioimmunoassay for their hCG (Benveniste et al., 1979) and progesterone (Auletta et al., 1978) content. The cell sheet remaining in the flask was washed with 0.9 percent sodium chloride and solubilized in 0.5 N sodium hydroxide; an aliquot of each cell digest was used for protein determination (Lowry et al., 1951). Each determination represents the mean ± S.E.M. of hCG or progesterone secreted per milligram of cellular protein per day in 3-4 flasks. The F-test was used for statistical analysis (Snedecor, 1956).

Iodination grade mouse EGF (M.W. 6,045) was purchased from Collaborative Research Inc., Waltham, MA. The following enzymatic effectors and metabolites of the arachidonic acid pathway purchased from Sigma Chemicals Co., St. Louis, MO, were used: phorbol myristate acetate (12-0-tetradecanoyl phorbol- 13 acetate, M.W. 617) which stimulates phospholipase activity (Levine et al., 1978; Mufson et al., 1979), indomethacin (M.W. 358) an inhibitor of cyclooxygenase activity (Samuelsson et al., 1975), NDGA (nordihydroguairetic acid, M.W. 302) a lipoxygenase inhibitor which blocks the conversion of arachidonic acid into various hydroperoxy fatty acids (Tappel et al., 1953; Kelly et al., 1979), imidazole, a thromboxane inhibitor (Hsin-Hsiung and Yuan, 1978), prostaglandin E_1 (M.W. 354), E_2 (M.W. 353), $F_{2\alpha}$ (M.W. 476), arachidonic acid (M.W. 304). Figure 1 illustrates the metabolic pathway of arachidonic acid and the loci of action of phorbol, indomethacin, and NDGA.

RESULTS

The effect of phorbol on hCG secretion by JEG-3 cells is shown in Figure 2. The stimulation of hCG by phorbol was dose-related and a significant increase was observed at a dose of 10 ng/ml; at a dose of 20-40 ng/ml the maximum stimulation represented 300-400 percent increase relative to basal hCG secretion. In contrast to its marked stimulatory effect on hCG secretion, phorbol had little or no effect on the secretion of progesterone. Similar results on hCG and progesterone secretion were obtained with EGF. The effect of phorbol and EGF in three representative experiments which differ in the levels of basal secretion is shown in Table 1. Only in experiment number 2, did phorbol have a stimulatory effect on progesterone secretion, just reaching 5 percent significance.

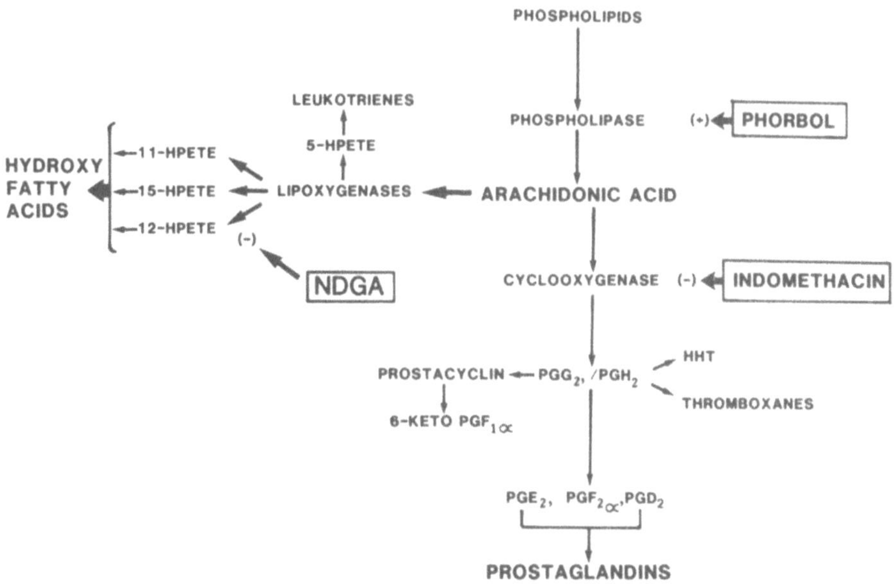

Figure 1. The metabolism of arachidonic acid; the sites of action of phorbol, indomethacin and nordihydroguairetic acid (NDGA) are indicated.

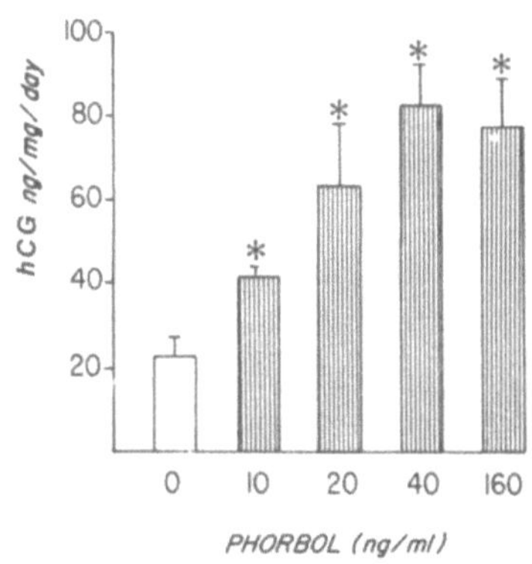

Figure 2. Effect of phorbol on hCG secretion by JEG-3 cells. After 2 days in serum-free Dulbecco's modified Eagles medium (DMEM), media were replaced by fresh DMEM alone or DMEM + phorbol and collected 24 h later. Each bar represents the mean ± S.E.M. of hCG (ng/mg protein/day) in three culture flasks; $p < 0.025$ is *.

Table I

Progesterone and hCG (ng/mg cellular protein/day) in-media from JEG-3 cell cultures incubated with either Dulbecco's modified Eagles medium (DMEM) alone (CT), DMEM + epidermal growth factor (EGF, 20 ng/ml) or DMEM + phorbol (40 ng/ml). The data shown are those of 3 representative experiments with different basal secretion (CT). Each value represents the mean of three flasks ± S.E.M.; $p<0.05$ is *; $p<0.005$ is **.

		ng/mg cellular protein/day			
		hCG		Progesterone	
Exp #1					
	CT	107.8 ± 12.2	–	53.2 ± 6.6	–
	EGF	310.0 ± 8.1	**	58.7 ± 0.5	NS
	PHORBOL	461.6 ± 39.3	**	61.5 ± 4.8	NS
Exp #2					
	CT	61.7 ± 2.9	–	53.5 ± 2.3	–
	EGF	189.6 ± 9.5	**	53.5 ± 2.7	NS
	PHORBOL	339.5 ± 58.2	**	80.4 ± 7.1	*
Exp #3					
	CT	19.3 ± 1.8	–	29.8 ± 8.7	–
	EGF	90.9 ± 17.2	**	38.5 ± 2.7	NS
	PHORBOL	79.7 ± 18.1	**	29.1 ± 7.1	NS

The dose-related stimulatory effect of arachidonic acid on progesterone secretion was maximal (150-200 percent from basal secretion) at a dose of 10 µg/ml. In the same experiment, at the various concentrations we used, arachidonic acid was ineffective in altering hCG secretion (data not shown). The effect of arachidonic acid alone (0.5 µg/ml) or in the presence of either EGF (20 ng/ml) or phorbol (40 ng/ml) on hCG secretion is shown in Figure 4. Arachidonic acid significantly potentiated the effect of EGF, inducing a secretion of hCG comparable to the maximal stimulatory effect obtained with phorbol.

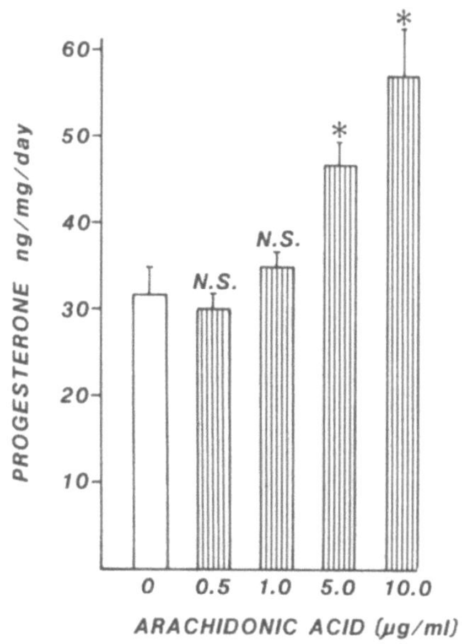

Figure 3. Effect of arachidonic acid on progesterone secretion. Collection of media as in Figure 2. Each bar represents the mean ± S.E.M. of progesterone (ng/mg protein/day) in three culture flasks; $p < 0.01$ is *.

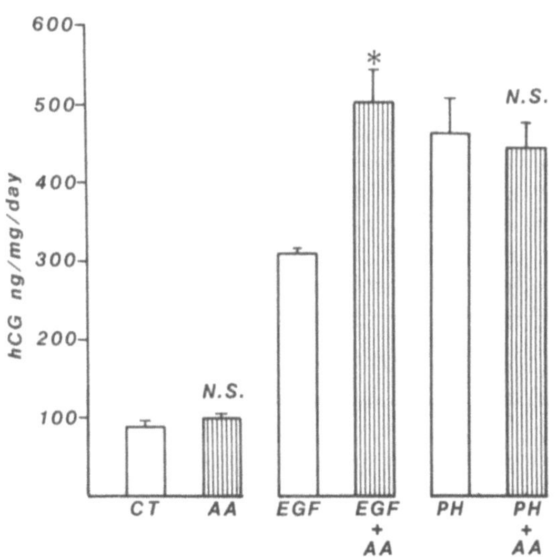

Figure 4. Effect of arachidonic acid (0.5 μg/ml) on hCG secretion by JEG-3 cells in DMEM alone (CT), DMEM + EGF (20 ng/ml), and DMEM + phorbol (40 ng/ml). Collection of media as in Figure 2. Each bar represents the mean ± S.E.M. of hCG (ng/mg protein/day) in 4 culture flasks; $p < 0.005$ is *.

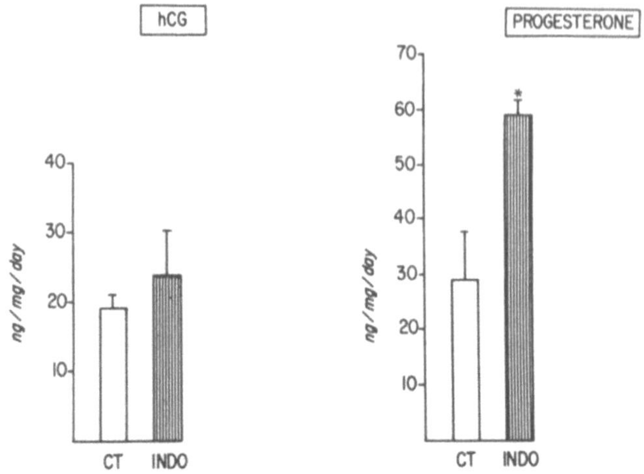

Figure 5. Effect of indomethacin (50 µg/ml) on hCG (left panel) and progesterone (right panel) secretion by JEG-3 cells. Collection of media as in Figure 2. Each bar represents the mean ± S.E.M. of hCG or progesterone (ng/mg protein/day) in 3 culture flasks; $p < 0.025$ is *.

Table II

Progesterone and hCG (ng/mg of cellular protein/day) in media of JEG-3 cell cultures incubated for 3 hours with Dulbecco's modified Eagles medium (DMEM) used in control cultures (CT) or DMEM + 20 µg/ml nordihydroguairetic acid, NDGA (Exp); at that time, culture media were replaced by fresh DMEM and media collected 24 hours later (Day 1); at that time, culture media were replaced once more by fresh DMEM and media collected 24 hours later (Day 2); $p<0.05$ is *; $p<0.005$ is **.

	Day 1		Day 2	
	CT	Exp	CT	Exp
hCG	114.1±11.1**	9.6±0.6	75.8±6.8*	122.2±10.12
Progesterone	33.8±3.2**	146.8±8.1	28.8±1.4 N.S.	32.8±7.1

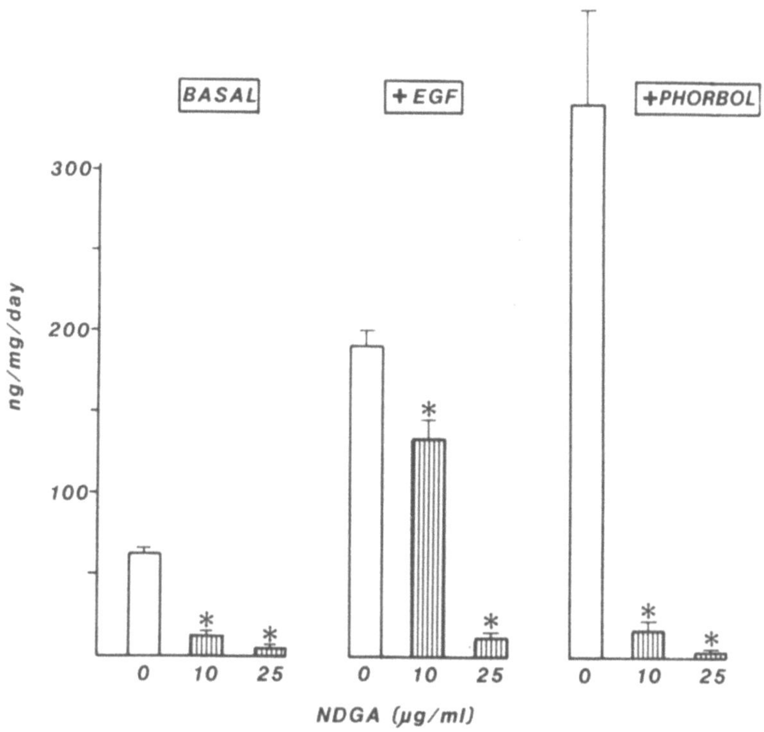

Figure 6. Effect of NDGA on hCG secretion by JEG-3 cells in DMEM alone (left panel), DMEM + 20 ng/ml EGF (middle panel), and DMEM + 40 ng/ml phorbol (right panel). Collection of media as in Figure 2. Each bar represents the mean ± S.E.M. of hCG (ng/mg protein/day) in 4 flasks; $p < 0.025$ is *.

Indomethacin was used to inhibit the metabolism of arachidonic acid via cyclooxygenase activity (Figure 1). Indomethacin stimulated progesterone secretion in a dose-related manner. A maximum effect on progesterone (about 200 percent from basal secretion) was obtained at a dose of 50 μg/ml (Figure 5, right panel), a dose of indomethacin which had no significant effect on hCG secretion (Figure 5, left panel). The stimulatory effect of indomethacin on progesterone secretion could not be reversed with the simultaneous addition of prostaglandin E_1, E_2, or $F_{2\alpha}$ used to a dose of 1 μg/ml (data not shown).

A lipoxygenase inhibitor, NDGA, was used to block the conversion of arachidonic acid into hydroperoxy fatty acids (Figure 1). Figure 6 shows the inhibitory effect of NDGA on basal hCG secretion (left panel) and on the secretion of hCG stimulated either by EGF (middle panel) or by phorbol (right panel). In contrast to the inhibitory effect on hCG secretion, NDGA stimulated the secretion of progesterone. Similar results to those shown in Figure 6 (a 24 hour exposure to NDGA) were obtained after only 3 hours of exposure to NDGA. However, in both protocols of incubation, there was a decrease in the number of attached cells as indicated by a decrease in cellular protein per flask. Table II shows the results obtained after 3 hours exposure to NDGA (20 µg/ml). A change to fresh media and measurement of hCG in the 24 hour collection demonstrated an inhibition of hCG secretion (about 90 percent) and a stimulation of progesterone secretion (about 400 per cent); incubation for an extra-day in fresh DMEM showed that the reduced number of cells pre-exposed to NDGA were able to recover their secretion of hCG and progesterone to levels comparable to control cultures.

DISCUSSION

As an exploratory model, the JEG-3 cell offers an opportunity to address several important questions related to the endocrinology of the trophoblast, which include a possible relation between steroidogenesis and the production of chorionic gonadotropin. In addition, the presence on the cell surface of EGF receptors allows one to study pathways involved in the transduction of a message initiated by EGF which leads to hormonal secretion. Finally, the finding of a receptor to a tumor-promotor (phorbol) on the JEG-3 cell reaches beyond endocrinology and provokes new questions when a comparison is made between the characteristics of the embryonic trophoblast and those of malignant tissues.

Extract from JEG-3 cells revealed that these cells store less than two percent of the hCG found in the 24 hour culture media (Benveniste et al., 1978b) and herein we considered hCG secretion as reflecting the state of hCG synthesis. The ability of JEG-3 cells to grow, secrete and multiply in a simplified serum-free medium is advantageous when evaluating the cell response to an effector. The results presented in Figure 2 and Table I demonstrate the stimulatory effect of both EGF and phorbol on hCG secretion. As we indicated earlier, there is also an interplay between phorbol and EGF at the receptor level, since the exposure of the cell to phorbol rapidly reduces the binding of EGF. It is possible that the increase in hCG secretion (which follows phorbol and EGF occupancy of their respective receptors) is coupled to a pathway which down-regulates receptors, thus limiting the stimulation on hCG. This hypothesis would be consistent with the results (not shown) obtained from the simultaneous exposure of JEG-3 cells to EGF and phorbol and the absence of an additive stimulatory effect on hCG secretion. Further work is necessary to unravel those mechanisms of action common to the growth factor and the tumor promotor.

While our study was in progress, Shupnik (1982) reported that in osteosarcoma cells, EGF (like phorbol in other cells) increases arachidonic formation. In order to evaluate the influence of the metabolites of the arachidonic acid pathway on hCG secretion, we used agents recognized in other cell types to inhibit cyclooxygenase and lipoxygenase pathways. Indomethacin had no significant effect on hCG secretion (Figure 5, left panel), thus suggesting that none of the cyclooxygenase products have a major role in hCG secretion. In contrast to the effect of indomethacin the inhibition of lipoxygenase activity by NDGA was effective in modulating hCG secretion. NDGA inhibited hCG secretion and this contrasted to the stimulatory effect induced by either EGF or phorbol. This inhibition was not due to a decrease in cell viability; indeed, the media from culture flasks exposed to NDGA contained 48 hours later even more hCG than the media from control cultures (Table II). Thus, the lipoxygenase products may be important for the secretion of hCG by JEG-3 cells. The additional property of NDGA to inhibit in some cells the formation of thromboxanes (Hammarstrom and Fallardeau, 1977) does not seem to have a role in the inhibition of hCG, since neither the thromboxane inhibitor imidazole (Ilekis and Benveniste, unpublished) nor indomethacin (Figure 5) were capable of duplicating the effect of NDGA on hCG secretion by JEG-3 cells.

Addition of arachidonic acid alone to JEG-3 cell cultures did not significantly affect hCG secretion. However, at a dose of 0.5 µg/ml, arachidonic acid potentiated the stimulatory effect of EGF (Figure 4). Thus, a hypothetical model is proposed in which (1) the stimulatory effect of both EGF and phorbol on hCG secretion is not solely induced by an increase in arachidonic acid but also requires the stimulation of enzymes beyond those involved in arachidonic acid formation, and (2) the enzymes activated by EGF or phorbol belong to the lipoxygenase system since NDGA inhibits the stimulatory effect of both EGF and phorbol. Given this construct, the stimulation of hCG secretion would result from the concomitant stimulation by EGF or phorbol of both the formation of arachidonic acid and the stimulation of lipoxygenases capable of using the newly formed arachidonic acid. Although other fundamental pathways may be implicated, our objective in formulating the foregoing hypothesis is solely to organize our results into a working model for further investigation.

The stimulation of progesterone secretion by indomethacin (Figure 5) at first suggested that prostaglandins have a role in inhibiting progesterone secretion, inasmuch as the inhibition of progesterone by prostaglandins has been suggested in other steroid-secreting cells, including the luteal cell (Auletta et al., 1978). In JEG-3 cells, however, this notion could not be documented since (1) the addition of either PGE_1, PGE_2 or $PGF_{2\alpha}$ was unable to reverse the effect of indomethacin, and (2) the addition of arachidonic acid, a substrate for PGs formation, stimulated progesterone secretion (Figure 3). Instead, we speculated that the increase of arachidonic acid was responsible for the stimulatory effect on progesterone. The absence or mild effect of phorbol and EGF on progesterone secretion, (Table I) despite their ability to increase arachidonic acid formation, may be explained by their concomitant stimulation of certain lipoxygenases which actively shunt arachidonic acid toward pathways involved in hCG formation. In our model, the progesterone increase after exposure to NDGA would reflect (1) an accumulation of arachidonic acid due to the block NDGA induces on those EGF- and phorbol-sensitive lipoxygenases involved in hCG secretion, and (2) the use of arachidonic acid by different lipoxygenases important for progesterone secretion but not for the secretion of hCG.

The relatively recent and expanding field of prostaglandins, hydroperoxy fatty acids, leukotrienes and other metabolites of the arachidonic acid pathway already has a considerable impact on several medical disciplines, particularly immunology and obstetrics. Arachidonic acid metabolites may, in fact, represent generalized cellular intermediates in the metabolic cascade initiated by the activation of receptors and the ensuing changes in membrane- bound phospholipids (Hirata et al., 1978). The role of the arachidonic acid pathway in modulating steroid and protein hormones secretion has been reported (Samuelsson et al., 1975; Handwerger et al., 1981). The results of the present investigation suggest that the arachidonic acid pathway has a role in the control of hCG and progesterone secretion, an important notion which warrants further study.

SUMMARY

The relationship and control of hCG and progesterone secretion by the trophoblast is not known. The cultured human choriocarcinoma JEG-3 cell, an extensively used model of the trophoblast biochemistry, secretes both hormones. We first observed that binding of Epidermal Growth Factor (EGF) to the JEG-3 cell was followed by an increase in hCG secretion. Then, we observed that a diester derivative of phorbol (a tumor promoter) binds to the JEG-3 cell, affects the binding of EGF to its own receptor, and also stimulates hCG secretion. Since both EGF and phorbol have been related to the formation of arachidonic acid, we further investigated the role of the arachidonic acid pathway in the control of hCG and progesterone secretion. The results showed (1) the involvement of the arachidonic acid pathway in both hCG and progesterone secretion (2) various effectors of the arachidonic acid pathway can differentially modulate hCG secretion, and (3) hCG secretion can be inhibited in a situation where the secretion of progesterone is stimulated. Discussion of the results leads to a hypothesis in which hCG and progesterone secretion is dependent on the activity of different enzymes belonging to the lipoxygenase system, and the lipoxygenases involved in the control of hCG secretion are stimulated by EGF or phorbol.

ACKNOWLEDGMENT

It is a pleasure to thank Ms. Mary Ann Linderman for her excellent assistance in cell culture and hormonal measurement, and Ms. Francine Marcelle for her dedicated secretarial help. Research was supported in part by a grant from M.R.H. School of Health Sciences.

REFERENCES

Auletta, F.J., Agins, H.J., and Scommegna, A. (1978) Prostaglandin F mediation of the inhibitory effect of estrogen on the corpus luteum of the Rhesus monkey. *Endocr.*, 103, 1183-1189.

Benveniste, R., Speeg, K.V., Carpenter, G., Cohen, S., Lindner, J. and Rabinowitz, D. (1978a) Epidermal growth factor stimulates secretion of human chorionic gonadotropin by cultured human choriocarcinoma cells. *J. Clin. Endocr. Metabol.* 46, 169-172.

Benveniste, R., Speeg, K.V., Long, A., and Rabinowitz, D. (1978b) Concanavalin-A stimulates human chorionic gonadotropin (hCG) and hCG-alpha secretion by human choriocarcinoma cells. *Biochem. Biophys. Res. Commun.*, 84, 1082-1087.

Benveniste, R., Lindner, J., Puett, D., and Rabin, D. (1979) hCG alpha- subunit from cultured choriocarcinoma (JEG) cells: Comparison of the subunit secreted free with that prepared from secreted hCG. *Endocr.*, 105, 581-587.

Benveniste, R. and Scommegna, A. (1981) Human chorionic gonadotropin (hCG) and free alpha-subunit secreted by cultured human choriocarcinoma (JEG-3) cells. In *Placenta: Receptors Pathology and Toxicology* (ed.) Miller, R.K. and Thiede, H., pp. 241-248. London: W.B. Saunders Company.

Cohen, S. and Taylor, I.M. (1974) EGF: Chemical and biological characterization. *Symp. Soc. Develop. Biol.*, 30, 25-42.

Gregory, H. (1975) Isolationand structure of urogastrone and its relationship to epidermal growth factor. *Nature* 257, 325.

Hammerstrom, S. and Fallardeau, P. (1977) Resolution of prostaglandin endoperoxide synthase and thromboxane synthase of human platelets. *Proc. Nat. Acad. Sci.* USA 74, 3691-3695.

Handwerger, S., Barry, S., Barrett, J., Markoff, E., Zeitler, B., Cwikel, B. and Siegel, M. (1981) Inhibition of the synthesis and secretion of decidual prolactin by arachidonic acid. *Endocr.*, 109, 2016-2021.

Hirata, F., Viveros, H.O., Diliberto, Jr., E.J. and Axelrod, J. (1978) Identification and properties of two methyltransferases in conversion of phosphatidylethanolamine to phosphatidylcholine. *Proc. Nat. Acad. Sci.* USA, 75, 1718-1721.

Hsin-Hsiung, T. and Yuan, B. (1978) On the inhibitory potency of imidazole and its derivatives on thromboxane synthetase. *Biochem. Biophys. Res. Commun.*, 80, 236-242.

Kelly, J.P., Johnson, H.C. and Parker, C.W. (1979) Effect of inhibitors of arachidonic acid metabolism on mitogenesis in human lymphocytes: possible role of thromboxane and products of the lipoxygenase pathway. *J. Immunol.*, 122, 1563-1571.

Kohler, P.O. and Bridson, W.E. (1971) Isolation of hormone-producing clonal lines of human choriocarcinoma. *J. Clin. Endo. Metabol.*, 32, 683-687.

Levine, L. and Ohuci, K. (1978) Retinoids as well as tumor promoters enhance deacylation of cellular lipids and prostaglandin production in MDCK-cells. *Nature*, 276, 274-275.

Lowry, O.H., Rosenbrough, N.J., Farr, A.L. and Randall, R.J. (1951) Protein measurement with the Folin phenol reagent. *J. Biol. Chem.*, 193:265-275.

Mufson, R.A., Laskin, J.D., Fisher, P.B. and Weinstein, I.B. (1979) Melittin shares certain cellular effects with phorbol ester tumor promoters. *Nature*, 280, 72-74.

Salomon, D.S. (1981) Inhibition of epidermal growth factor binding to mouse carcinoma cells by phorbol esters mediated by specific phorbol esters receptor.

Samuelsson, B., Granstrom, E., Green, M., Hamberg, M. and Hammarstrom, S. (1975) Prostaglandins. *Ann. Rev. Biochem.*, 44, 669-695.

Shupnik, M.A. (1982) Involvement of calcium in epidermal growth factor and phorbol ester stimulated production of prostaglandins by osteosarcoma cells. Sixty-fourth Annual Meeting of the Endocrine Society, San Francisco, California.

Snedecor, G.W. (1956) *Statistical Methods*, p. 394-398. Ames: Iowa University Press.

Tappel, A.L., Lundberg, W. and Boyer, P.D. (1953) Effect of temperature and antioxidants upon the lipoxidase catalyzed oxidation of sodium linoleate. *Arch. Biochem. Biophys.*, 42, 293-304.

Trophoblast Research 1:301-304, 1983

METABOLISM REPORTS

Aromatase Activity in the Human Placenta

(Brownscheidle et al., 1982)

Steroid synthesis by the trophoblast continues to be an area of investigation requiring substantial resolution. Carol Brownscheidle presented an important preliminary evaluation for the biochemistry and morphology of the normal placenta and its regional differences in synthetic capacity for steroids.

Ten percent homogenates of normal term placentae (N = 6) were evaluated for aromatase I and aromatase II in four different regions: decidua, cotyledon, chorionic plate, and amnion. Aromatase I is the enzyme which converts 16α-hydroxyandrogen precursors ([1,2-^{3}H, 4-^{14}C] 16α-hydroxyandrostenedione) to estriol. Aromatase II is the enzyme which converts [1-^{3}H, 4-^{14}C] androstenedione to estrone and estradiol.

In the placenta, values for aromatase I and II were comparable being in the range of 63-91 pmol/min/mg protein, while the values for the amnion were much lower (4-15 pmol/min/mg protein). Ratios of aromatase I/II were calculated to be 0.65-1.0 for the placenta and 5.2 for the amnion. Large variations in the activites for both aromatases were noted within specific regions of the placentae. Such information leads one to speculate that different extraembryonic membranes may have different supportive roles in estrogen synthesis. Dr. Brownscheidle indicated that antibodies to aromatase II have recently been isolated in their laboratories (Osawa and Nakamura, 1982) and will be used to localize aromatase in specific cell types by immunocytochemical technics.

Stimulation of Estrogen Synthetase Activity by Hemin in Trophoblast Cultures from Human Choriocarcinoma

(Bellino and Hussa, 1982)

At the Eight Rochester Trophoblast Conference in 1980, Frank Bellino introduced some preliminary data concerning the interesting question of heme interaction with estrogen synthesis by the trophoblast and at the Ninth Conference established these relationships. As noted previously, cyclic AMP stimulates estrogen synthetase in the human trophoblast cell culture (JAr line). This stimulation is responsive to inhibitors of protein and RNA synthesis. Since the cytochrome P_{450} component of estrogen synthetase requires heme, if heme biosynthesis is rate-limiting and if the cells possess sufficient estrogen synthetase apo- cytochrome P_{450}, then hemin should increase the activity of estrogen synthetase.

Conversion of [1 B-^{3}H, 4-^{14}C] androstenedione into tritiated water was used as a measure of estrogen synthetase activity in these studies. Exposure to hemin at about 25 uM for 24 h optimally stimulated estrogen synthetase activity by 165-260%. In addition, heme content was increased by 58% following treatment of trophoblastic cells with cyclic AMP and theophylline for 72 h. Thus, the regulation of estrogen synthesis by cyclic AMP appears to involve the biosynthetic pathway for heme.

Initiation of Labor: Possible Role of Lysosomal Enzymes and Phagocytosis in the Chorioamniotic Membrane

(Sbarra et al., 1982)

The role of prostaglandins in labor has been known for a number of years. However, how labor is initiated has been an enigma. Anthony Sbarra reported a number of interesting experiments regarding the release of lysosomal enzymes by the chorioamnion from term pregnancies following labor and vaginal delivery and after Cesarean section delivery and no labor.

Previous studies have documented that lysosomal enzymes are activated by phagocytosis of surface-active agents. Some of these enzymes are N-acetylglucosamidase (NAG) and phospholipase A_2, which hydrolyze glycerophospholipids to arachidonic acid. The availibility of arachidonic acid is usually the limiting factor in prostaglandin synthesis.

Under in vitro incubation conditions, using a mounted chorioamniotic membrane, Sbarra described a dramatic increase in the release of NAG when labor was active. Latex particles also increase the release of NAG in membranes only from patients not in labor. Centrifuged in contrast to noncentrifuged amniotic fluid as an incubation medium did not induce a release of NAG. The authors presume this was due to the removal of surface active agents, e.g., phospholipids in the noncentrifuged amniotic fluid. This was confirmed by adding lysolecithin to the medium. Lechithin did not increase NAG release.

From these important preliminary observations, Sbarra and associates hypothesized that the lysosomal enzymes from the chorioamnion can be activated by a phagocytosis-like process, which may be a component in the onset of labor.

Lack of Human Placental Lactogen in Serum and Placental Tissue from an Apparently Normal Pregnancy

(Sideri et al., 1982, 1983)

Human placental lactogen (hPL) has been routinely utilized to determine the growth of the placenta. Mario Sideri presented a fascinating case report of a pregnancy resulting in a normal term delivery of a female, where hPL was undetectable. Normal values of human chorionic gonadotropin, prolactin, human growth hormone and urinary estriols were observed. However, serum levels of hPL were <0.06 µg/ml as measured by two different RIA procedures. In addition, hPL values for the placenta were <0.5 µg/g as measured by RIA in tissue extracts and SDS-PAGE.

These analyses of hPL via both immunological and non-immunological technics in combination with the four previously reported cases (Gaede et al., 1978; Nielsen et al., 1979; Borody et al., 1981; Alexander et al., 1982), and the recent demonstration that a gene deletion is responsible for the absence of hPL (Wurzel et al., 1982), support the conclusion that the production of this protein, hPL, is not essential for a normal pregnancy.

The Opiate Receptor from Human Placentae

(Ahmed, 1982)

Mahmoud Ahmed first reported his exciting work concerning opiate receptors to us at the Eighth Rochester Trophoblast Conference (Ahmed et al., 1981). Since that Conference, he has continued to purify and characterize this macromolecular complex. Narcotics may be involved in a number of different placental functions; however, they have been primarily implicated in the modulation of amino acid transport by the human placenta (Barnwell et al., this volume). Such functions may be normally regulated by endogenous substrates which interact with this receptor complex.

Ahmed has solubilized the receptor and demonstrated that it is truly soluble because it does not sediment at 160,000 x g after 90 min of centrifugation. In addition, it migrates on Sepharose CL-6B column with an apparent Stokes radius of approximately 7 nanometers and with a molecular rate of approximately 300,000 daltons. Further investigations by Ahmed are in progress to purify this receptor with covalent chromatography and to determine any relationship between opiate receptor activity and the mode of delivery as well as maternal drug history.

REFERENCES

Ahmed, M.S. (1983) Characterization of Solubilized Opiate Receptors from Human Placenta, *J. Membrane Biochem.* 5, 35-47.

Ahmed, M.S. (1982) Partial Purification and Characterization of the Opiate Receptor from Human Placenta, *9th Rochester Trophoblast Conference* Abstracts, p. 32.

Ahmed, M.S. (1981) Solubilization of Opiate Receptors from Human Placenta, *Placenta Suppl.* 3, pp. 115-121.

Alexander, I., Anthoni, F. and Letchworth, A. T. (1982) Placental Protein Profile and Glucose Studies in a Normal Pregnancy with Extremely Low Levels of Human Placental Lactogen. Case Report. *Brit. J. Obst. Gynecol.* 89, 241.

Bellino, F. L. and Hussa, R. O. (1980) Mechanism of the regulation of estrogen biosynthesis by cyclic AMP in the trophoblastic cell culture. *8th Rochester Trophoblast Conference Abstracts,* Abstract #27.

Bellino, F. L. and Hussa, R. O. (1982) Hemin stimulation of estrogen synthetase activity in human trophoblast culture from choriocarcinoma. *9th Rochester Trophoblast Conference Abstracts,* p. 28.

Borody, I.D. and Carlton, N. A. (1981) Isolated Defect in Human Placental Lactogen Synthesis in a Normal Pregnancy. Case Report. *Brit. J. Obstet. Gynecol.* 88, 447.

Brownscheidle, C. M., Yarborough, C., and Osawa, Y. (1982) A Regional analysis of human placental aromatase activity. *9th Rochester Trophoblast Conference Abstracts*, p. 39.

Gaede, T., Trolle, D., and Pedersen, H. (1978) Extremely Low Placental Lactogen Hormone (hPL) Values in an Otherwise Uneventful Pregnancy Preceeding the Delivery of a Normal Baby. *Acta Obstet. Gynecol. Scand.* 57, 203.

Nielsen, P. B., Pedersen, H., and Kampmann, E. M. (1979) Absence of Human Placental Lactogen in an Otherwise Uneventful Pregnancy. *Amer. J. Obstet. Gynecol.* 135, 322.

Osawa, Y. and Nakamura, T. (1982) Anti-human placental aromatase II cytochrome P_{450} antibody and immunochemical study of estrogen biosynthesis, *Endocrinology* 110, (Suppl.), A31.

Sbarra, A., Selvaraj, R., Cetrulo, C., Thomas, G., Louis, F. and Kennison, R. (1982) Phagocytosis and onset of human labor, *9th Rochester Trophoblast Conference Abstracts*, p. 31.

Sideri, M., deVirgiliis, G., Guidobono, F., Borgese, N., Sereni, L.P., Nicolini, U. and Remotti, G. (1982) Absence of Human Placental Lactogen in Serum and Placenta from an Otherwise Normal Pregnancy, *9th Rochester Trophoblast Conference*, p. 26.

Sideri, M., deVirgiliis, G., Guidobono, F., Borgese, N., Piecni Sereni, L., Nicolini, U., and Remotti, G. (1983) Immunologically Undetectable Human Placental Lactogen in Normal Pregnancy. Case Report. *Brit. J. Obstet. Gynecol.* 90, 771-773.

IMMUNOLOGY

Trophoblast Research 1: 307-314, 1983

ANTIBODY INDUCED ABORTION IN pp WOMEN IN THREE DIFFERENT STUDIES

- A Review-

Philip Levine

Ortho Research Foundation, Route 202, Raritan, New Jersey 08869 and
Memorial Sloan Kettering Cancer Center, 1275 York Avenue, New York, NY 10021
U.S.A.

The immunology and genetics involved in the pathogenesis of Rh hemolytic disease of the newborn (HDN) stimulated a renewed interest in abortions induced in group O women by ABO incompatibility (Levine, 1943). This was confirmed in several but not all studies of group O women with two or more spontaneous abortions. A statistical analysis of nine such American and European studies revealed a high degree of heterogeneity and it was concluded that there was some overall tendency for ABO incompatibility to increase the risk of abortions (Levene and Rosenfield, 1961).

Of the three main rbc antigenic systems, the ABO-P are linked together because biochemically their terminal determinants are nonreducing sugars and their antigens are present also in tissue cells. The determinants of MNSs antigens are amino acids while Rh (Kell and Duffy) are lipoproteins and both systems are limited to the red blood cell membrane only. Accordingly, it is the ABO-P system with their normally present antibodies which is associated with antibody-induced abortions.

The lesion immediately responsible for abortion in group O women is exerted by the action of maternal IgG molecules on A and/or B sites in fetal tissues and the only guide to the number of such sites on fetal tissue can be derived from corresponding values of A and B sites on cord rbc as compared to those on adult rbc (Race and Sanger, 1975) as given below:

	Adult	10^6	Cord
A1	0.81 - 1.17		0.25 - 0.37
A2	0.24 - 0.29		0.14

This loss by abortion is not excessively large because the number of A or B sites even in the 3 month old fetal rbc and tissue cells may exceed the limit which can be disposed of by the variable IgG content in maternal group O serum.

A and B sites have been demonstrated in numerous adult tissues as glycoproteins (GP) but more significantly as glycosphingolipids (GSP). Presumably these sites are also represented in the tissues of the 3 month old fetus when antibody induced abortion occurs even though experimental data on the actual number A and B sites are not yet available. Only the number of A_1 sites on cord or fetal rbc is significant because the affinity of IgG anti-A_1 to A_2 sites is very low and by the same token ABO HDN is very rarely observed in A_2 infants (Race and Sanger, 1975).

The first variant of the P system was described in a 66 year old patient suffering from gastric cancer (Levine et al., 1951). Initially termed Tj(a-), this rbc property was found to be very rare with a random incidence of about 1:150,000 with higher incidences in isolates such as an Amish sect with a high rate of consanguinity (Obregon and McKeever, 1980). This variant was indeed part of the P system and at first it was identified as the "phenotype p" and later as the homozygous genotype pp (Race and Sanger, 1975). But it was already suggested that pp women tend to lose their pregnancies by abortion at the first trimester (Levine and Koch, 1954). Although there were exceptions in the initial study - mainly in all 7 offspring of the compatible sib of the 1951 proposita, it was already obvious that (a) all individuals with this rare property were homozygous, (b) their antibodies probably contained IgG molecules and (c) the fetal loss in pp women was far in excess of that in ABO incompatibility (Levine and Koch, 1954). One may well be guided by the assumption that the rare genotype pp is quite analogous to the very frequent homozygous recessive group O.

When methods became available for solubilizing the glycolipid rbc membrane, the sequence of the sugars in the chain of carbohydrates with the specific determinants for the various antigens of the ABO-P system were fully described (Hakomori and Kobata, 1974; Marcus et al., 1976). The antigens of the P system are derived from 2 metabolic pathways - one from globoside and another from paragloboside. The sequence of the sugars in both pathways for the P system is presented in Table 1.

Paragloboside acquires A and B specificity provided that fucose (α1-2) is attached to its terminal galactose. Blood group A specificity results from the action of a transferase which deposits the nonreducing N-acetylgalactosamine as its terminal

Table 1. The series of glycosphingolipids from ceramide dihexoside to end products of the P blood group system

CDH	Gal (β,1 →4)Glc-Cer
CTH (Pk)	Gal(β,1 →4)Gal(β,1 →4)Glc-Cer
Globoside (P_2)	GalNAc(β,1 →3)Gal(α,1 →4)Gal(β,1 →4)Glc-Cer
Forssman (Fs)	GalNAc(α,1 →3)GalNAc(α,1 →3)Gal(α,1 →4)Gal(β,1 →4)Glc-Cer
Paragloboside	Gal(β,1 →4)GlcNAc(β,1 →3)Gal(β,1 →4)Glc-Cer
P_1	Gal(α,1 →4)Gal(β,1 →4)GlcNAc(β,1 →3)Gal(β,1 →4)Glc-Cer
p	Gal(β,1 →4)GlcNAc(β,1 →3)Gal(β,1 →4)Glc-Cer | Neu

monosaccharide. Similarly an allelic transferase deposits galactose (α,1-3) as its nonreducing terminal monosaccharide to determine group B specificity.

The similarities in the biochemical structure of the ABO and P blood group systems are so striking that one may well predict that whatever has been previously shown to characterize the antigens of the ABO system should also apply to the P system. It was the lack of potent human antibodies for antigens of the P system, particularly those of the IgG variety, which explains the failure to search for soluble P substances soon after ovarian cyst fluid became a rich source for biochemical studies of A and B soluble substances (Morgan and VanHeyningen, 1944).

Although the history and clinical data suggested the presence of IgG antibodies in the sera of pp individuals (Levine et al., 1951), a period of 20 years elapsed before proof that each of the three antibodies, anti-P_1PP^k, contained IgG components (Wurzel et al., 1971; Pollack et al., 1977). That antigens of the P system are present also on tissue cells is evident from their association with at least one striking example of cancer (Levine et al., 1951), antibody induced abortion in pp women (Levine and Koch, 1954) and a Japanese woman of the very rare genotype P^kP^k, whose remarkable history of 8 abortions will be described below.

The biochemical structures of the several antigens found in the lyophilized gastric tumor which confirmed the results of the absorption tests (Levine et al., 1951) have been in part defined and a basis for remarkably successful immunotherapy which prevented metastasis has been proposed (Kannagi et al., 1982).

The findings in three independent studies of antibody induced abortion in pp women are presented in Table 2. The first study (Levine and Koch, 1954) was carried out prior to the description of the sequence of the several sugars in globoside and paragloboside metabolic pathways of the P system.

The 18 abortions of unknown origin in 5 families from each of the 5 continents were referred to the author in the interval of 1952-1954 for testing with anti-Tj^a. In each of the 5 women (ages 19 to 37 years), their rbc were shown to be Tj^{a-} (pp) and their sera contained the characteristic high incidence anti-Tj^a, using the terminology of the index family (Levine et al., 1951). In this family with no abortions, the 66 year old proposita was later shown to have 4 P_2p children and her 45 year old compatible sib had 7 exceptional P_1p children.

In the second study in the Västerbottom area of North Sweden, the incidence of pp was 70 times more frequent than in random populations but with a low incidence of consanguinity in contrast to the third study of an agricultural Amish isolate not far from Cleveland, Ohio, with a high incidence of pp individuals resulting from a high rate of consanguinity.

In each of the 3 groups, most of the surviving children were of genotype P_2p in which gene P_2 determines the presence of antigen P which is the globoside tetrasaccharide. Although anti-P is one of the antibodies in the serum of pp individuals - anti-P_1PP^k - the cytotoxicity is exerted by the anti-P_1 component and specifically directed to P_1p pregnancies at the first trimester. An explanation is then required for the failure of some P_1p pregnancies to abort.

A possible explanation for the survival of the exceptional P1p pregnancies is based on an analysis of the experimental data reported in a brief communication on the varying agglutinability of fetal rbc of slightly differing ages when tested with human anti-P_1 (Ikin et al., 1961). On testing 403 fetuses of ages between 12 and 28 weeks the data showed "the incidence of P_1 to be below the adult level; however, it was found to be considerably higher in young than in old foetuses. Moreover, in the early foetus the strength of the agglutination also tended to be greater" (Ikin et al., 1961). The data on the varying agglutinability of 403 fetal rbc represented in Table 3 are divided in terms of crown-rump length as 86 less than 10 cm. and 317 more than 10 cm. and the distinction of the two is "highly significant" (Figure 1 and Table 3).

It would appear then that in the great majority of the pregnancies the number of P_1 sites on fetal rbc gradually diminish until sufficiently low levels of P_1 sites remain and stimulate production of IgG anti-P_1. Thus the increased antibody response is sufficient to induce cytotoxicity directed to the ever diminishing number of P_1 sites in fetal tissues.

In the exceptional cases however P1p pregnancies escape abortion and it is assumed that the number of P_1 sites fail to diminish and remain at sufficiently high levels to absorb the IgG anti-P_1 of the anti-P_1PP^k complex. Accordingly, the greatly diminished antibody can no longer exert its cytotoxic effect on the numerous P_1 sites in the fetal tissue cells. Because of the 7 surviving P_1 children of the compatible sib of the 1951 patient with gastric adenoca and more than one example in several other families (Race and Sanger, 1975), one may assume that the persistence of high numbers of P_1 sites in fetal rbc (and presumably also in tissue cells) is probably controlled by a dominant genetic property (Figure 1).

Table 2. Antibody induced abortion in pp women

	1. Levine and Koch (1954)	2. Cedergren (1980)	3. Obregon and McKeever (1980)	Total
Pregnancies	29	51	75	155
Abortions	18	33	33	80
Surviving Children	11	14	46	71
Genotypes				
P2p	4	10	27	41
P1p	7	4	6	17
pp	0	0	12	12

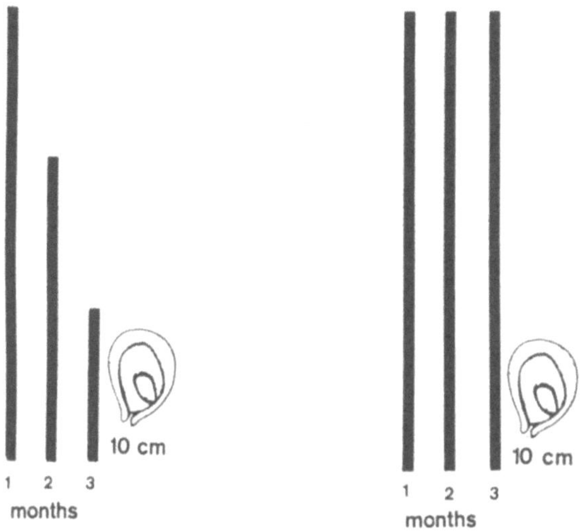

Figure 1. P_1 sites on fetal RBC (see Table 3).

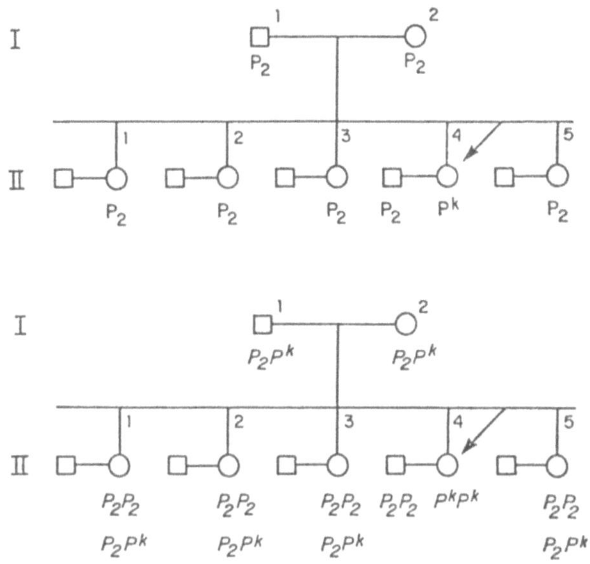

Figure 2. Upper: The pedigree of family Kom as given by the authors in terms of P phenotypes. Lower: The pedigree of family Kom given in terms of P genotypes to explain the 8 antibody induced abortions (adapted from Furukawa et al., 1974).

Table 3. Tests of 403 fetal RBC with human anti-P_1
from Ikin, Kay, Playfair and Mourant, 1961

	P_1+	P_1	Total	%P+
Crown-rump Length				
Less than 10 cm	50	36	86	58.14
More than 10 cm	67	250	317	21.14
Adults	1984	641	2625	75.58

In contrast to ABO antigens, the failure to demonstrate P_1 glycoprotein and glycolipid antigenic sites in adult or fetal tissue cells can be associated in general with their far fewer antigenic sites and the absence until 1951 of suitably potent IgG anti-P_1 antibodies in sera of pp individuals stimulated in this patient by a mini transfusion of P_1 incompatible blood

Eight antibody induced abortions in a P^kP^k Japanese women

Reference to Table 1 indicates that the rbc antigen pk is a precursor to globoside, a tetrasaccharide, and by analogy with the homozygous recessive group O, pk when recognized serologically is homozygous and recessive, i.e. P^kP^k. As such it contains an antibody specific for globoside or antigen P with its determinant which is β-GalNAc.

In the remarkable Kom family (Furukawa et al., 1974) the proposita (#4 in Figure 2A) had 8 consecutive early abortions. The pedigree in Figure 2A yields no significant information because it is given in phenotypes; the rbc of the proposita is shown to contain antigen P^k because it reacted with anti-P^k derived from pp serum absorbed with P_1 (a pentasaccharide derived from paragloboside). It is therefore obvious that the genotype of the proposita can be represented as P^kP^k so that the genotype of each of her parents, not known to be related to each other, should be P_2P^k (Figure 2B).

The husband's genotype in view of the 8 consecutive abortions had to be P_2P_2 or homozygous for antigen P so that the genotype of the fetuses had to be P_2P^k. Thus the maternal anti-P exerted its cytotoxic effect on antigen P in the tissue cells of the young fetus. Actually anti-P was clearly demonstrated in the serum of the proposita. Each of her 4 sisters had several children and their genotypes could be either P_2P_2 or P_2P^k. The presence of anti-P in their sera tested at lower temperature would suggest the presence of genotype P_2P_2.

It is noteworthy that another "Japanese woman of group P^k reported by Hayashida had the history of four miscarriages at fourth to sixth month" (Furukawa et al., 1974). Apparently this woman's genotype was also P^kP^k and her serum contained IgG anti-P molecules (Hayashida, 1968). The observations confirm the higher rate of consanguinity especially in rural and mountainous Japan (Hirschhorn, 1982).

SUMMARY

Loss of P_1p pregnancies in pp women is much higher than that of A_1 pregnancies in the incompatible A_1xO mating. This may be associated with a much higher incidence of A_1 (or B) antigenic sites in rbc or tissue cells than P sites. Actually there are no data whatever on the number of P sites in rbc or tissue cells and also no data on the presence of P_1 in secretions such as saliva or ovarian cyst fluid.

In P_1P_1 x pp matings not all P_1p pregnancies end in abortions and these exceptions were observed in each of the three independent studies. In two families with the very rare P^kP^k genotype - rare because the common transferase which converts P^kP^k to the frequent P antigen (globoside), was absent. The two proposita had 8 and 3 abortions each; the sera of all p^kp^k individuals contain IgG molecules of anti-P specificity and their husbands were of genotype PP so that the PP^k fetus was subject to the action of maternal cytotoxic anti-P. Table 1 shows the sugar deteminants of the P system to be almost identical to that of the ABO system but the structure of the very rare pp rbc differs from all others in that it resists the hemolysis by the Donath/Landsteiner antibody in paroxysmal cold hemoglobinuria. This may be due to the fact the pp is the only rbc antigen which contains neuraminic (sialic) acid which prevents the hemolysis.

ACKNOWLEDGMENTS

This research was supported in part by NCI Grant #1 RO1 CA 28448.

REFERENCES

Furukawa, K., Takizawa, H., Takizawa, H., and Iseki, S. (1974) Examples of Blood Groups p and P^k in Japanese Families. *Jap. J. Human Gen.* 19, 1377-1450.

Hakomori, S., and Kobata, A. (1974) Blood Group Antigens. In *The Antigens II* (ed.), M. Sela, pp. 79-140.

Hayashida, Y. (1968) An Example of Blood Group P^k. *J. Japan Soc. Blood Transf.* 15, 181-183.

Hirschhorn, K. (1982) Oral communication.

Ikin, E., Kay H.E.M., Playfair, J.H.L., and Mourant, A.E. (1961) P_1 Antigen in the Human Foetus. *Nature* 192, 883.

Kannagi, R., Levine, P., Watanabe, K., Hakomori, S. (1982). Recent Studies of Glycoprotein Profiles and Characterization of the Major Glycolipid Antigen in Gastric Cancer of a Patient of Blood Group Genotype pp. (Tj^{a-}) First studied in 1951. *Cancer Res.* 42, 5249-5254.

Levene, H., and Rosenfield, R.E. (1961) ABO Incompatibility. In *Progress in Medical Genetics* (ed.), A.G. Steinberg, New York: Grune and Stratton Inc., pp. 120-157.

Levine P. (1943) Serological Factors as Possible Causes in Spontaneous Abortions. *J. Heredity* 34, 71-80.

Levine, P., Bobbitt, O.B., Waller, R.K., and Kuhmichel, A. (1951) Isoimmunization by a New Blood factor in Tumor Cells. *Proc. Soc. Exp. Biol. Med.* 77, 403-405.

Levine, P., and Koch, E.A. (1954) The Rare Human Isoagglutinin Anti-Tj[a] and Habitual Abortion. *Science* 120, 239- 241.

Marcus, D., Naiki, M., Kundu, I.K. (1976) Abnormalities in the Glycosphingolipid Content of Human P^k and p Erythrocytes. *Proc. Nat. Acad. Sci.* 73, 3263-3267.

Morgan, W.T.J. and Van Heyningen, R. (1944) The Occurrence of A, B and O Blood Group Substances in Pseudo-Mucinous Ovarian Cyst Fluids. *Brit. J. Exp. Path.* 25, 5-15.

Obregon, E. and McKeever, B.G. (1980) Studies on Offspring of pp Mothers. Abstract in *Transfusion* 20, 621.

Pollack, M., Levine, P. and Cedergren, B. (1977) IgG as Well as IgM Activity in Sera of Individuals of Genotype PP. Implications for Antibody Induced Abortions. *Blood* 50, 299.

Race, R. and Sanger, R. (1975) *Blood Groups in Man.* 6th Ed. Oxford: Blackwell Pub. Scient. pp. 169.

Wurzell, H.A., Gottlieb, A.J. and Abelson, N.M. (1971) Immunoglobulin Characterization of Anti-Tj[a] Antibodies. *Transfusion* 11, 1037.

Trophoblast Research 1:315-322, 1983

A CELL-MEDIATED IMMUNE DEFECT IN RECURRENT SPONTANEOUS ABORTION

John A. McIntyre[1] and W. Page Faulk[2]

[1]Department of Obstetrics and Gynecology, Southern Illinois University, School of Medicine, Springfield, Illinois 62708 U.S.A.
[2]Department of Immunology, University of Nice, School of Medicine, Chemin de Vallombrose, 06034, Nice, Cedex, France

INTRODUCTION

Recurrent spontaneous abortion in certain women is associated with an increased frequency of histocompatibility (HLA) antigen sharing with their husbands (Komlos and Halbrecht, 1979; McIntyre and Faulk, 1982a). Our studies of the HLA profiles of spontaneous aborting women and their husbands have revealed couples who do not share common HLA types, yet their clinical histories do not differ remarkably from those who do share. In an attempt to identify some of the immunological characteristics of abortion-prone couples, we have studied the response of husband and wife lymphocytes to each other as well as to controls in one-way mixed lymphocyte culture (MLC) reactions. In this report, we confirm that many aborting couples share HLA antigens. Furthermore, we provide additional data to show that spontaneously-aborted pregnancies can be ascribed to some women who do not share HLA identity with their husbands when measured by the standard complement-dependent cytotoxicity assays, but these women demonstrate a sub-optimal or total lack of cellular responsiveness to their mates in one-way MLC reactions. These data suggest that many abortion-prone couples may share the HLA-D locus antigens without sharing at the HLA-DR locus.

PATIENTS AND METHODS

Patients

Seventeen abortion-prone couples with no children were evaluated. No gynecological or hormonal abnormalities were found in these women to account for their miscarriages, and all had experienced three or more abortions, usually during the first twelve weeks of pregnancy. Twelve age-matched couples with one or more children and no known history of spontaneous abortions served as controls. Third-party control lymphocytes were obtained from volunteer hospital and university staff members.

Methods

Peripheral blood samples were collected in citric acid/sodium citrate/dextrose (ACD) solution and mononuclear leucocytes separated by Ficoll/Hypaque density gradient centrifugation, washed and re-suspended to 2 x 10^6 cells per ml in RPMI medium (GIBCO) containing 100 mg of streptomycin per ml, 25 mM HEPES buffer and 15% autologous plasma, serum or normal goat serum (NGS) as previously described (McIntyre, 1976). Stimulator cells received 3000 rads in a ^{137}cesium irradiator (Gammacell Model C, AEC of Canada) to abolish their capacity proliferate.

To study the MLC reactivity of spontaneous aborting couples, the following combinations were tested: Wife (W) responding to husband (H), W responding to third-party control (C), H responding to W, H responding to C, C responding to W, and C responding to H. Each culture consisted of 200,000 responder cells (0.1 ml) cultured with 200,000 stimulator cells (0.1 ml) in flat-bottom microtiter trays (Falcon 3040). Cultures were plated in triplicate and incubated in an air/5% CO_2 humidified incubator for six days at 37°C. Eighteen hours before termination, each culture received 2 µCi (^{3}H)-thymidine (Amersham). Harvest was done with a MASH II (Microbiological Associates, Walkersville, Maryland), and the degree of (^{3}H)-thymidine uptake measured by an LKB liquid scintillation counter. Microtechniques for HLA-typing and complement-dependent cytotoxicity have been described in detail (McIntyre, 1976). Because prelminary observations showed the aborting wives' MLC responses to their husbands were less than their responses to controls, the wife-husband pairs were used as denominators to obtain the relative response (RR) ratio according to the equation

$$RR = \frac{WCr\,(cpm)}{WHr\,(cpm)}$$

For example, if a wife's response to her husband, WHr was 1000 cpm, and her response to a randomly selected third-party control, WCr was 10,000 cpm, then her RR would be 10. In short, she responded 10 times better to the third- party cells, than to her husband's cells.

RESULTS

The shared HLA antigens between seventeen aborting wives, their husbands and randomly selected controls are shown in Table 1. The number of shared antigens ranged from none to five between the husband-wife pairs, and none to three between wife-control pairs. Similar HLA tissue typing data are presented for childbearing couples in Table 2 and show that wife-husband pairs share two or less antigens, while wife-control combinations shared none to three. In no case could MLC reactivity clearly be correlated with the degree of HLA antigen sharing. Indeed, for both groups the sharing of a common DR locus (the antigens of which are related to the D locus antigens thought directly responsible for initiating MLC responses) could not forecast the magnitude of the MLC response, since the intensity of the reactions was often the same in combination that shared as in a pair that did not. Screening the wife's serum for the presence of complement-dependent cytotoxicity to her husband's cells included assays for both warm and cold antibodies, and although such activity was noted in four aborting wives and one childbearing wife, in only one instance did it appear that these antibodies were responsible for MLC inhibition. That such antibody activity could not predict MLC outcome was often demonstrated by observing optimal MLC responses in cultures where the husband's lymphocytes served either as responder or stimulator to third-party lymphocytes in the presence of his wife's serum.

An underlying deficiency in allogeneic recognition exists between aborting husband-wife pairs as the composite data in Table 3 demonstrate. In both NGS and the wife's autologous sera the responses by either the wife's or husband's cells to a third-party control stimulator cells was 2.09 to 3.18 times better than their responses

Table 1
HLA antigens shared between aborting wives, their husbands and controls

Aborting Patients	Antigens Shared with Husband	Antigens Shared with Control
1	B18	A3, DRw4
2	None	DRw1
3	DRw2	None
4	A1	None
5	None	None
6	None	Cw3
7	DRw7	None
8	None	None
9	None	A2; DRw1
10	Aw30	A11; DRw5
11	B8	None
12	B5; Bw44; DRw1, DRw2	Bw44
13	Cw3;DRw7	A3
14	A2; B7; B5; Cw7	None
15	A1; B15	A1; B8; DRw3
16	A3; DRw2	None
17	A1; A2; Bw44; Cw5, DRw1	None

to each other. When these MLC combinations are performed in the presence of the wife's autologous plasma, there was a dramatic effect as shown by a 6.92 to 8.12-fold increase in the wife's or husband's response to the control compared to each other. The plasma effect is specific, as evidenced by the values (combinations 5 and 6 in Table 3) which resulted when the wife and husband are not together in the equation as denominator. Under these experimental conditions, no plasma effect was observed; thus the MLC relative response ratio approached unity. For comparison, MLC experiments were done with the same wife-husband and wife-control combinations with lymphocytes from fertile couples, and regardless of the combinations tested of the plasma or serum employed, in these women there was no indication of suppressed MLC reactivity as evidenced by the observation that all the MLC relative response ratios approached unity (Table 4).

Table 2
HLA antigens shared between child-bearing women, their husbands and controls

Normal Patients	Antigens Shared with Husband	Antigens Shared with Control
1	None	Bw35; Cw4; DRw4
2	None	B18; DRw3
3	A3; Cw3	None
4	B27	A2
5	A2	A2; Bw44
6	DRw7	B12, DRw7
7	A1, B17	None
8	None	None
9	None	None
10	A2, B5	A2
11	A2, B12	A2, DRw2
12	B40, Cw3	None

DISCUSSION

From the above results it appears that some couples who experience recurrent spontaneous abortions manifest an intrinsic cellular recognition deficiency which is characterized by an absent or weak allogeneic response when their cells are cultured together. Their lymphocytes seem to be otherwise immunologically normal, for either partner stimulates and responds to control lymphocytes. Identical and parallel studies of childbearing couples showed that the husbands and wives responded the same or better to each other as compared with their reactions to control cells. Another characteristic of the aborting wives was the presence in their plasma of a factor which inhibited MLC reactions with their husbands but not with controls, and this factor was present when the patients were not pregnant. A similar allogeneic plasma blocking effect was reported in normal pregnancy blood, (McIntyre and Faulk, 1979) but this activity was apparent only during the latter half of gestation and was not identified in non-pregnant plasma from fertile females. Incompatible allotypic trophoblast-lymphocyte cross reactive (TLX) antigens (McIntyre and Faulk, 1982b) could cause the mother to mount specific recognition factors which normally protect extra-embryonic membranes at the materno-fetal interface (Faulk and McIntyre, 1981; 1983). Failure to recognize paternally derived trophoblast allotypes due to shared allotypy between the mating partners may lead to an aberrent response in the female which disallows successful implantation and is clinically apparent as recurrent abortion. This hypothesis is supported by the results of clinical studies

Table 3
Composite MLC reactions between aborting couples and controls

MLC Combination		MLC relative responses* in: Normal goat serum	Maternal Plasma	Maternal Sera
1	$\frac{C_r:W}{H_r:W}$	3.18 ± 1.07	8.12 ± 4.38	2.75 ± 0.70
2	$\frac{C_r:H}{W_r:H}$	2.14 ± 0.51	6.92 ± 2.90	2.09 ± 0.57
3	$\frac{W_r:C}{W_r:H}$	2.50 ± 0.71	12.27 ± 5.72	2.70 ± 0.88
4	$\frac{H_r:C}{H_r:W}$	6.07 ± 2.93	2.51 ± 0.64	2.03 ± 0.63
5	$\frac{H_r:C}{C_r:H}$	1.47 ± 0.34	1.13 ± 0.25	0.93 ± 0.19
6	$\frac{W_r:C}{C_r:W}$	1.20 ± 0.22	1.46 ± 0.36	1.23 ± 0.32

*To obtain each MLC relative response, the Wife (W) Husband (H), or Control (C) responder cells were co-cultured with irradiated (r) W_r; H_r; and C_r; stimulator cells. For preliminary observations the assumption was made that the aborting wive's responses to their husbands or the husbands' responses to aborting wives were less than their relative responses to the controls, thus husband-wife combinations were subsequently used as denominators to obtain these MLC response ratios. For example, if the responses to husbands by wives were the same as to the controls, the ratio would equal 1. In combination 1, the wives responded to controls 3.18 times better than to their husbands in normal goat serum, 8.12 times better in autologous plasma and 2.75 times better in autologous serum. The data are expressed as the mean relative response ± standard error of the mean.

(Taylor and Faulk, 1981) which show that some recurrent aborters can conceive and deliver normal babies at term following multiple intravenous infusions of HLA incompatible leukocytes; the idea being that HLA mismatched cells would provide incompatible TLX stimulation for the mother, resulting in her production of the necessary protective factors. In addition to HLA sharing, whether blocking factors in maternal plasma and selective MLC unresponsiveness are involved in the same or different syndromes is not presently clear, but they do seem to be emerging as parts of the pathophysiology of recurrent spontaneous abortion (McIntyre and Faulk, 1983).

SUMMARY

Serological examinations of couples with histories of habitual spontaneous abortions do not always reveal an increased incidence of HLA A, B, C, DR antigen sharing between husband and wife. MLC studies of mating couples to compare the wives' responses to their husbands versus third-party controls demonstrated that

Table 4
Composite MLC reactions between child-bearing and controls.*

	MLC Combination	Normal Goat Serum	Maternal Plasma	Maternal Sera
1	$\frac{C_r:W}{H_r:W}$	0.93 ± 0.07	0.75 ± 0.12	0.93 ± 0.10
2	$\frac{C_r:H}{W_r:H}$	0.89 ± 0.10	0.94 ± 0.14	1.14 ± 0.11
3	$\frac{W_r:C}{W_r:H}$	1.24 ± 0.34	1.10 ± 0.23	1.01 ± 0.34
4	$\frac{H_r:C}{H_r:W}$	1.14 ± 0.30	0.64 ± 0.03	1.05 ± 0.26
5	$\frac{H_r:C}{C_r:H}$	1.44 ± 0.33	1.40 ± 0.53	1.42 ± 0.56
6	$\frac{W_r:C}{C_r:W}$	0.98 ± 0.20	1.21 ± 0.32	1.01 ± 0.13

*Calculations and code as detailed in legend for Table 3.

most abortion-prone women responded less well to their mates than to controls, especially when the wife's autologous plasma was used to supplement the culture media. Wives of childbearing couples showed no such MLC anomalies.

ACKNOWLEDGEMENTS

Supported in part by the Medical Research Council, Grant 1-732 from the March of Dimes Birth Defects Foundation, Dialysis Clinic Inc., Charleston, S.C. and the Human Embryology and Pregnancy Foundation.

REFERENCES

Faulk W.P., and McIntyre J.A. (1981) Trophoblast Survival. *Transplantation*, 32,1-5.

Faulk,W.P. and McIntyre J.A. (1983) Immunological studies of human trophoblast: markers, subsets and functions. *Immunological Reviews*, 75, 372-408.

Komlos, L. and Halbrecht, I. (1979) Repeated abortions and histocompatibility antigens. *Medical Hypothesis*, 5, 901-908.

McIntyre, J.A. (1976) Laboratory Techniques. In: *Surgical Immunology*. A.M. Munster, (ed.) Grune and Stratton, New York, pp. 288-306.

McIntyre, J.A and Faulk, W.P. (1979) Maternal blocking factors in human pregnancy are found in plasma, not serum. *Lancet* ii, 821-823.

McIntyre, J.A. and Faulk, W.P. (1982a) HLA and the generation of diversity in human pregnancy. In: *Immunological Aspects of Placental Proteins*. Placenta, Suppl. 4, W. Saunders, Eastbourne, pp. 1-11.

McIntyre, J.A. and Faulk, W.P. (1982b) Allotypic trophoblast-lymphocyte cross reactive (TLX) cell surface antigens. *Human Immunology*, 4, 27-35.

McIntyre, J.A. and Faulk, W.P. (1983) Recurrent spontaneous abortion in human pregnancy: Results of Immunogenetical, cellular and humoral studies. *Am. J. Reprod. Immunol. 75,* (in press).

Taylor, C. and Faulk, W.P. (1981) Prevention of recurrent abortion with leucocyte transfusions. *Lancet*, ii,68-70.

Trophoblast Research 1: 323-334 1983

PREGNANCY-ASSOCIATED PLASMA PROTEIN-A (PAPP-A) IS A SPECIFIC INHIBITOR OF THE THIRD COMPONENT OF HUMAN COMPLEMENT

Paul Bischof and Antoine Geinoz

Division of Clinical Biology of Growth and Reproduction
Department of Obstetrics and Gynecology
University of Geneva, 1211 Geneva 4, Switzerland

INTRODUCTION

Pregnancy-associated plasma protein-A (PAPP-A) was discovered in the plasma of pregnant women by Gall and Halbert (1972). It was later shown by Lin et al. (1974a) that PAPP-A was indeed a new pregnancy protein, immunologically different from other known pregnancy proteins.

PAPP-A has been purified to homogenicity (Bischof, 1979, Sutcliffe et al., 1980, Folkersen et al., 1981a) and characterized biochemically. It is a macromolecular glycoprotein with an α2 electrophoretic mobility. Its structure is a dimer of 800,000 molecular weight (MW), each monomer being composed of 2 apparently identical subunits of 200,000 MW.

PAPP-A increases in the maternal circulation during pregnancy, reaching a peak around parturition (Lin et al., 1974b, Smith et al., 1979, Folkersen et al., 1981b, Bischof et al., 1982a). Using a radioimmunoassay, Bischof et al.(1981) demonstrated the presence of PAPP-A in the circulation of non-pregnant females. Thus PAPP-A is not specific to pregnancy but associated with human pregnancy.

Immunohistochemical studies demonstrated the presence of PAPP-A in the syncytiotrophoblast (Lin and Halbert 1976, Wahlstrom et al., 1981), and it was concluded that PAPP-A is probably of trophoblastic origin (Lin et al., 1976). Very recently, Schindler et al. (1983) localized PAPP-A also in decidualized endometrium so that the tissue origin of PAPP-A in pregnant and non-pregnant women awaits further experimentation.

The biological function of PAPP-A is unknown, but in vitro PAPP-A exerts immunosuppressive effects by inhibiting mitogen induced lymphocyte transformation (Bischof et al., 1982b) and by inhibiting the activity of complement (Bischof, 1981). Because of the affinity of PAPP-A for heparin (Sinosich et al., 1981) it has been argued that the inhibitory effect of PAPP-A (purified from heparin plasma) on complement activity might be due to the heparin moiety bound to PAPP-A since heparin is known as an inhibitor of complement (Dr. Teisner, personal communication).

It is the purpose of the present study to determine if inhibition of complement induced hemolysis is due to PAPP-A or to heparin, and to determine on which subunit this effect is exerted.

MATERIALS AND METHODS

Purification of PAPP-A

PAPP-A was purified by 2 different techniques and from 2 different sources:

A) By ion exchange, affinity chromatography and gel filtration as reported previously (Bischof, 1979) starting from a pool of heparinized late pregnancy plasma.

B) By ion exchange chromatography on DEAE Sephadex A50 (elution with NaCl gradient from 0.2 to 1M in phosphate buffer 0.05 M pH 7.0) and affinity chromatography on heparin-Sepharose (elution with NaCl 0.6 M in phosphate buffer 0.05 M pH 7.0) starting from a pool of ethylenediamine tetraacetate (EDTA 2 mg/ml) treated late pregnancy plasma.

Both preparations were electrophoretically pure by SDS polyacrylamide gel electrophoresis.

Radioiodination of C3

Functionally pure human C3 (Cordis Laboratories, Miami) was iodinated with 1 mCi of ^{125}I according to the lactoperoxidase technique or Thorell and Johansson as modified by Aubert (1977).

Chromatography on sepharose Cl4B

Preswollen Sepharose Cl4B (Pharmacia Uppsala, Sweden) was extensively washed with buffer A (0.05 M phosphate, 0.2 M NaCl, 0.5% bovine serum albumin pH 7.4), and packed into a column (2.5 x 84 cm).

Samples applied to the column had a volume of 5 ml and elution with buffer A was conducted under standardized conditions (persistaltic pump setting and volume of fractions collected: 5 ml). The column was calibrated with proteins of known molecular weights (α2 macroglobulin, urease, immunoglobulin G and bovine serum albumin).

Preparation of immunosorbant

Rabbit anti-human PAPP-A (Bischof, 1979) was bound to Protein-A-Sepharose (Pharmacia, Uppsala, Sweden) according to the manufacturer's instructions. The gel was then dispersed in buffer A.

Hemolytic assays

Heparin (0.03 to 2 IU, Liquemin Roche, Basel, Switzerland), EDTA (3 to 33 µg/ml, Merck, Darmstadt, Germany) or PAPP-A (4.8 and 11.3 µg/ml solutions were prepared with assay buffer and tested for their ability to modify the hemolytic activity of human complement according to the method of Reid et al. (1972). The protocols of the hemolytic assays used are given in Table 1. All reagents were purchased from Cordis laboratories (Miami, Florida). Before each assay, serial dilutions of the complement subcomponent under investigation were tested in order to determine the concentration of complement needed to obtain a 50% lysis of the sensitized sheep red blood cells (CH 50). The subsequent assay was performed at this dilution of complement.

After incubation, the remaining non-hemolysed cells are centrifuged, and the optical density of the supernatant measured at 415 nm. The results are expressed as percentage of inhibition (or stimulation) of hemolysis and calculated as follows:

$$100 \times \frac{\text{E415 in absence of inhibitors} - \text{E415 in presence of inhibitors}}{\text{E415 in absence of inhibitors}}$$

Thus, the higher the percentage of inhibition, the more suppressed the activity of complement.

RESULTS

Inhibition of hemolysis: effects of heparin and EDTA

Increasing the concentration of heparin (0.03 to 0.4 IU/ml) in the assay buffer has a marked inhibitory effect on Cl-9 (whole complement) induced hemolysis (Figure 1). The maximal effect (100% inhibition) is obtained with a concentration of 0.13 IU/ml. In sharp contrast, EDTA (3 to 33 µg/ml) has no inhibitory effect (Figure 1).

Inhibition of hemolysis: effects of PAPP-A

Both PAPP-A preparations (isolated from heparin plasma or from EDTA plasma) exert a statistically significant inhibition on whole complement induced hemolysis (Table 2).

The effect of PAPP-A isolated from heparin plasma is partially masked by the inhibitory effect of phosphate buffer alone (Table 2).

To investigate the effect of PAPP-A on the hemolytic activty of isolated complement subunits, PAPP-A had to be removed after preincubation. Heparín-free PAPP-A in phosphate buffer (11.3 µg) was preincubated with the complement subunit

Table 1. Protocols of hemolytic assays

Assay for	Reagents and incubation conditions (total volume 1.2 ml)
C1	1 X CH_{50} of Cl + EA[a] C4 (30°C, 20 min) + C2 (30°C, 10 min) + EDTA - GVB[b] + C - EDTA[c] (37°C, 60 min)
C2	1 X CH_{50} of C2 + EACl,4 (30°C, 2.5 min) + EDTA - GVB + C - EDTA (37°C, 60 min)
C3	1 X CH_{50} of C3 + C2, 5, 6, 7 + EACl,4 (30° C, 30 min) + C8,9 (37°C, 60 min)
C4	1 X CH_{50} of C4 + EACl (30°C, 20 min) + C2 (30°C, 10 min) EDTA - GVB + C - EDTA (37°C, 60 min)
C5	1 X CH_{50} of C5 + C2,3,6,7 + EACl,4 (30°C, 30 min) + C8,9 (37°C, 60 min)
C6	1 X CH_{50} of C6 + C2,3,5,7 + EACl,4 (30°C, 30 min) + C8,9 (37°C, 60 min)
C7	1 X CH_{50} of C7 + C2,3,5,6 + EACl,4 (30°C, 30 min) + C8,9 (37°C, 60 min)
C8	1 X CH_{50} of C8 + C2,3,5,6 + C9 + EACl,4,7 (37°C, 90 min)
C9	1 X CH_{50} of C9 + C2,3,5,6 + C8 + EACl,4,7 (37°C, 90 min)
C1-9	1 X CH_5 of Cl-9 + EA + GVB^{++} (37°C, 60 min)

a) EA: sheep erythrocytes-anti-sheep erythrocyte complexes (10^8cells/ml)
b) EDTA-GCB: 0.04M EDTA in 0.03 M veronal containing 0.1% gelatin
c) C-EDTA: guinea pig complement (1:12.5) in EDTA-GVB
Assay buffer: Glc-GVB^{++}:2.5% glucose, 0.015 M veronal, 0.015 mM Ca^{++}, 0.5 mM Mg^{++}, 0.05% gelatin

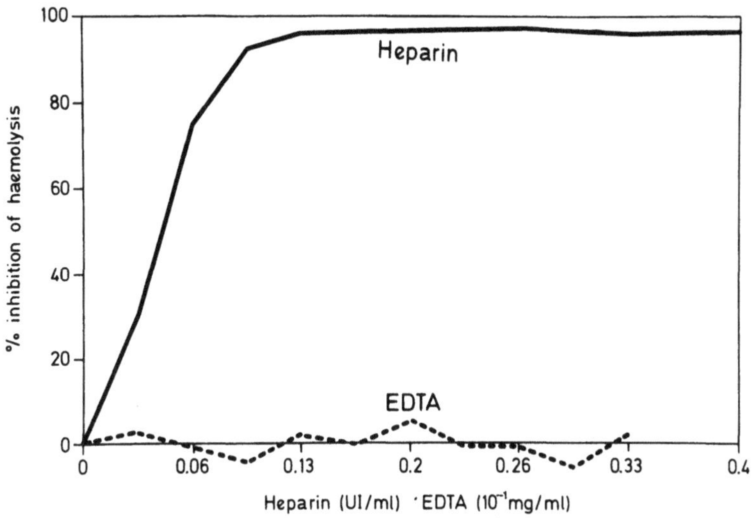

Figure 1. Effect of heparin and EDTA on whole complement (Cl-9) induced hemolysis.

Table 2. Inhibition of whole human complement induced hemolytic activity in % at CH50

	Inhibition in %	
0.05 PO_4 (200 µl) 4.8 µg PAPP-A[a] in 200 µl PO_4	51.8 ± 17.6[c] 77.3 ± 6.1	$p < 0.05$
0.05 PO_4 (30 µl) 11.3 µg PAPP-A[b] in 30 µl PO_4	36.0 ± 14.7 88.8 ± 20.5	$p < 0.01$

a) PAPP-A isolated from heparin plasma
b) PAPP-A isolated from EDTA plasma by heparin-Sepharose column
c) mean ± SD, n = 4

under study. After incubation (30 min at 30°C) anti-PAPP-A bound to protein-A-Sepharose (immunosorbant) was added, the mixture agitated (10 min) and centrifuged. The supernatant was then transferred to the respective hemolytic assays.

The immunosorbant alone exerted marked inhibitory effects, except on Cl and C3 (Figure 2). Immunosorbant alone stimulated Cl induced hemolysis up to 100%. C3 induced hemolysis was moderately stimulated by immunosorbant alone (20%) whereas in presence of heparin-free PAPP-A and immunosorbant a 60% inhibition was observed. This means that the net effect attributable to PAPP-A alone must be approximately 80% inhibition for 11.3 µg. This corresponds to what was found on whole complement (Table 2).

Elution profile on sepahrose Cl 4B

Radiolabeled C3, when submitted to a standardized Sepharose Cl 4B column, eluted in 3 peaks: one peak in the void volume (MW > 2 x 10^6) which represents aggregation products, one large peak with 170,000 MW (Figure 3) and one smaller peak at fraction nb. 150 which is free iodine (not shown in Figure 4). When ^{125}I-C3 was incubated in 5 ml of pregnancy plasma before submitting it to the column, there was still a peak in the void volume, but the second peak eluted earlier with a MW of around 10^6, the peak of free iodine remained unchanged (Figure 3).

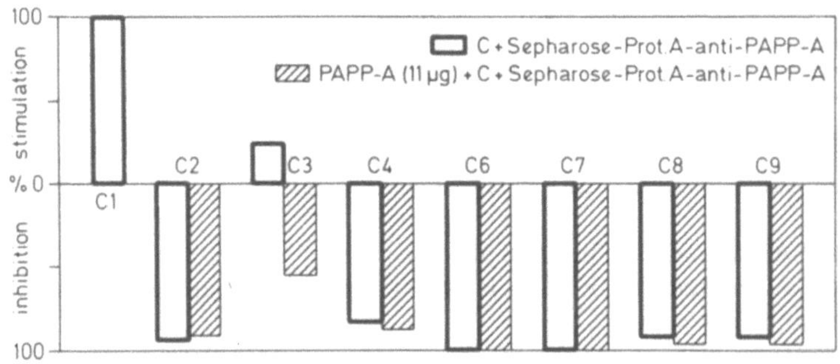

Figure 2. Complement induced hemolysis, effect of PAPP-A and immunosorbant on complement subcomponents.

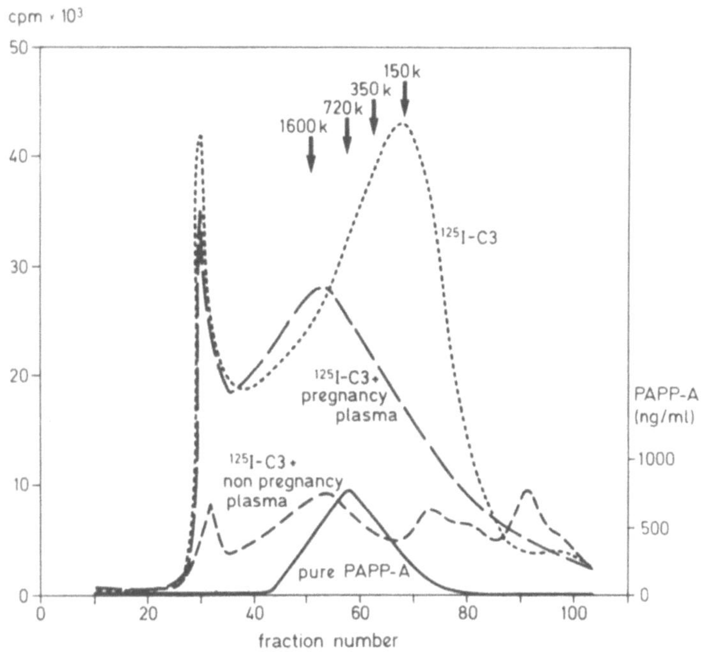

Figure 3. Elution profile on Sepharose C14B of pure PAPP-A and of ^{125}I-C3 with or without preincubation with pregnancy plasma.

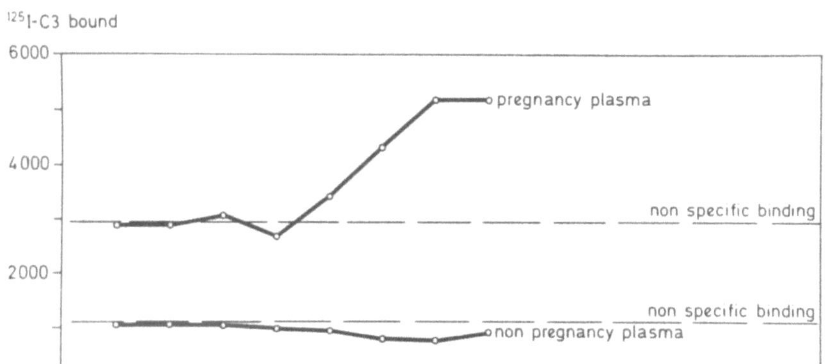

Figure 4. Binding of ^{125}I-C3 to immunoprecipitable PAPP-A in pregnancy plasma or non-pregnancy plasma.

The preincubation mixture of ^{125}I-C3 and normal human plasma, was resolved into 5 peaks: one peak in the void volume, one peak with MW of 10^6, one peak with MW 170,000, another peak with MW around 60,000, and the peak of free iodine at fraction 150 (not shown in Figure 4).

Pure PAPP-A on the same column was eluted with MW 720,000.

Binding experiments

Radioiodinated C3 was incubated overnight with rabbit anti- PAPP-A and with serial dilutions of pregnancy plasma or normal human plasma.

After incubation the mixture was agitated in presence of cellulose bound goat anti-rabbit immunoglobulins, centrifuged and the supernatant counted. Non specific binding was measured in tubes not containing anti-PAPP-A. ^{125}I-C3; specifically bound to PAPP-A anti-PAPP-A complexes in pregnancy plasma, whereas in identical dilution of non-pregnancy plasma no binding could be detected (Figure 4). Anti-PAPP-A alone did not bind ^{125}I-C3, the radioactivity associated with the pellet was of the same order as for the non-specific binding.

DISCUSSION

PAPP-A purified from heparin plasma inhibits complement induced hemolysis (Bischof 1979, Bischof 1981).

It was recently reported by Sinosich et al. (1981) that heparin reversibly binds to PAPP-A. Thus, PAPP-A isolated from heparin plasma could well have the anticoagulant bound to it. Since heparin exerts inhibitory effects on complement, it could be that the described inhibitory effect of PAPP-A is in fact due to the heparin bound to it.

According to the present results, heparin exerts a marked inhibitory effect on whole complement induced hemolysis. PAPP-A, purified form heparin-plasma, is also inhibitory. The fact that PAPP-A isolated from EDTA plasma and purified on a heparin column (thus heparin free PAPP-A) is also markedly inhibitory on whole complement activity, seems to rule out the possibility of heparin being the active inhibitor of the PAPP-A molecule. Clearly, PAPP-A is inhibitory by itself and seems to "specifically" inhibit C3 induced hemolysis. It must be said that our approach did not permit to evaluate properly the effect of PAPP-A on all subunits because the immunosorbant used to separate free and bound PAPP-A exerted inhibitory effects per se.

The inhibition of PAPP-A on C3 seems to be due to a binding of PAPP-A to C3, since the apparent molecular weight (MW) of C3 when incubated with pregnancy plasma is increased by a factor corresponding to the MW of PAPP-A, and since radiolabeled C3 binds to PAPP-A antiserum only in presence of PAPP-A (pregnancy plasma).

This means that PAPP-A acts on C3 itself and not on C3 convertase (C4,2) as does C3 inactivator.

Although complement inhibition has been obtained in this study with physiological concentrations of PAPP-A, it is unknown if the observed in vitro effect of PAPP-A is at all relevant in the in vivo situation.

It is, of course, tempting to speculate that PAPP-A inhibits C3 in vivo and reduces by this mechanism complement mediated lysis and phagocytosis of fetal cells and antigens, contributing in that way to the survival of the fetal allograft in an immunocompetent mother.

SUMMARY

PAPP-A is a macromolecular glycoprotein associated with pregnancy, which was shown to inhibit complement induced hemolysis and to reversibly bind heparin. Because of the inhibitory effect of heparin on the complement cascade, it was not clear if the inhibition of complement activity observed with PAPP-A (isolated from heparin plasma) was attributable to the heparin moiety bound to PAPP-A.

The present work demonstrates that heparin exerts an inhibitory effect on complement activity, but that heparin free PAPP-A is also inhibitory. PAPP-A specifically inhibits C3 by binding to this complement subcomponent and not by inhibiting C3 convertase as demonstrated for C3 inactivator.

ACKNOWLEDGMENTS

We thank Mrs. L. Haenggeli and M.T. Sizonenko for technical help and Mrs. D. Roiron for typing the manuscript. This work was supported by a grant from the Swiss National Fund for Scientific Research No. 3.931.0.80.

REFERENCES

Aubert, M.L. (1977) Radioimmunoassay for human prolactin. In: *Handbook of Radioimmunoassay*, Abraham G.E. (ed.), pp. 179-208, New York: M. Dekker.

Bischof, P. (1979) Purification and characterization of pregnancy-associated plasma protein-A (PAPP-A), *Arch. Gynecol.* 227, 315-326.

Bischof, P. (1981) Pregnancy-associated plasma protein-A (PAPP-A): An inhibitor of the complement system. *Placenta* 2, 29-34.

Bischof, P., Haenggeli, L., Sizonenko, M.T., Herrmann, W.L. and Sizonenko, P.C. (1981) Radioimmunoassay for the measurement of pregnancy-associated plasma protein-A (PAPP-A) in humans. *Biol. Reprod.* 24, 1076-1081.

Bischof, P., DuBerg, S., Herrmann, W.L. and Sizonenko, P.C. (1982a), Amniotic fluid and circulating levels of pregnancy-associated plasma protein-A (PAPP-A) throughout pregnancy. *Brit. J. Obstet. Gynaecol.* 89, 358-363.

Bischof, P., Lauber, K., de Wurstemberger, B. and Girard, J.P. (1982b) Inhibition of lymphocyte transformation by pregnancy- associated plasma protein-A (PAPP-A). *J. Clin. Lab. Immunol.* 7, 61-65.

Folkersen, J., Grudzinskas, J.G., Hindersson, P., Teisner, B. and Westergaard, J.G. (1981a) Purification of pregnancy-associated plasma protein-A by a two step affinity chromatograhic procedure. *Placenta* 2, 11-18.

Folkersen, J., Grudzinskas, J.G., Hindersson, P., Teisner, B. and Westergaard, J.G. (1981b) Pregnancy-associated plasma protein- A: Circulating levels during normal pregnancy. *Amer. J. Obstet. Gynecol.* 139, 910-914.
Gall, S.A. and Halbert, S.P. (1972) Antigenic constituents in pregnancy plasma which are undetectable in normal non-pregnant female or male plasma. *Int. Arch. Allergy* 42, 503-515.
Lin, T.M., Halbert, S.P., Kiefer, D. and Spellacy, W.N. (1974a) Three pregnancy-associated plasma proteins: Purification monospecific antisera and immunological identification. *Int. Arch. Allergy* 47, 35-53.
Lin, T.M., Halbert, S.P. and Spellacy, W.N. (1974b) Measurements of pregnancy-asociated plasma proteins during human gestation. *J. Clin. Invest.* 54, 576-582.
Lin, T.M. and Halbert, S.P. (1976) Placental localization of human pregnancy-associated plasma proteins. *Science* 193, 1249- 1252.
Lin, T.M., Halbert, S.P. and Kiefer, D. (1976) Quantitative analysis of pregnancy associated plasma proteins in human placenta. *J. Clin. Invest.* 57, 466-472.
Reid, K.B., Lowe, D.M. and Porter, R.R. (1972) Isolation and characterization of Clq and subcomponents fo the first component of complement from human and rabbit sera. *Biochem. J.* 130,749-763.
Schindler, A.M., Bordignon, P. and Bischof, P. (1983) Immunohistochemical localization of pregnancy-associated plasma protein-A in decidua and trophoblast. Comparison with hCG and Fibrin. *Placenta,* In press.
Sinosich, M.J., Teisner, B., Davey, M. and Grudzinskas, J.G. (1981) Pregnancy-associated plasma protein-A: Interaction with heparin in crossed affinity immunoelectrophoresis. *Australian New Zealand J. Med.* 11, 429-433.
Smith, R., Bischof, P., Hughes, G. and Klopper, A. (1979) Studies on pregnancy-associated plasma protein-A in the third trimester of pregnancy. *Brit. J. Obstet. Gynaecol.* 86, 882-887.
Sutcliffe, R.G., Kukulska-Langlands, B.M., Coggins, J.R., Hunter, J.B. and Gore, G.H. (1980) Studies on pregnancy-associated plasma protein-A. Purification by affinity chromatography and structural comparison with α2-macroglobulin. *Biochem. J.* 191, 799-809.
Wahlstrom, T., Teisner, B. and Folkersen, J. (1981) Tissue localization of pregnancy-associated plasma protein-A (PAPP-A) in normal placenta. *Placenta* 2, 253-258.

DISCUSSION

BENVENISTE (Chicago): PAPP-A consists of two parts, a carbohydrate and a protein constituent. If you degrade PAPP-A with pronase, do you see a disappearance of binding to complement?

BISCHOF (Geneva): That would be an interesting experiment but we have not pursued it.

FAULK (Nice): In the preparation of your plasma, you use EDTA to remove calcium. For the convertase system to work, calcium is required. Do you recalcify your plasma before you test for the hemolytic properties of the plasma? It has certainly been well established that the kinetics of complement binding to anything, including red cell membranes coated with the antibodies such as you have used, are known to be inhibited by very small amounts of EDA. Therefore, it may be essential to recalcify your medium to have a functional level of calcium for C'-1 fixation and transfer testing.

BISCHOF (Geneva): No, we have not recalcified the medium and no inhibition could be observed with EDTA up to 33 mg/ml.

Trophoblast Research 1:335-346, 1983

THE EMBRYOPATHOLOGIC EFFECTS OF TERATOGENIC YOLK SAC ANTISERUM

Robert L. Brent,[1] David A. Beckman, Marcela Jensen, Thomas R. Koszalka and Ivan Damjanov

Departments of Pediatrics, Radiology, Anatomy and Biochemistry
Jefferson Medical College, Philadelphia, PA, USA
and Department of Pathology, Hahneman Medical College,Philadelphia, PA, USA

INTRODUCTION

In 1961, our laboratory reported that the injection of rabbit anti-rat kidney serum into pregnant rats resulted in a high incidence of congenital malformations in the offspring (Brent et al., 1961). Attempts to demonstrate an indirect mechanism of teratogenesis secondary to maternal immunologic or metabolic disease were not successful (Brent, 1964, 1966a, 1966b). It was demonstrated that the teratogenic factor was IgG and that the teratogenic process following exposure to kidney antibody was not dependent on complement fixation (Brent, 1966b; Bragonier et al., 1970). Furthermore, pretreatment with cortisone or antihistamines did not prevent the teratogenic effect of the kidney antiserum (Brent, 1966b). In 1966, Slotnick and Brent demonstrated that teratogenic antisera prepared against rat kidney or chorioplacenta localized in the developing yolk sac placentae of the rat. These results indicated that the mechanism of action of teratogenic antisera was not due to an indirect effect of induced maternal disease or a direct effect on the embryo, but possibly the induction of yolk sac dysfunction. In 1971, Brent and associates demonstrated that antiserum prepared against yolk was a more potent teratogen than was kidney antiserum. Yolk sac antiserum also localized in the visceral and parietal yolk sac (Brent et al., 1971). A direct primary effect was further supported by the work of New and Brent (1972). In their experiments, rat embryos were dissected from the embryonic sites on the 9th day of development and were cultured for 48 hours. The culture media contained various concentrations of teratogenic yolk sac antisera or normal rabbit serum. The ectoplacental cone was unaffected by the presence of yolk sac antibody, but the yolk sac was markedly affected. If the dose of antiserum was high enough, the yolk sac could be severely growth retarded or destroyed. Yet, direct injections of teratogenic antiserum into the amnionic cavity or the yolk sac cavity was innocuous to the embryonic site. Other laboratories confirmed that teratogenic antisera could be prepared against rat or mouse kidney and that teratogen-stimulating antigens were present in other tissues (Mercier-Parot et al., 1963; David et al., 1963; Barrow and Taylor, 1971; Eyquem et al., 1968; Gebhardt et al., 1970; Mikhailov, 1967; Vaillancourt and McCallion, 1972). The following experiment was designed to evaluate the histopathologic effects of teratogenic yolk sac antiserum on the developing embryo, as well as on the visceral and parietal yolk sac and the chorioplacenta.

[1]send reprint requests to:
Robert L. Brent, M.D., Ph.D., Jefferson Medical College, Stein Research Center, 920 Chancellor Street, Philadelphia, PA 19107

METHODS

Teratogenic antisera was prepared against rat visceral yolk obtained at term. Whole rat visceral yolk sacs were removed from rat fetuses obtained by cesarean section at term. The yolk sacs were homogenized in a Virtis microhomogenizer in phosphate buffered physiologic saline. One half milliliter of yolk sac solution containing 10 mg of yolk sac protein was homogenized with 0.5 ml of incomplete Freund's adjuvant. Rabbits were immunized with 0.2 ml of antigen into the hindpaw digits with a total dose of 1 ml. Three intramuscular biweekly injections of antigen were followed by harvesting of the antiserum. The experiments reported in this paper were performed utilizing antiserum from a large pool. The antiserum utilized in these experiments had an LD_{50} dose of 125 mg/kg when administered to pregnant rats on the 9th day of gestation. This dose is innocuous to the mothers and results in a 50 percent mortality to the embryos. Doses of 150 mg/kg result in a higher resorption rate with no effect on the mother. All of the surviving embryos are malformed. Fifty percent of surviving embryos are malformed with a dose of 100 mg/kg.

Thirty-two pregnant rats were utilized in this study. Pregnancy was determined by the presence of vaginal sperm on the morning after mating. At 9 AM on that morning, the pregnancy was designated as the beginning of the first day. On the morning of the 9th day, a rat was injected with nothing, normal sheep serum, 100, 125 or 150 mg/kg of sheep anti-rat yolk sac teratogenic serum (see Table 1). Uterine horns were removed at 4, 8, 12, 24, 48 and 72 hours. Since each rat has two uterine horns, a pregnant rat could provide embryonic sites for two time periods. In order to accomplish this, the pregnant rats were lightly anesthetized and a small incision was made in the abdomen. The uterine artery and ovarian artery were ligated on one side, and that uterine horn was surgically removed. The abdominal incision was closed with silk sutures, and the skin incision was closed with Michelle wound clips. When the other horn was removed from 4 to 72 hours later, a similar procedure was used. After removing the second uterine horn, the animal was killed.

The uterine horns were placed in Bouins fixative. After fixation, the embryonic sites were imbedded in paraffin, serially sectioned and stained with hematoxylin and eosin. Photomicrographs were made with an American Optical microscope and Olympus OM-2 automatic camera.

RESULTS

One hundred and forty-seven embryonic sites were serially sectioned (Table 1). All of the specimens included the complete embryo. There was no difference discernible between those embryonic sites that were exposed to normal sheep serum and those from animals that received nothing.

Following the injection of teratogenic antiserum there were no changes visible in the yolk sac (visceral or parietal) at 4, 8, 12 or 24 hours post-injection (Figures 1, 2). The height of the visceral yolk sac endodermal cells, the vascularity of the visceral yolk sac, and the size of the amniotic and yolk sac cavities were all comparable to control embryos at the same stage of development. Similarly, the Reichert's membrane and parietal endodermal cells could not be distinguished from the control embryos during the first 12 hours of exposure. The formation of the ectoplacental cone developed exactly the same in the control and antiserum exposed embryos. Even after 96 hours, the developing chorioplacenta was normal in surviving embryos in the control and exposed embryos.

The first evidence of pathology at the light microscope level was observed, not in the yolk sac placentae, but in the embryo at 48 hours after exposure (Figure 3). The signs of embryopathology were increased cell death (as evidenced by cell necrosis or cell pyknosis), embryonic maldevelopment and/or growth retardation. At 48 hours, obvious embryonic death was observed in six embryonic sites at the higher dosage (150 mg/kg) of teratogenic antiserum. At lower dosages (100 mg/kg), embryopathology was readily discernable (Figure 3 (B)).

Embryos exposed to antiserum for 72 hours exhibited gross malformations (Figure 4B) as compared to control embryos (Figure 4A). It was obvious that some of the embryos given the higher doses of antiserum (125 mg and 150 mg/kg) had such serious disorganization that they would not survive.

Since we had the advantage of having embryonic sites from the same pregnancy at two different times, it was possible to examine and compare the yolk sac placentae, chorioplacentae and mortality at 48 and 72 hours post-injection and at an earlier stage. Granted, they were not the same embryonic sites, but they were embryonic sites that were of a comparable embryonic age at the time of exposure and embryonic sites that received a similar exposure of antiserum. In none of the litters containing embryos with obvious embryotoxic effects was their antecedant histopathologic effects evidence in the yolk sac.

Table 1. Number of embryos serially sectioned and examined

Exposure (9 days)	9 days 4 hours	9 days 8 hours	9 days 12 hours	10 days	11 days
control	6	7	6	5	5
sheep serum 300 mg/kg	6	6	6	5	6
teratogenic yolk sac antiserum 100 mg/kg	7	6	7	6	5
125 mg/kg	6	7	6	4	5
150 mg/kg	6	6	7	6	5

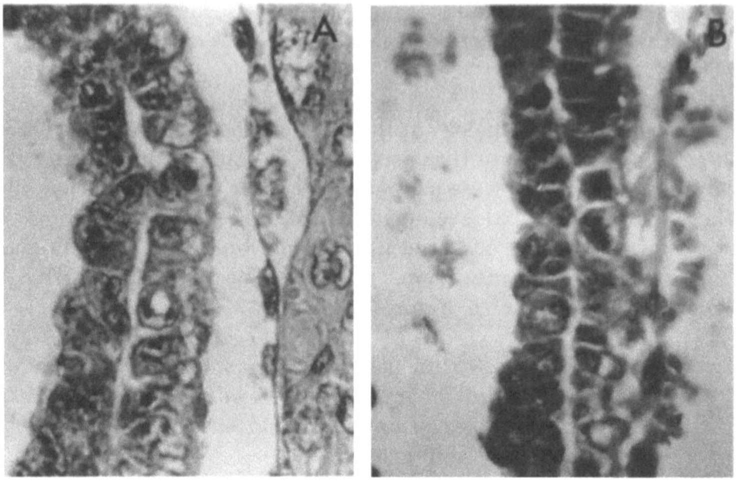

Figure 1. Rat embryonic sites 8 days and 12 hours old, obtained from pregnant rats administered (A) normal sheep serum or (B) sheep anti-rat whole visceral yolk sac serum 12 hours previously. Reichert's membrane and the embryonic endodermal cells and yolk sac cells are similar in both embryos. There is no sign of embryonic damage or excessive cell death in the embryo or the visceral yolk sac hematoxylin and eosin (X640).

When embryotoxic effects were manifested in the embryo, histopathological changes became apparent in the yolk sac. In the presence of a dying embryo exposed to teratogenic antiserum, there was a decrease in vascularity of the vitelline circulation in the visceral yolk sac and, regardless of the doses of teratogenic antiserum, histopathologic changes were always visible in the embryo before they were observed in the yolk sac placentae.

DISCUSSION

Recent studies with rabbit anti-rat yolk sac serum have demonstrated that this antiserum can decrease the pinocytosis of proteins by the visceral yolk sac (Freeman et al., 1982). The mechanism of teratogenesis suggested is that the reduction in pinocytosis decreases the uptake of maternal serum proteins by the yolk sac and therefore the availability of amnio acids for the yolk sac and embryo is also decreased.

Teratogenic antibody is present only on the distal portion of the visceral yolk sac endodermal cell and is never localized in the central or proximal portion of the endodermal cell. Furthermore, the antibody is never identified in the other areas of the yolk sac or in the embryo (Brent et al., 1971). Thus, the biochemical lesion produced by teratogenic antiserum in the visceral endodermal cell results in a

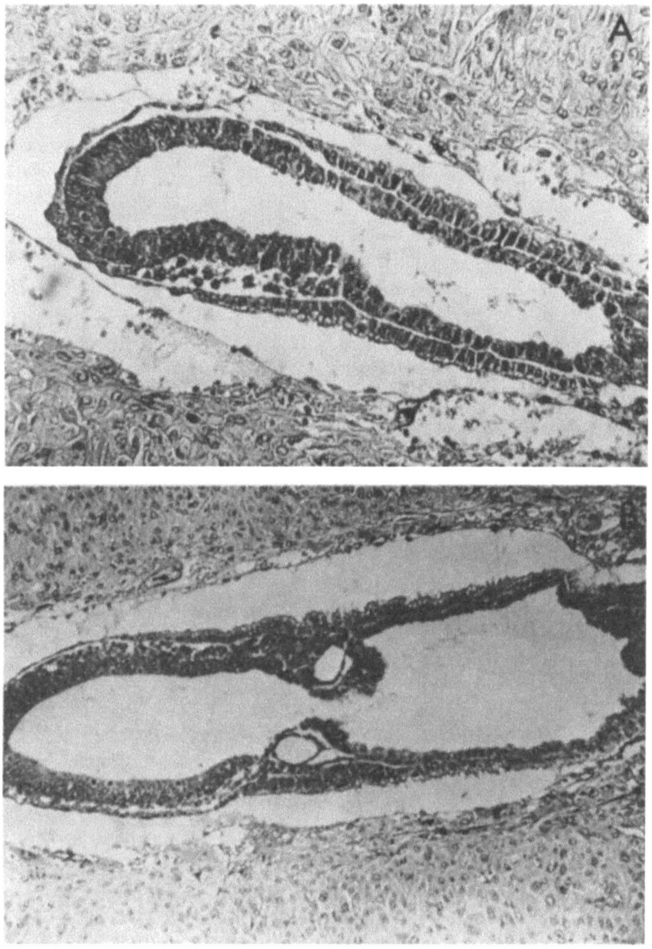

Figure 2. Rat embryonic sites 9 days old obtained from pregnant rats administered (A) normal sheep serum or (B) sheep anti-rat visceral yolk sac serum 24 hours previously. After 24 hours, there is no significant damage in the antibody-treated embryo (X320).

Figure 3. Rat embryonic sites 10 days old obtained from pregnant rats administered (A) normal sheep serum or (B) sheep anti-rat visceral yolk sac serum 48 hours previously. The antibody exposed embryonic site has an embryo with a distorted neural tube, disaggregated somites, slight retardation and some treated embryos given the highest dose exhibited early signs of embryonic death. Although there was no difference between Reichert's membrane in the control (C) and antiserum exposed embryos, there was marked reduction in the vascularity of the visceral yolk sac of the embryos exposed to antiserum for 48 hours (D). *Figure overleaf* ⟶

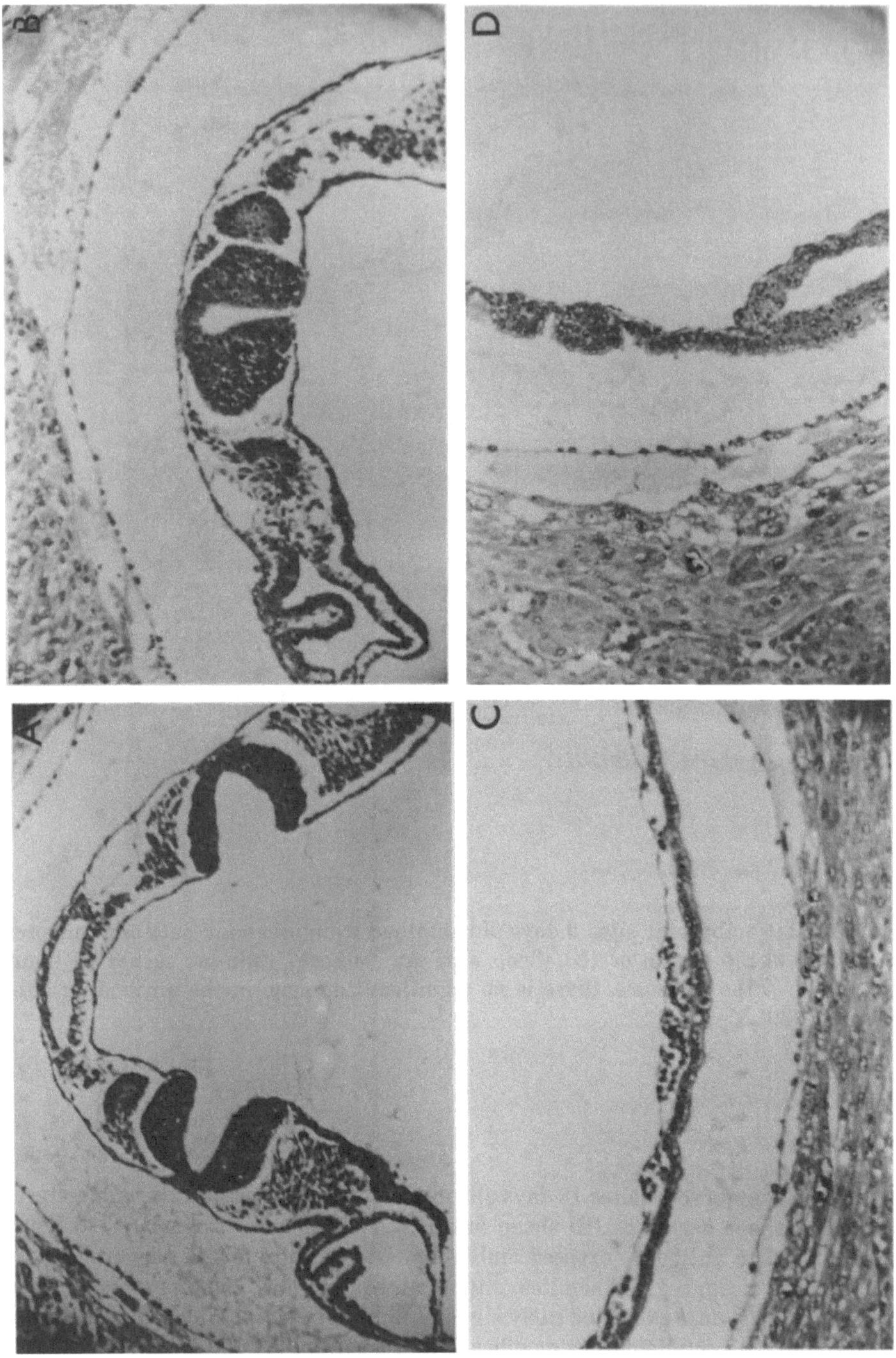
B
D
A
C

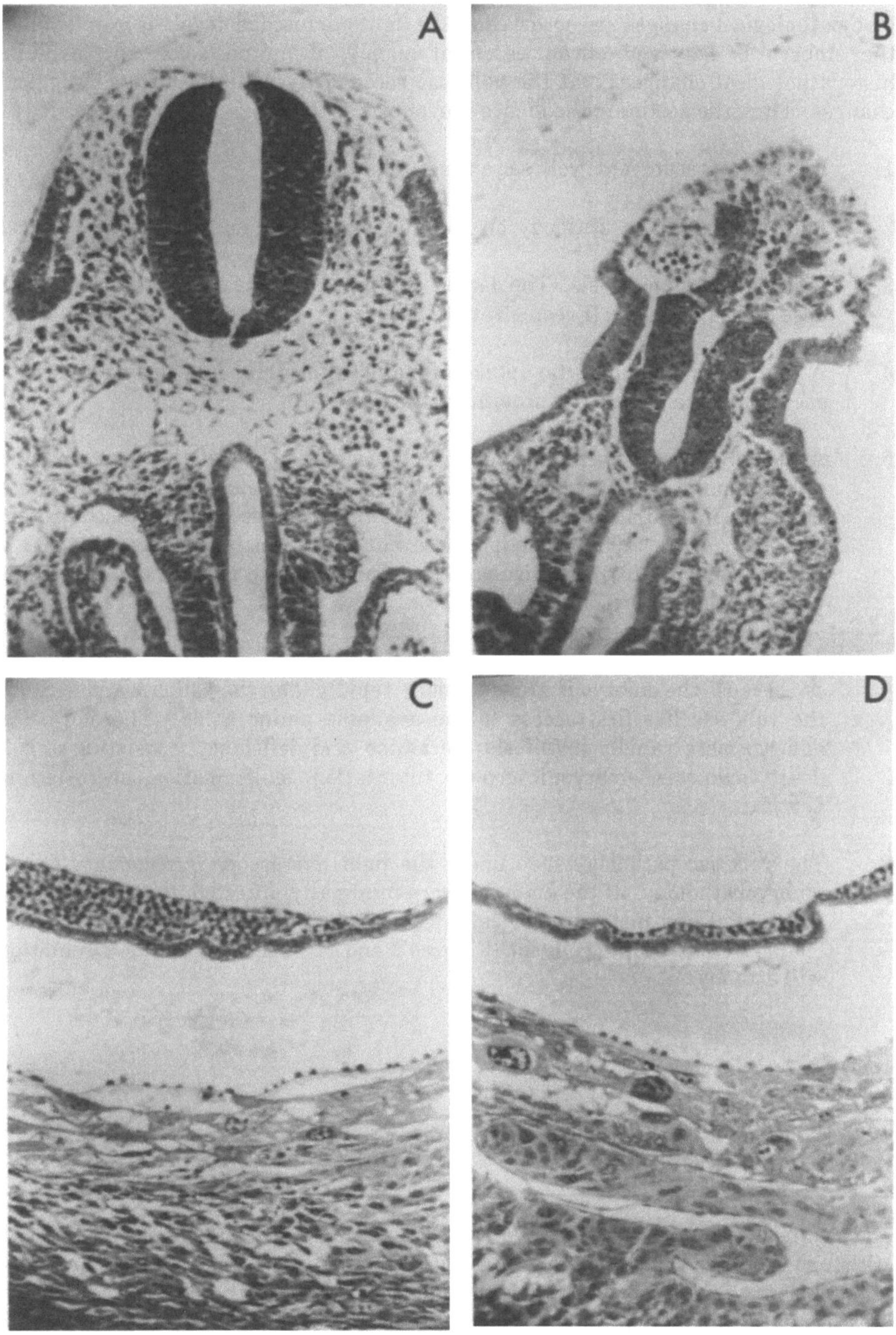

Figure 4. Rat embryos 11 days old administered normal sheep serum (A,C) or antiserum (B,D) 72 hours previously. The treated embryo (B) exhibits neural tube
(Continued on page 342)

functional change, namely a reduction in pinocytosis, but no immediate histopathological changes are observed at the light microscope level. It is only when the embryo is deprived of an essential supply of amino acids and exhibits histopathological changes, that the yolk sac secondarily exhibits histopathological changes. Thus, the postulated sequence of events is as follows:

1. Injection of teratogenic yolk sac antiserum.

2. Localization of the antibody on the distal pole and surface of the visceral endodermal cell.
3. Reduction in pinocytosis. The decrease in pinocytosis is directly related to the dose of the antiserum (Freeman et al., 1982).

4. A decrease in the pinocytic uptake of maternal proteins into the visceral yolk sac results in a decrease of proteins in the lysosomes.

5. Although there is no inability of the lysosomes to digest the proteins and release amino acids for embryonic and yolk sac protein synthesis, there is a reduction in available amino acids due to the decrease in pinocytosed protein (Freeman et al., 1982). Under these circumstances, the embryo retains a normal capacity to synthesize proteins if an adequate amount of amino acids were present (Kobrin and Brent, 1973).

6. The reduction in available amino acids affects the embryo sooner than the yolk sac because the embryo is growing more rapidly than the yolk sac and because the yolk sac has first access to the available amino acids. Therefore, the embryo more rapidly manifests the amino acid deficiency, consisting of cell death, pyknosis, embryonic growth retardation, malformation, necrosis and death.

7. The yolk sac pathology seen under the light microscope is secondary to the embryopathology. If the embryos were minimally affected, the yolk sac does not exhibit any histopathological effects. If the embryo dies, then, of course, changes occur in the yolk sac (Figures 3 and 4) since the vitelline circulation will atrophy.

---

and somite disorganization. It is obvious that this embryo (B) will not survive to term. Although there is a reduction in vascularity of the yolk sac in the treated embryo, the embryo is much more affected than is the yolk sac. Although there appeared to be an increase in the amount of proteinaceous material in the yolk sac cavity in antiserum embryos, this observation could be a secondary effect. Even after 72 hours Reichert's membrane appeared identical in the control and treated embryos, as did the developing chorioplacenta.

The accumulation of proteinaceous material between the parietal and visceral endodermal cells may be a physiologic phenomenon rather than pathologic. One explanation might be that the atrophy of the vitelline circulation (due to the death of the embryo) prevents the visceral yolk sac from delivering the substrates to the embryos (Figure 4D). Therefore, the material passing through the parietal yolk sac cannot be processed by the visceral yolk sac and accumulates between the two yolk sacs. Thus, while a reduction in pinocytosis is the primary pathological process, it does not alone account for the end pathological state observed in Figure 4B.

It is likely that examination of these tissues by electron microscopy may reveal pathological changes in the yolk sac that would correlate with the biochemical lesion. This observation would not alter the fact that the major effect of the yolk sac antibody is first observed in the embryo and is literally due to amino acid deprivation. Thus, the model of teratogenesis utilizing yolk sac antibody, first described in 1961 (Brent et al.), appears to be an experimental model of nutritional teratogenesis that is unique because it can produce a nutritional deprivation in the embryo without causing significant nutritional alterations in the mother.

SUMMARY

Pregnant rats were administered teratogenic yolk sac antiserum on the 9th day of gestation. Embryonic sites were removed at 4, 8, 12, 24, 48 and 72 hours after injection of the antiserum and examined histologically. The first evidence of histopathological effects appeared in the embryo in spite of the fact that the primary action of yolk sac antiserum is a reduction in pinocytosis in the yolk sac endodermal cell. Histopathological changes in the yolk sac occur only after extensive pathology has occurred in the embryo. All previously reported in vivo experiments of nutritional teratogenesis involve simultaneous nutritional deprivation or toxicity in the maternal organism. It is believed that this immunological model of teratogenesis, first described in 1961, is a unique model of nutritional teratogenesis with minimal alteration of the maternal organism.

ACKNOWLEDGMENTS

Supported by NIH. Grant # 13411

REFERENCES

Barrow, M.V., and Taylor, W.J. (1971) The production of congenital defects in rats using antisera. *J. Exp. Zool.* 176,41-60.

Bragonier, J.R., Frank, M.M., and Brent, R.L. (1970) Production of congenital malformations using tissue antisera. VIII. Effectiveness of reduced alkylated and digested anti-Kidney antibodies. *J. Immunol.* 105, 1175-1180.

Brent, R.L. (1964) The production of congenital malformations using tissue antisera. II. The spectrum and incidence of malformations following the administration of kidney antiserum to pregnant rats. *Amer. J. Anat.*115, 525- 542.

Brent, R.L. (1966a) The production of congenital malformations using tissue antisera. IV. Evaluation of the mechanism of teratogenesis by varying the route and time of administration of anti-rat kidney antiserum. *Amer. J. Anat.* 119, 555-562.

Brent, R.L. (1966b) Some biologic properties of teratogenic antisera. *Offic. J. Congr. Anat. Res. Assoc. Jap* 6, 12-14.

Brent, R.L., Averich, E., and Drapiewski, V.A. (1961). Production of congenital malformations using tissue antibodies. I. Kidney antisera. *Proc. Soc. Exp. Biol. Med.* 106, 523-526.

Brent, R.L., Johnson, A.J., and Jensen, M. (1971). The production of congenital malformations using tissue antisera. VII. Yolk sac antiserum. *Teratology* 4, 255-276.

David, G., Mercier-Parot, L., and Tuchman-Duplesis, H. (1963). Action teratogene d'heteroanticorps tissulaires, I. Production de malformations chez le rat par action d'un serum antirein. *C.R. Soc.* Biol. 157, 939.

Eyquem, A., Gutman, G., Bisson, J., Mercier-Parot, L., David, G., and Tuchmann-Dpulessis, H. (1968). Etude en immunofluorescence et cytotoxicite des immunserums teratogenes. *Ann. Inst. Pasteur* (Paris) 115, 841-854.

Freeman, S.J., Brent, R.I., and Lloyd, J.B. (1982). The effect of teratogenic antiserum on yolk-sac function in rat embryos cultured in vitro. *J. Embryol. exp. Morph.* 71, 63-74.

Gebhardt, D.O.E., Baart de la Faille-Kuyper, E.H., and Nagel, J. (1970). The embryolethality and localization of anti-kidney serum in the pregnant mouse, Mus musculus. *Teratology* 3, 143-152.

Kobrin, L.E. & Brent, R.L. (1973). Effect of yolk sac antiserum on the passage of free and bound [^{14}C] leucine across the rat yolk sac. *Fed. Proc.* 32(3), 831.

Mercier-Parot, L., David, G., and Tuchmann-Duplessis, H. (1963). Action teratogene d'heteroanticorps tissulaires. II. Etude de l'action teratogene chez la souris de serums anti-rein. *C.R. Soc. Biol.* 157, 974.

Mikhailov, V.M. (1967). Pathogenic action of nephrocytotoxic serum on embryonic development of albino rats. *Biull. Eksp. Biol. Med.* 63, 97-100.

New, D.A.T. & Brent, R.L. (1972). Effect of yolk sac antibody on rat embryos grown in culture. *J. Embryol. exp. Morph.* 27, 543-553.

Slotnick, V. & Brent, R.L. (1966). The production of congenital malformations using tissue antisera. V. Fluorescent localization of teratogenic antisera in the maternal and fetal tissues of the rat. *J. Immunol.* 95, 606-610.

Vaillancourt, P., and McCallion, D.J. (1972). Inhibitory effects of nephrotoxic antisera on the growth of rat fetuses. *Amer. J. Obstet. Gynecol.* 114, 225-231.

DISCUSSION

KLOPPER (Aberdeen): How does your antiyolk teratogenic antiserum affect the rodent mothers? Do they develop albuminuria and retroplacental hemorrhages? Besides a nutritional model, could this also be a model for preeclamptic toxemia?

BRENT (Philadelphia): The original antiplacental antiserum model was first reported in 1902, but it was popularized in modern embryo pathology by Beatrice Segal at Columbia University. She actually developed the antiplacental and antikidney model to uncover the pathophysiology of eclampsia in her animals. They developed a Masugi nephritis, hematuria, hypertension and liver necrosis. Our effort to further develop the model has been to eliminate the basement membrane antigens of the kidney. In fact, the antigens in the kidney, which we have not spoken about, are not basement membrane antigens. We originally felt the teratogenic antigen was in the glomerulus; however, it turns out to be a very rare antigen in the soluble fraction of tubules. If you isolate the antigen from the kidney and eliminate the basement membrane component, you will obtain a nonnephrotoxic teratogenic antiserum. Work by Leung et al. (*J. Immunol.* 1974, 133:885-895) demonstrated that teratogenic stimulating antigen from the kidneys does not alter the foot processes in the glomerulus or any aspect of the kidney function.

FAULK (Nice): Does the teratogenic antiserum from the yolk sac localize to any renal antigen?

BRENT (Philadelphia): No. Some antigens which we now obtain from isoelectric focusing will no longer localize in the kidney.

FAULK (Nice): Will it localize in the gut?

BRENT (Philadelphia): No, it will not localize in the gut. We originally thought that we could obtain similar reactivity in the gastrointestinal tract because the embryonic gastrointestinal tract is so similar to the visceral yolk sac. However, there are no antigens in common in the embryonic rat gut and the visceral endoderm. This is embryologically speaking quite fascinating. Why should the kidney have an antigen in common with the visceral yolk sac and not the embryonic gut?

SANYEL (New Haven): We have performed similar experiments using a micromanipulator. The antiserum was placed directly into the amniotic yolk sac cavity. These experiments were performed on day 11 embryos. When we place a teratogen such as phosphoramide mustard into the yolk sac cavity, the teratogenic effect is enormous; however, if we place the teratogen into the amniotic cavity, the teratogenic effect is much, much lower. Thus, there is a differential effect of the teratogen when it is placed in the yolk sac cavity vs. the amniotic cavity. So the teratogenic effect as you are demonstrating with antisera could be mediated via the yolk sac.

BRENT (Philadelphia): If you place a protein, which is what our antibody is, into the amniotic cavity or the yolk sac cavity, there is no way for it to get to the surface of the visceral yolk sac. If you place a small molecule like cyclophosphamide or methotrextate in those cavities, they are going to diffuse into the embryo. The embryo has no way to obtain a protein or serum protein from the distal portion of the yolk sac cell. I believe what you are reporting agrees with our observations and would be predictable.

WINICK (New York): It is fascinating to note that the embryo is able to obtain amino acids presumably from the protein solution. If the mechanism you propose is correct, would it be possible to demonstrate that by adding amino acids to the solution, you can prevent the kinds of malformations that do occur?

BRENT (Philadelphia): We believe we are studying in embryo culture, the effects of antisera on quantitatively decreasing the ability for the yolk sac to endocytose micromolecules. We would not expect such a decrease for small molecules necessarily. Thus, using this model, we can modulate the importance of serum amino acids or free amino acids and proteins. The limiting factor may be concentration. Nature has performed a magnificent thing by making proteins because for every millimole of protein you obtain a thousand millimoles of amino acids to the embryo. In order to get a thousand millimoles of amino acids for the embryo, you would destroy the whole system because your osmolarity is three times the osmolarity that the organism can sustain. Thus, with proteins, there is a most efficient way for the embryo who is rapidly taking up amino acids to obtain them in appropriate size packages. This does not mean though that 5, 10, or 20 percent of amino acids that are necessary could not be obtained via free small molecule transfer. We currently have not answered that question but will be trying to do so.

MCINTYRE (Springfield): How species specific is your antibody?

BRENT (Philadelphia): Yolk sac carcinoma from the mouse does contain a mixture of antigens that includes the visceral yolk sac. It will produce malformations in the rat. But if you examine other species, they do not appear to work. The only species that might work would be the rat, the mouse, perhaps the guinea pig and rabbit. However, this work has not been done. I do know that the ferret does not work.

MILLER (Rochester): In trying to extrapolate to the trophoblast, do you believe there is any relationship between visceral yolk sac protein utilization and the actual amino acid and protein supply in the hemochorial placenta?

BRENT (Philadelphia): I do not have an exact answer for your question. However, we have tried to develop an equivalent antisera against the trophoblast and were unsuccessful (Placenta Supplement 3, 75-84).

FAULK (Nice): Since the yolk sac is the progenitor of the hemopoietic stem cells, following the passive deliverance of your anti-yolk sac antibody, do you observe any changes in hematopoesis?

BRENT (Philadelphia): We have never examined this question post-partum. At the right dose of antisera though, we can produce almost a 75 percent incidence of hydrocephalus. This is the only post partum evaluation we have made. Your question is certainly a pertinent one.

Trophoblast Research 1:347-360, 1983

ANALYSIS OF SERA FROM MONKEYS WITH HISTORIES OF FETAL WASTAGE AND THE IDENTIFICATION OF TERATOGENICITY IN SERA FROM HUMAN CHRONIC SPONTANEOUS ABORTERS USING RAT EMBRYO CULTURES

Sean W. Carey[1], Norman W. Klein[1,5], W. T. Fredrickson[2], Gene P. Sackett[2], Robert M. Greenstein[3], Probat Sehgal[4] and Martha Elliott[4]

[1]Department of Animal Genetics and the Genetics and Cell Biology Section, The University of Connecticut, Storrs, CT 06268 U.S.A. and
[2]Regional Primate Research Center, The University of Washington, Seattle, WA 98195 U.S.A. and
[3]Department of Pediatrics, Genetics Section, The University of Connecticut Health Center, Farmington, CT 06032 U.S.A.and
[4]New England Regional Primate Research Center, Harvard Medical School, Southboro, MA 01772 U.S.A.

INTRODUCTION

The use of whole rat embryo cultures to detect teratogenicity in serum was first demonstrated by culturing embryos on sera taken from rats that had been previously injected with cadmium or cyclophosphamide (Klein et al., 1980). This approach was then extended to the testing of human subjects, and we found that sera from subjects receiving drug treatments for cancer or epilepsy were teratogenic (Chatot et al., 1980). In another application of the cultured rat embryo teratogenicity test, the ability to culture rat embryos on monkey sera was evaluated with the hope of incorporating primate metabolism into the test. During the course of this study, serum samples from 18 untreated Rhesus (M. mulatta) monkeys were tested and 16 of the samples supported excellent rat embryo growth and development (Klein et al., 1982). An examination of the breeding records indicated that the two teratogenic samples came from the only two monkeys that had failed to become pregnant in two years of breeding trials. An additonal 14 pigtailed (M. nemestrina) monkeys with histories of reproductive failures and 12 with excellent breeding records were then tested (Klein et al., 1982). Serum from the 14 monkeys with histories of fetal wastage, stillbirths and neonatal deaths were teratogenic at a greater frequency (12 of 14 tested for 86 percent) than sera from the 12 excellent reproducers (4 of 12 tested for 33 percent).

[5] Reprint requests should be addressed to:
N.W. Klein, Department of Animal Genetics, U-39, The University of Connecticut, Storrs, CT 06268

In this paper, we report recent studies concerned first, with the identification of teratogenic substances in the sera from monkeys with histories of reproductive failure and second, with the extent to which the rat embryo culture test might be applied to the identification of sera from human subjects with histories of fetal wastage.

MATERIALS AND METHODS

Embryo culture

Embryos were isolated from CD strain rats (Charles River Breeding Laboratory, Inc., Wilmington, MA) at 9.5 days of gestation. Only mid head fold stage embryos (Klein et al., 1980) removed from 10-15 rats were pooled and distributed at random among the various experimental groups. Embryos were cultured with intact visceral yolk sacs and ectoplacental cones but Reichert's membranes were removed (New, 1966). Culture bottles contained either 3 embryos in 2.0 ml of media or 2 embryos in 1.3 ml of media and were rotated at 30 rpm in a room maintained at 37.5°C. Cultures were gassed with 5 percent CO_2 but with different percentages of O_2 and N_2 as follows: pregas, zero time and after 3 hr. O_2(5 percent), N_2(90 percent); 20 hr. O_2(15 percent), N_2(80 percent); 27 hr. O_2(30 percent), N_2(65 percent) and 44 hr. O_2(40 percent), N_2(55 percent).

Media preparation

Human and monkey blood were drawn by syringe from the forearm and leg veins respectively, centrifuged immediately (Steele and New, 1974), and the serum was frozen at -20°C. Prior to use all samples were thawed, the clots were removed, sera were heat inactivated at 56°C for 30 minutes and then filtrated for sterility with a Millipore type HA filter. Sera glucose concentrations were determined by the glucose oxidase method (Bergmeyer and Bernt, 1974). The final media consisted of 90 percent serum and 10 percent water. The water contained 0.66 mg/ml streptomycin sulfate, 0.006 mg/ml penicillin-G-potassium and enough glucose to adjust final media levels to 3 mg/ml.

Embryo analysis

After 48 hours of culture, embryos were first examined for heart pulsations and yolk sac circulation. They were then removed from the surrounding extraembryonic membranes, photographed, examined for abnormalities, and somites and pharyngeal pouches were counted. Embryo protein contents were determined by the method of Lowry et al. (1951). In the fetal wastage study using human serum the few samples that gave ambiguous results (i.e. the embryos cultured at one time on a sample were not similar) were retested and considered teratogenic if a total of 50 percent or more of the embryos were abnormal.

Ammonium sulfate fractionation and dialysis

Saturated ammonium sulfate solution (room temperature, pH7) was added to serum until a concentration of 30 percent was reached. The precipitate was then removed by centrifugation at 5900 x g for 10 minutes. This procedure was repeated after the supernatant was brought to 50 percent saturation and again to 70 percent saturation. The three precipitates were then dissolved in Cockroft's balanced salt solution and dialyzed at 4°C against this salt solution for 48 hr. Fractions were filtered for sterility prior to testing. For dialysis of whole serum, 2 ml of monkey serum were dialyzed against 8 ml of rat serum for 24 hours at 4°C.

Analytic electrophoresis

Ammonium sulfate fractions were analyzed in discontinuous 7 1/2 percent, 10 percent and 12 1/2 percent polyacrylamide slab gels containing sodium dodecylsulfate at a current of 20mA (Laemmli, 1970). Gels were stained in 0.2 percent Coomassie Brilliant Blue R in 50 percent trichloroacetic acid and destained in an aqueous solution containing (v/v) 10 percent acetic acid and 25 percent methanol.

RESULTS

Serum analysis of a human control subject

In an early study (Chatot et al., 1980) we noted that 21 percent of the human serum samples obtained from a control (untreated) group of human subjects were teratogenic to cultured rat embryos. Although multiple samples from these subjects were not tested, a variety of factors could have contributed to the temporary presence of embryo toxic substances in the serum. We felt, therefore, that it was important to analyze control sera for some of the possible causes. In this initial study, we chose to study the serum from a 20 year old nulliparous female (subject 23). The serum produced the most extreme teratogenic response of any tested in our control group as the serum was lethal to cultured embryos. All samples examined over a two year period retained the embryo lethal activity.

When a mixture of 5 percent serum from subject 23 was mixed with 95 percent human control serum (v/v), the protein content of embryos was reduced by 43 percent of control values (Table 1) and the embryos were exencephalic and dorsiflexed. This implicated the presence of a toxic factor rather than a deficiency in the serum from subject 23 as a comparable dilution of control serum with a salt solution was not detrimental to cultured embryos. Nutrient supplementation, ultraviolet irradiation or dialysis of the lethal serum did not alter the embryo lethal activity (Table 1). However, the activity was removed by treating the serum with trypsin which indicated that the lethality was associated with a protein. To localize the activity, serum proteins were then fractionated with a saturated ammonium sulfate solution to yield 3 fractions corresponding to proteins precipitated at 0-30 percent, 30-50 percent and 50-70 percent saturation. Using the fractions from subject 23 serum, the precipitate obtained at 0-30 percent saturation caused the exencephaly, abnormal body rotation and reduction in embryo size characteristic of the whole serum. The 50 percent precipitate caused exencephaly but rotation and embryo size were not adversely affected, while embryos cultured in the presence of the 70 percent precipitate were normal (Fig. 1 A-C). Embryo growth and development were not adversely affected when these fractions were prepared from human control serum. Sodium dodecylsulfate polylacrylamide gel analysis revealed that the active 0-30 percent ammonium sulfate fraction contained two polypeptides of apparent molecular weights of 52,000 and 25,000 daltons (Fig. 1 a-c). Based on their characteristic precipitation patterns with ammonium sulfate and molecular weight estimations, these polypeptides appeared to represent the heavy and light chain of IgG. Thus, IgG was then purified using DEAE-Affi Gel Blue chromatography and purified IgG from subject 23 caused the same abnormalities in cultured embryos as that produced both by the 30 percent ammonium sulfate fraction and whole serum (Table 1). Human control serum IgG tested at the same levels was non-toxic.

Table 1. Protocol used in the analysis of serum from human subject 23.

Media		Embryo analysis: Abnormalities,[a] abnormal/total	Embryo analysis: Protein content µg/embryo[b]
Serum mixtures (% v/v)[c]			
Subject 23	Human control[d]		
100	0	3/3	20.8
50	50	3/3	40.0
15	85	3/3	37.1±6.7
5	95	3/3	73.8±7.5
0	100	0/3	129.3±16.0
Vitamin supplementation[e]		3/3	41.0
Ultraviolet irradiation[f]		3/3	17.8
Trypsin treated sera (10% v/v) added to human control sera (80% v/v)[g]			
Human control serum[h]		0/3	130.3±7.9
Trypsin treated human control serum		0/3	113.0±3.6
Subject 23 serum[h]		3/3	47.7
Trypsin treated subject 23 serum		0/3	117.0±3.5
Ammonium sulfate cuts added to human control serum[i]			
No addition		0/3	167.7±4.9
0-30% cut of human contol serum		0/3	162.5±11.5
0-30% cut of subject 23 serum		3/3	76.0±21.2
30-50% cut of subject 23 serum		2/3	142.3±10.2
50-70% cut of subject 23 serum		0/3	184.7±24.2
Purified IgG added to human control serum			
No addition		0/3	163.0±10.0
0.6 mg/ml human control serum IgG		0/3	178.0±10.0
0.6 mg/ml human control serum IgG		3/3	52.0

[a] Embryo abnormalities consisted of one or more of the following: anophthalmia, exencephaly or anterior-posterior neural fold fusion.

[b] Mean ± SEM. When embryos were too small for individual determinations they were combined for single determinations and SEM could not be calculated.

[c] Media consisted of 90% (v/v) serum and 10% water with glucose and antibiotics. Mixture percentages represent the contribution of each sera type to the total sera volume (1.8ml = 100%).

[d] Control serum was obtained from a male volunteer.

[e] Vitamin supplementation as described by Cockroft, 1979.

[f] Serum was treated with 6 ergs/mm^2/sec for 10 minutes.

[g] Media consisted of 80% (v/v) human control serum, 10% serum treated as indicated, and 10% water with glucose and antibiotics.

[h] Serum was incubated as in the trypsin treated group, but without trypsin.

[i] Media consisted of 90% (v/v) human control serum and 10% balanced salt solution containing fractions as indicated with glucose and antibiotics. The ammonium sulfate cuts are the reconstituted precipitates formed at the designated saturations with ammonium sulfate, and were added to human control serum at 1.7 mg protein/ml.

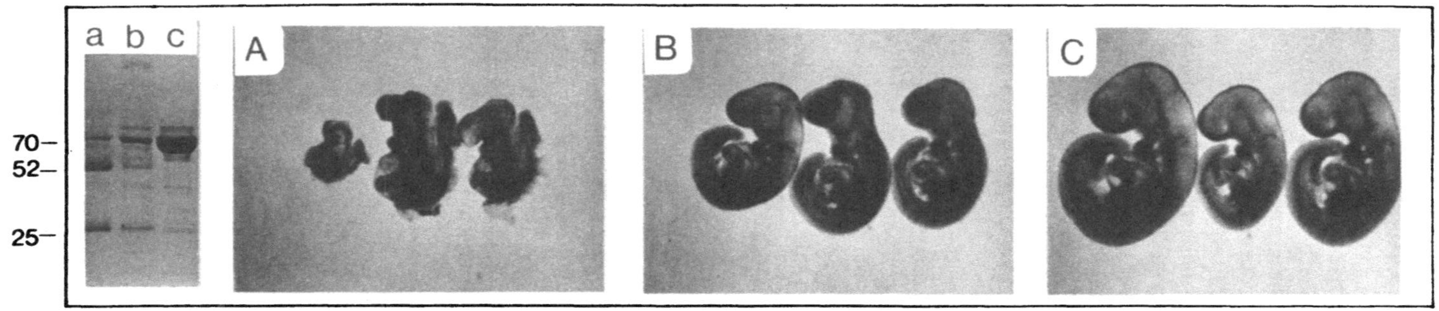

Figure 1. Embryos cultured for 48 hr in the presence of ammonium sulfate fractions of serum from human subject 23. Figures at the left (a-c) represent sodium dodecylsulfate polyacrylamide gel patterns of the ammonium sulfate fractions, while figures at the right represent embryos cultured with the corresponding fractions (A-C). (a, A) 0-30 percent cut; (b, B) 30-50 percent cut; (c, C) 50-70 percent cut. Culture media contained 1.8 ml human control serum with 0.2 ml of a balanced salt solution containing 3.4 mg of the appropriate fraction.

Analysis of sera from monkeys with histories of fetal wastage

Concurrent with the studies of serum from human subject 23, several monkeys were identified that also provided teratogenic sera. In addition, they possessed known histories of reproductive failure. Sera from three of these monkeys have been studied to date. Monkey 71333 (M. nemestrina) had a reproductive record which included a spontaneous abortion, a neonatal death and two normal pregnancies. Embryos cultured on this serum were exencephalic, anophthalmic and were abnormally curved (dorsiflexed) with anterior-posterior neural tube fusion (Fig. 2A). Monkey 73209 (M. nemestrina) had three spontaneous abortions and a neonatal death in five pregnancies. Sera from this animal produced embryos characterized by exencephaly, anophthalmia and microcephaly (Fig. 2B). Monkey 482-79 (M. fasicularis) had not achieved a successful pregnancy in over a year of breeding trials but because she was not individually housed, the nature of her reproductive problem (i.e. primary infertility or fetal wastage) could not be determined. Embryos cultured on this sera were exencephalic, anophthalmic and dorsiflexed with anterior-posterior neural tube fusion (Fig. 2C).

Using the protocol developed in the case study of human subject 23, various amounts of the teratogenic sera were mixed with control sera. Levels of less than 50 percent (v/v) of sera from 71333 and 482-79 were sufficient to cause severe abnormalities in cultured rat embryos but even at higher levels (60 percent (v/v)) only slight reduction in embryo brain size was observed with the serum from 73209. This clearly suggested the presence of toxic substances in the sera from 71333 and 482-79, but with 73209 either a serum deficiency or a substance of low toxicity could explain the result.

In addition, sera from each of the three monkeys were individually dialyzed against control rat serum. For sera from 71333 and 482-79 this treatment failed to improve embryo development (Fig. 2 a, c). For 73209 however, this treatment abolished the teratogenicity of the sample and embryos cultured on dialyzed 73209 serum developed normally and accumulated a protein content comparable to control rat serum (Fig. 2b). It remains to be determined if dialysis of 73209 removes a toxic factor or contributes an essential nutrient, but the problem with this serum is clearly associated with a small molecule (less than 5,000 daltons).

For animal 482-79, the high molecular weight nature of the embryo toxic factor has been confirmed using ultrafiltration membranes. Additions of serum components excluded by a 10,000 dalton membrane to control serum caused cultured embryo abnormalities comparable to whole serum from this animal. With animal 71333, the serum analysis has been extended to the localization of toxicity by ammonium sulfate fractionation. Similar to the human subject 23 study, the 0-35 percent fraction produced the exencephaly and dorsiflexion characteristic of whole 71333 serum (Fig. 3 A). The 35-55 percent fraction was slightly toxic (Fig. 3 B) while the 55-75 percent fraction had no adverse effects on cultured embryo development (Fig. 3 C). Fractions prepared from a control monkey were not toxic to cultured embryos.

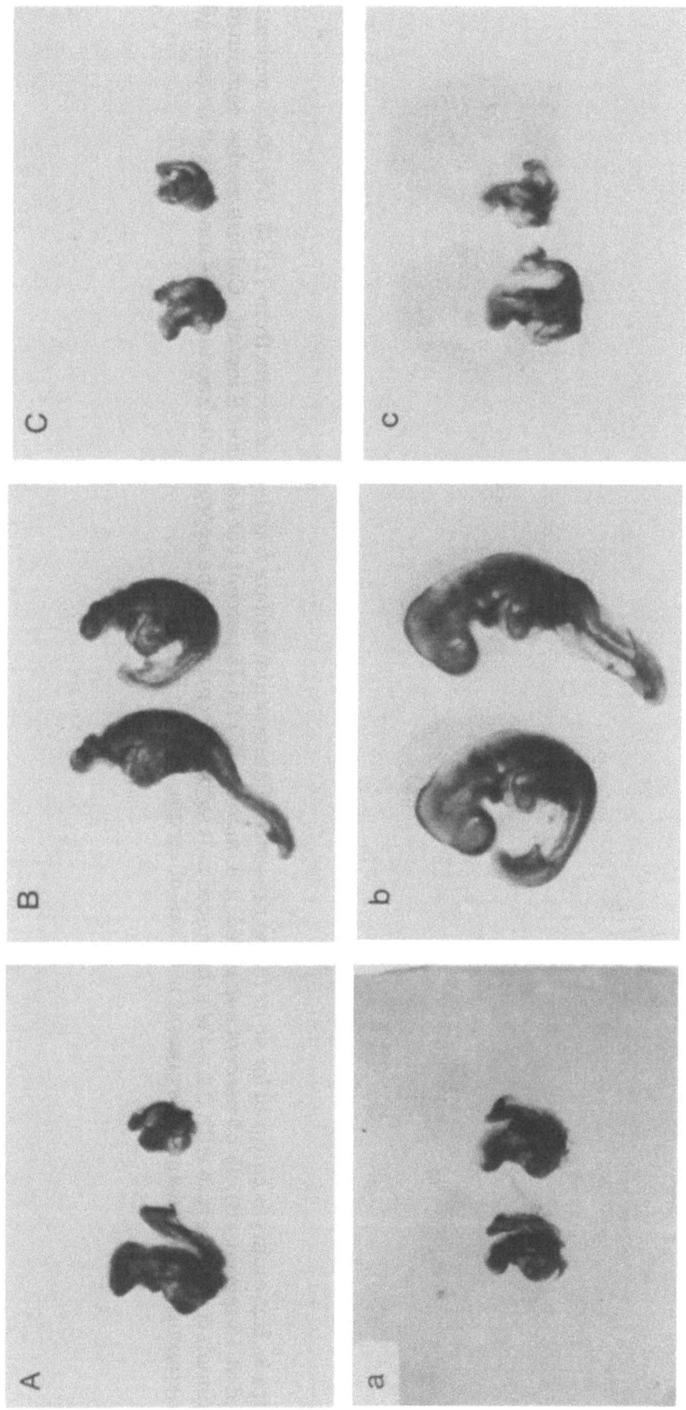

Figure 2. Rat embryos cultured for 48 hr on monkey sera before and after dialysis against rat serum. The top three figures represent embryos cultured on untreated monkey sera (A-C), while the lower three figures represent embryos cultured on monkey sera dialyzed against rat serum (a-c). (A, a), 71333; (B, b), 73209; (C, c) 482-79. Two ml of monkey sera were dialyzed for 24 hr at 4°C against 8 ml of rat serum.

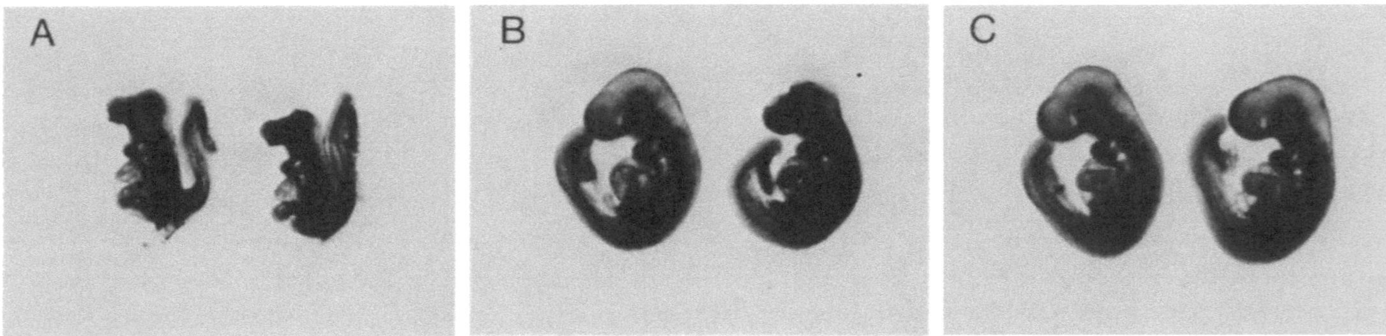

Figure 3. Rat embryos cultured for 48 hr in the presence of ammonium sulfate fractions of serum from 71333. (A), 0-35 percent cut added at 13 mg/ml; (B), 35-55 percent cut added at 8 mg/ml. (C) 55-75 percent cut added at 8 mg/ml. Culture media contained 1.1 ml human control serum with 0.2 ml of a balanced salt solution containing the appropriate fraction. The amounts of protein added were equivalent to the amounts present in 0.5 ml of serum.

Table 2. Teratogenicity of sera from humans and monkeys with histories of fetal wastage.

Serum Donor	Donor reproductive history[a]			Evaluation of initial serum sample (% teratogenic)[b]	
	AB	SB/ND	NS		
Humans[c]					
High risk females(n=16)	50	2	5	6NT,	10T(63)%
High risk males(n=13)	-	-	-	9NT,	4T (31%)
General control population(n=19)	NE[d]	NE	NE	15NT,	4T (21%)
Monkeys[e]					
High risk females(n=14)	30	20	13	2NT,	12T (86%)
Low risk females(n=12)	2	1	43	8NT,	4T (33%)

[a]AB, spontaneous abortions; SB/ND, still births and neonatal deaths; NS, neonatal survivors.
[b]NT, non-teratogenic; T, teratogenic.
[c]High risk human sera were obtained from the University of Connecticut Health Center, Farmington, CT. The general control population was used in a separate study and was selected without regard to reproductive histories (Chatot et al., 1980).
[d]NE, not established.
[e]High risk monkey sera were obtained from the Regional Primate Research Center, University of Washington, Seattle, WA.

Testing sera from human subjects with histories of fetal wastage

Rat embryos were cultured on serum samples from 16 women with histories of at least two pregnancy wastages and 13 of their husbands. This group of women has experienced an overall pregnancy wastage frequency of approximately 90 percent, with only 5 successful births out of 57 recorded pregnancies (Table 2). Based on the results obtained with the initial serum samples from these women, 10 of 16 sera were designated teratogenic. This frequency of 63 percent can be compared to the 86 percent observed in the previous study of high reproductive risk monkeys and to the 21 percent teratogenic frequency observed in a human control group (Chatot et al., 1980) (Table 2).

For the husbands, serum samples from 4 of the 13 tested were teratogenic. Of particular interest, for the 4 teratogenic samples, the wives' sera were also teratogenic and the cultured embryo abnormalities were similar for the related husband-wife pairs.

The reproducibility of the human data has been evaluated in 17 cases. For 12 subjects, both the first and second serum samples produced comparable results with cultured embryos. With the remaining 5, sera from 2 subjects produced normal embryos with the initial sample but were teratogenic on the second sample; for the remaining 3 subjects the opposite was observed (first samples were teratogenic and the second samples were non- teratogenic).

DISCUSSION

In order to determine the possible causes for teratogenicity in serum from control subjects used in the development of a human teratogenicty test we analyzed serum from one control subject in detail. Serum fractionation techniques used in conjunction with cultured rat embryos have identified an embryo-toxic IgG in this serum. The specificity of the antibody for embryonic antigens has not yet been determined, but some evidence indicates that sites on the yolk sac may be involved as absorption of the serum with intact rat yolk sacs but not whole embryos reduces the teratogenicity of the serum. Although the reproductive significance of this selected case could not be established (the subject lacks a reproductive history), the study led to the development of a general protocol for the use of rat embryo cultures in human sera analysis.

Concurrent with the analysis of teratogenic serum from "control" humans, we found in a separate study that serum from 2 of 16 "control" Rhesus monkeys also produced abnormalities in cultured rat embryos. The finding that these 2 sera were obtained inadvertently from monkeys with histories of reproductive failures provided the basis of a study which established the correlation of serum donor reproductive failure to the teratogenicity of the serum sample (Klein et al., 1982). Analysis of sera from three of these high risk monkeys has led to some preliminary findings. In serum from monkey 71333, a non-dialyzable rat embryo toxic substance has been isolated in the precipitate formed by a 0-35 percent saturation of the serum with ammonium sulfate. It appears likely that the presence of embryo toxic activity in this fraction of serum is indicative of toxic serum antibodies (similar to human subject number 23). Although it has yet to be shown that such an antibody has reproductive significance in vivo, the role of maternal circulating antibodies is of particular concern during pregnancy because the human placenta has receptors for the Fc portion of the IgG molecule and actively transports IgG antibodies from the maternal circulation into the fetal circulation (Kohler and Farr, 1966; Schlamowitz, 1976). Studies are currently underway to identify the antigen(s) of both rat embryos and monkey embryos which may react with such an antibody. A second monkey, 482-79 also has provided serum with a non-dialyzable embryo toxic activity. It has not yet been determined if the embryo toxic activity, as found in serum from 71333, may be antibody associated or whether activity is associated with other serum macromolecules. A third monkey, 73209, has provided teratogenic serum which, unlike the other two monkey sera, became nonteratogenic after dialysis against control serum. This finding demonstrated first that serum teratogenicity from all high reproductive risk monkeys is not caused by the same factors and second, that low molecular weight substances may be responsible for serum teratogenicity.

Our preliminary observations using rat embryos to evaluate human subjects with histories of fetal wastage have been encouraging. The frequency of teratogenic sera obtained from the reproductive failure group was greater (63 percent of the females) than the frequency found in a control population of human subjects tested in another study (21 percent of males and females combined). Furthermore, while the overall frequency of teratogenic sera from husbands in the study (31 percent) was similar to the controls, it may be significant that in all cases where the husbands' sera were teratogenic, the sera from the wives of these husbands were also teratogenic. In addition, the cultured embryo abnormalities were similar for the related husband-wife pairs. This observation suggests that some couples may share a common problem such as a dietary deficiency or hazardous environmental exposure. At present, we have not completed tests with comparable numbers of control humans matched for parity. These results will be essential to provide a statistical evaluation of the study. More important, however, we seek to establish the relationship of the causes for in vitro teratogenicity and the in vivo reproductive failure of the serum donor. Such a relationship, we hope, will be established through the analysis of serum.

SUMMARY

In vitro cultures of whole rat embryos have been used to evaluate the teratogenicity of sera and to identify specific teratogenic substances in serum. A general protocol for human serum analysis was developed using embryo lethal serum obtained from a nulliparous female subject. An IgG fraction which produced embryo abnormalities similar to her whole serum was identified. The analysis of sera has now been extended to three monkeys with histories of fetal wastage. The embryo toxic activity of serum from monkey 71333 was found associated with the 0-35 percent ammonium sulfate fraction of serum, which may indicate embryo toxic antibodies. The teratogenicity of sera from a second monkey, 482-79, was found associated with a substance in serum greater than 10,000 daltons. Sera from a third monkey, 73209, unlike the other two, became non-teratogenic after dialysis against control serum. Lastly, we report that rat embryo cultures may be used to identify some human subjects with histories of fetal wastage.

ACKNOWLEDGMENTS

Scientific contribution 937 Storrs Agriculture Experiment Station, University of Connecticut. This work was supported by Department of Energy contract EV03139 (Office of Health and Environmental Research) and National Institutes of Health grants RR00169 and RR00168 (Animal Resources Branch).

REFERENCE

Bergmeyer, H.U. and Bernt, E. (1974) Methods of Enzymatic Analysis. New York: p.1205 , Academic Press.

Chatot, C.L., Klein, N.W., Piatek, J. and Pierro, L.J. (1980) Successful culture of rat embryos on human serum: Use in the detection of teratogens. Science, 207, 1471-1473.

Cockroft, D.L. (1979) Nutrient requirements of rat embryos undergoing organogenesis in vitro. J. Reprod. Fert., 57, 505-510.

Klein, N.W., Vogler, M.A., Chatot, C.L. and Pierro, L.J. (1980) The use of cultured rat embryos to evaluate the teratogenic activity of serum: Cadmium and cyclophosphamide. Teratology, 21, 199-208.

Klein, N.W., Plenefisch, J.D., Carey, S.W., Fredrickson, W.T., Sackett, G.P., Burbacher, T.M. and Parker, R.M. (1982) Serum from monkeys with histories of fetal wastage causes abnormalities in cultured rat embryos. Science, 215, 66-69.
Kohler, P.F. and Farr, R.S. (1966) Elevation of cord over maternal IgG immunoglobulin: evidence for an active placental IgG transport. Nature 210, 1070-1071.
Laemmli, U.K. (1970) Cleavage of structural proteins during the assembly of the head of bacteriophage T4. Nature, 227, 680-685.
Lowry, O.H., Rosebrough, N.J., Farr, A.L. and Randall, R.J. (1951) Protein measurement with the folin phenol reagent. J. Biol. Chem., 193, 265-275.
New, D.A.T. (1966) Development of rat embryos cultured in blood sera. J. Reprod. Fertil., 12, 509-524.
Schlamowitz, M. (1976) Membrane receptors in the specific transfer of immunoglobulins from mother to young. Immunol. Commun., 5, 481-500.
Steele, C.E. and New, D.A.T. (1974) Serum variants causing the formation of double hearts and other abnormalities in explanted rat embryos. J. Embryol. Exp. Morphol., 31, 707-719.

DISCUSSION

WINICK (New York): Have you performed the in vivo experiment in your monkey population by adding serum and/or blood from the chronic aborters into normal monkeys? If so, do you produce abortions in these animals? Secondly, you indicated in your study that 20 percent of the humans (both male and female) in our society are carrying a factor in their serum that is at least significantly detrimental to the rat fetus? How specific then is this evaluation?

CAREY (Storrs): We have not performed the mixing study. This would be an interesting study; however, we have attempted to keep the populations separate at this point. In response to your second question, we certainly do pick up an abnormality frequency of approximately 20 percent in our control population. We are not sure of its etiology. It may be due to transient infections or problems of that sort.

WINICK (New York): Do you therefore believe that your species differences are important? Can you protect against damage in the human based upon the rodent alterations? Have you obtained a population of chronic aborters in rats and therefore removed the species differences?

CAREY (Storrs): All we have done to date is make a correlation, which is highly significant, 60 percent (experimental) vs. 20 percent (control). We cannot establish a cause and effect relationship in vitro to that in vivo at this point. That is what we are working on now. We have not found a select population of rats that would be considered to be chronic aborters. Therefore, we have not been able to pursue those studies.

MCINTRYE (Springfield): Have you performed any time related studies during the entire 48 hour period? Can the effect of the serum constituants be reversed?

CAREY (Storrs): The antibody from the human subject has been studied at two different time points: at the beginning of the culture, or at 24 hours when the embryos are at the 12-14 somite stage. Addition at both times will produce abnormalities; however, at the 24 hour period, the abnormalities are much less severe. This does not appear to indicate perhaps anything other than the first 24 hours having an uninhibited development. That is all we have performed to date. We do not know if this effect is reversable. We have not attempted to wash off the antibody to determine this effect. It would certainly be an interesting experiment.

METLAY (Rochester): In the human population that contains the habitual aborters, have you attempted to characterize it using the same criteria that both Drs. Faulk and Beer have used and presented at this meeting. This would be especially interesting for the mixed lymphocyte culture evaluations.

CAREY (Storrs): We currently do not know how the histocompatibility antigens do interact in this system when we are evaluating rat embryos vs. monkey embryos or human embryos. It is worth noting that in the monkey colony, there are a number of high risk monkeys that are males.

BRENT (Philadelphia): You have used the term, antibody, and I think you mean its just gammaglobulin. The fact is that if you isolate a protein on a sepharose column or another chromatographic column, this just tells you that it is a gammaglobulin. You are calling it an antibody. This is based upon the observation that it does localize by immunofluorence in the yolk sac. Such localization can be attributed to any serum protein. The difference will occur for specific antibody staining and attachment when they continue to be localized beyond 8 to 12 hours. Have you examined this issue?

CAREY (Storrs): We have not performed that exact study; however, we have purified an IgG. We did get quantitative staining differences between the control subjects and the embryolethal subjects; these were not just qualitative differences.

MCINTRYE (Springfield): Since you are working with an IgG molecule, what control absorptions have you undertaken? Since you may be utilizing a heterophilic antibody, have you absorbed against, for example, red blood cells?

CAREY (Storrs): We have only absorbed against embryos. We have not examined any adult tissue.

BEER (Ann Arbor): Have you absorbed the embryotoxic properties of this IgG fraction by preabsorption with embryos at various stages?

CAREY (Storrs): No, we have not performed those absorptions. We clearly have alot of characterization to perform.

Trophoblast Research 1:361-370, 1983

PROLONGED SURVIVAL OF HUMAN DECIDUAL GRAFTS IN A XENOGENEIC HOST

Hesham Arab, John A. McCoshen,* Marsha K. Leith, Agnes Wodzicki and John E. Tyson

Department of Obstetrics, Gynecology and Reproductive Sciences, University of Manitoba, Winnipeg, Manitoba R3E OW3, Canada

INTRODUCTION

Pregnancy is felt to represent a state of altered immunity consisting mainly of a suppression of host (maternal) versus allograft (fetal) reaction. Speculation on the nature of such suppression has included the uterus as an immunologically privileged site, fetal antigenic immaturity (Beer and Billingham, 1974; 1980), and alterations in the maternal immune system provoked by specific hormones secreted during pregnancy (Siiteri and Stites, 1982). Furthermore, placental hormones and/or factors may contribute to the immunology of pregnancy (Stimson, 1980).

Endometrium differentiates into hormone-producing decidua as early as the twenty-first day of the menstrual cycle (Maslar and Riddick, 1979). This event may in some way facilitate blastocyst implantation or possibly represent a preliminary change in endometrial antigenicity related to the anticipated immunologic challenge by an implanting fertilized ovum. Further evidence suggests that both decidua and amniotic fluid contain factors which suppress lymphocyte reactivity (Golander et al., 1981) and leukocyte migration (Gleicher et al., 1979) respectively. To evaluate several of these theories human decidual tissue was grafted to adult female and male rat hosts in order to determine the time of host rejection of the decidual implant. The results were compared to the rejection of grafts of both maternal and neonatal skin and fetal membrane including amnion and chorion.

MATERIALS AND METHODS

Tissue from 16 human placentae (9 male, 7 female) obtained at the time of elective Cesarean section was washed free of blood contaminants in 0.9% saline. Sections of reflected membrane including amnion, chorion, decidua or combinations of these tissues were prepared for transplantation to rat hosts. Adherent decidua (D) was scraped from the maternal surface of chorion, finely minced and weighed into 300 mg aliquots. Equivalent weights of amnion (A), chorio-decidua (CD) and amniochorion plus decidua (ACD) were similarly prepared. The tissues were suspended in 0.9% saline containing 10,000 IU/ml of penicillin G until time of grafting. Control tissue including sections of maternal skin obtained from the site of Cesarean section incision and prepuce obtained from newborn infants at the time of circumcision were treated in a similar manner.

*Address reprint requests to: Dr. John A. McCoshen, University of Manitoba, Department of Obstetrics, Gynecology and Reproductive Sciences, Winnipeg, Canada R3E 0W3.

Graft recipients

Mature male (26) and female (103) Sprague Dawley rats weighing approximately 250 grams each were used as graft recipients. The left dorsal thoracic region of each animal was used as the site for the tissue transplantation. This site was chosen principally because of the presence of a reasonable blood supply and the inability of the animals to tamper with the wounds.

The animals were anesthetized with ether and the skin shaved at the site of transplantation. The skin was then incised to approximately 1 cm and the graft of either D, A, CD, ACD or skin (S) was implanted subcutaneously. The wound was then closed with 000 polyethylene sutures. The animals were then observed until time of recovery and returned to their cages. Each series of animals representing a specific graft type was killed by ether overdose at 1, 2, 4, 6, 8 and 12 weeks post-operatively. The graft site was then excised and immersed in Bouin's fixative for 4 hours. Simultaneously 5-10 ml of whole blood was removed by cardiac puncture, the serum separated and stored at -20^{0}C until assayed for human prolactin (hPRL).

Methology

Tissues for histological evaluation were sectioned at 5-7 μ and stained with hematoxylin and eosin. Human PRL was iodinated for use in a double antibody radioimmunoassay for hPRL according to Thorell and Johansson (1971). Sections of decidua were obtained prior to and following 4 weeks post-transplantation and prepared for immunocytochemical localization of hPRL utilizing the immunoperoxidase technique of Sternberger (1978). Anti-human PRL antibody (Calbiochem) was used in a dilution of 1:20. As a control to this procedure the antibody was omitted from the selected sections. In addition, sections of fresh human decidua were tested for hPRL reactivity for control prior to their transplantation. Anti-human PRL (Friesen 27-8a) used for RIA shows no cross reactivity with rat PRL. Cross reactivity of both anti-hPRL antibodies with hGH, hFSH, hLH and TSH is less than one percent.

RESULTS

Tissue rejection was considered to have taken place when complete necrosis and/or cellular destruction of the graft was observed with the light microscope.

At the time of graft excision all tissues were found to be encapsulated by connective tissue. The implants were fixed to the base of the capsule which was filled with varying amounts of inflammatory exudate. The fibrocystic masses were occasionally found to reach a diameter of 2 cm during the second week post-grafting. Thereafter the amount of cystic fluid decreased and was in many instances absent at time of graft removal. The number of grafts and the time interval to complete rejection are presented in Table 1.

Microscopically the major features in the region of the graft included lymphocytic infiltration peripheral to the implant with varying degrees of penetration depending upon the type of graft. Control tissue (S) showed extensive

Table 1
Number of graft rejections (R) expressed per grafts transplanted (T) at various time intervals after subcutaneous transplantation of human tissues to rat hosts.

Day Post transplantation	Tissue Transplanted			
	Skin R/T	Amnion R/T	Chorion R/T	Decidua R/T
7	0/3	0/1	0/6	0/2
14	7/7	0/11	2/10	2/15
28	6/6	7/7	8/8	4/14
42	---	5/5	5/5	8/8
56	---	4/4	4/4	6/6
84	---	2/2	2/2	3/3

lymphocytic infiltration in both dermal and epidermal layers. Similar findings were observed where A and C were used. In the case of D tissue very little if any lymphocytic infiltration was encountered. Grafts of ACD revealed lymphocytic penetration into AC and within the interface between each of the three membranes, but not in D.

The appearance of D prior to grafting is presented in Figure 1a. Four weeks post-implantation D grafts retained the appearance of viable tissue and showed little host lymphocytic infiltration (Figure 1b). By 6 weeks post-transplantation all decidual grafts appeared to be in the process of disintegration (Figure lc), however, few lymphocytes had migrated into the tissue. Figure 2 represents the appearance of S grafts 2 weeks post-transplantation. At this time all grafts showed extensive lymphocytic infiltration with complete loss of cellular integrity in the epidermis. The appearance of A (Figure 3) 2 weeks post-transplantation indicates a high degree of loss of the amniotic epithelium, however, epithelial folds remained reasonably intact. Figure 4 represents amnion 4 weeks post-transplantation. In this instance there is a complete loss of the lining epithelium and extensive lymphocytic infiltration into the collagen layer of the membrane. There were no differences in rejection between male and female hosts nor time for rejection of skin from mother and prepuce.

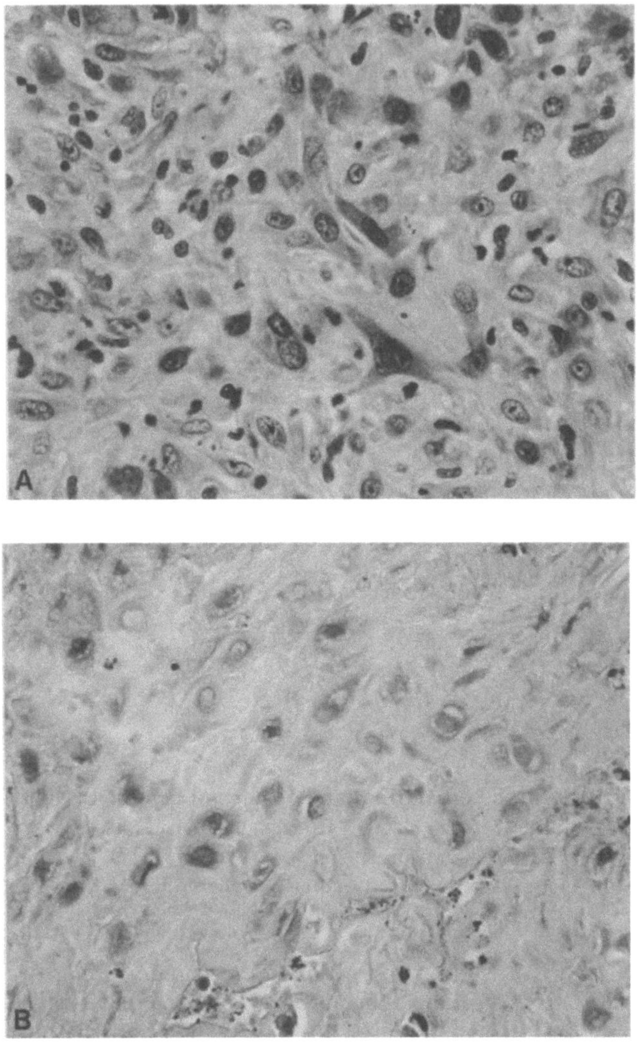

Figure 1A. Histological appearance of human decidua scraped free from the maternal surface of reflected chorion obtained at 39 weeks of gestation following Cesarean section. Stained with hematoxylin(H) and eosin(E), photographed at 400x. B. The histological appearance of decidua obtained four weeks post-implantation indicates cell viability and little host lymphocytic infiltration. Stained with H and E, photographed at 400x.

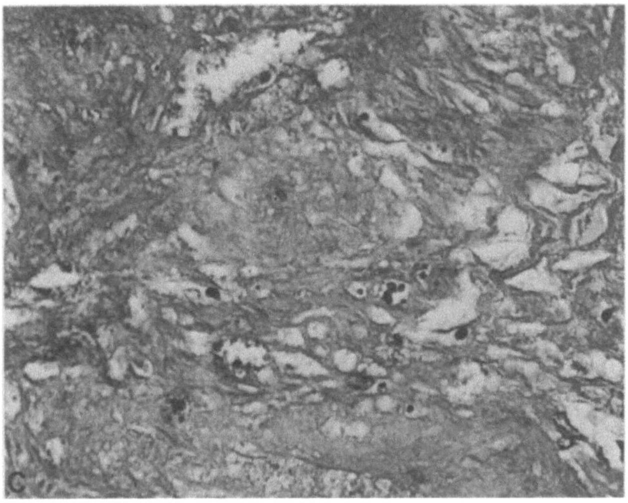

Figure 1C. Decidua six weeks post- transplantation has the appearance of complete cellular destruction with minimal infiltration of host lymphocytes. Stained with H and E, photographed at 400x.

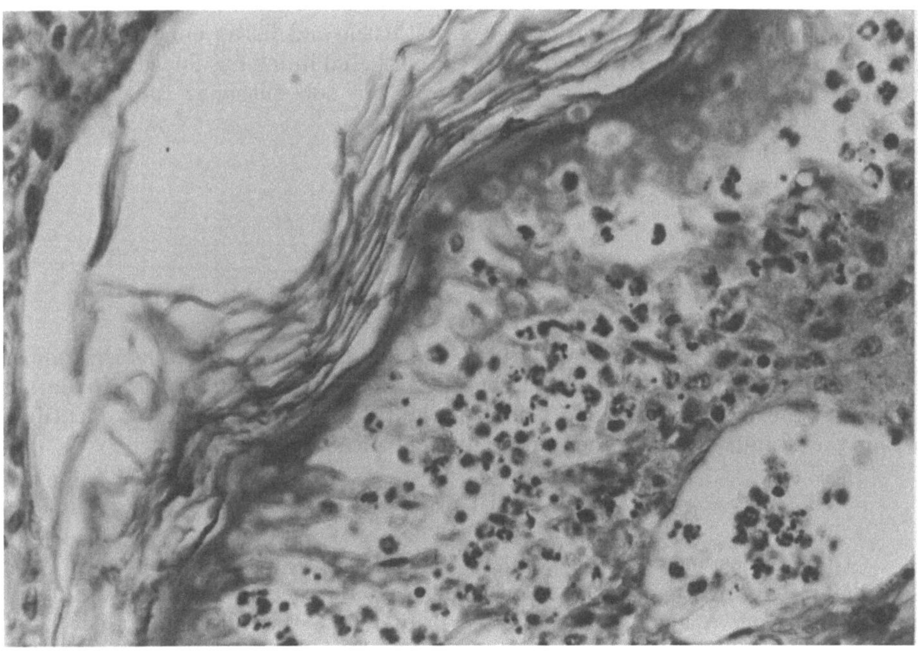

Figure 2. Photomicrograph of a section of maternal skin, obtained at time of Cesarean section, and transplanted for one week. Apparent is the loss of epidermal nuclei and extensive infiltration of host lymphocytes. Stained with H and E, photographed at 400 x.

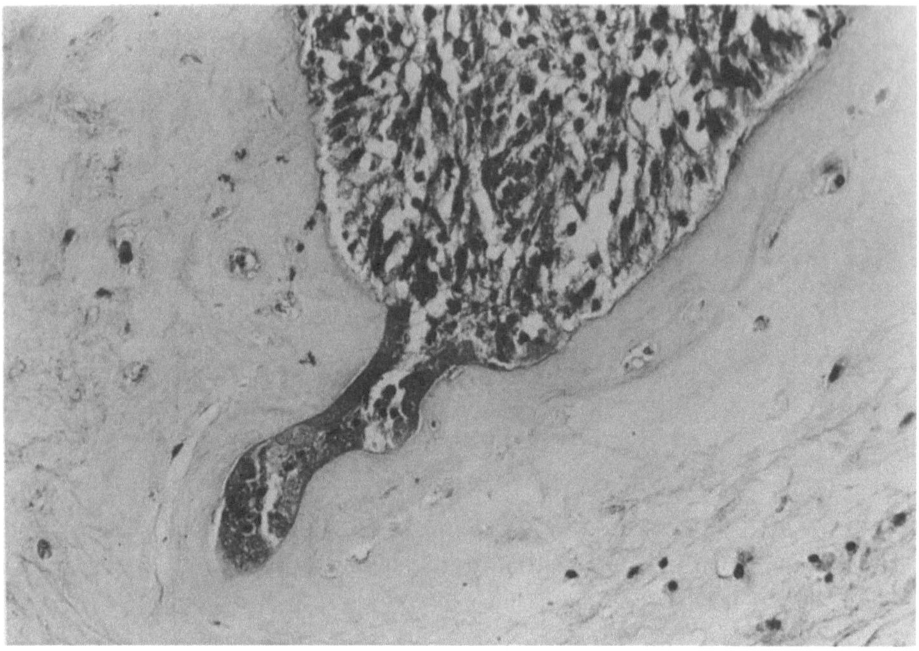

Figure 3. Representation of the appearance of human amnion following two weeks of transplantation. Apparent is infiltration of host tissue and disruption of the amniotic epithelium except in a small region where the epithelial lining has folded upon itself. Some host lymphocytes have infiltrated into the sub-epithelial collagen layer. Stained with H and E, photographed at 200 x.

RIA of host serum hPRL and attempts at immunohistochemical localization of hPRL in grafts failed to identify the hormone as being present in the circulating plasma of the host animal. No hPRL of significant concentration was identified within the decidual grafts by the immunohistochemical procedure.

DISCUSSION

Our studies indicate that human decidua possesses a unique property of survival when grafting occurs in a xenogeneic host. Furthermore, while human fetal tissues including A and C were rejected prior to the time of maternal decidual rejection, fetal tissue survived longer than human skin. Thus, grafts from both D and S obtained from the same pregnancy were genetically identical but differed in their rejection time. These findings suggest that human decidua contains factors delaying the host/graft rejection phenomenon.

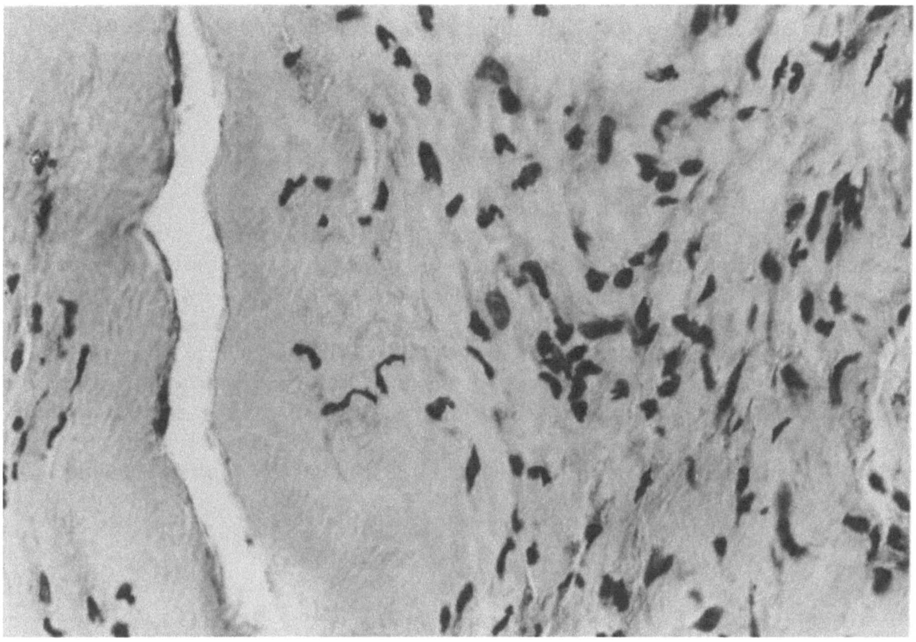

Figure 4. Following four weeks post-transplantation, complete removal of the epithelial layer of amnion had taken place with extensive infiltration of host lymphocytes into the collagen layer of the tissue. Stained with H and E, photographed at 400 x.

Human tissue survival in xenogeneic hosts has been studied by others. Douglas et al. (1954) reported that human chorionic membrane will survive an average of 13 days when transplanted to the mouse. Human skin, however, was rejected in 6 days. Human amnion and chorion have been shown to survive up to 14 days in rats and mice (Avery and Hunt, 1967; Payne and Payne, 1961). Following subcutaneous grafting of hamster skin to rats, Siiteri et al. (1977) reported rejection at 9-10 days. On the other hand, the injection of cultured human endometrial cells into hamster uteri resulted in complete rejection within a few days following discontinuance of steroid maintenance (Moriyama and Sugawa, 1972). Our studies support the prolonged survival of human decidua when transplanted to the rat. Thus, decidua is either immunologically inert or is capable of inhibiting the host rejection process. However, failure to detect hPRL in host serum or in decidual grafts may indicate that decidual hPRL production is unessential in the process of prolonged survival and inhibition of lymphocyte infiltration. Thus, the hPRL product of decidua may be coincidental to the establishment of pregnancy specific immune mechanism(s). In this regard, Golander et al. (1981) have suggested that a soluble human decidual factor suppresses lymphocyte reactivity that may be unrelated to hPRL secretion whereas Karmali et al. (1974) earlier reported on suppressive activity specific to hPRL. Recent observations in our laboratory have led us to favor the conclusions of Golander et al. (1981) since concentrations of hPRL and hGH (0 - 500 ng/ml) were unable to suppress human lymphocyte proliferation even after 6 days in vitro (unpublished observations).

SUMMARY

Human term decidual tissue displays a prolonged rate of survival when placed in a xenogenic host environment. In studies utilizing human skin and various segments of fetal membrane, the subcutaneous grafting of such tissue to adult male and female rats provoked significant histologic changes between 1 and 2 weeks after the grafts had been implanted. Human decidua survived for at least 4 weeks in the xenogeneic environment compared to 2 weeks or less for sections of skin and human fetal membrane including the amnion and chorion. Host lymphocyte infiltration into the graft tissue was seen in all but the decidual transplants. These studies imply that human decidua contains some factor(s) which accounts for the failure of host lymphocytic infiltration into graft tissue and the prolongation of graft survival in an immunologically alien environment.

ACKNOWLEDGMENTS

We are grateful to Dr. N. Pettigrew, Department of Pathology, University of Manitoba, for his assistance. This study was supported in part by the Medical Research Council of Canada.

REFERENCES

Avery, G.B., C.V. Hunt (1967) The fetal membranes as a barrier to transplantation immunity. *Transplantation* 5, 444-454.

Beer, A.E. and R.E. Billingham (1974) Host responses to intrauterine tissue, cellular and fetal allografts. *J. Reprod. Fertil. Suppl.* 21, 59-88.

Beer, A.E. and R.E. Billingham (1980) Mechanisms of non- rejection of fetoplacental allografts. *Folia Biol.* 26, 225-243.

Douglas, B., H. Conway, R.B. Stark, D. Joslin, G. Neito-Cano (1954) The fate of homologous and heterologous chorionic transplants as observed by the transparent tissue chamber technique in the mouse. *Plast. Reconst. Surg.* 13, 125-129.

Gleicher, N., C. Cohen, T. Kerenyi and S. Gusberg (1979) A blocking factor in amniotic fluid causing leukocyte migration enhancement. *Amer. J. Obstet. Gynecol.* 133, 386-390.

Golander, A., V. Zakuth, Y. Shechter and Z. Spirer (1981) Suppression of lymphocyte reactivity in vitro by a soluble factor secreted by explants of human decidua. *Eur. J. Immunol.* 11, 849- 851.

Karmali, R.A., I. Launder, D.F. Horrobin (1974) Prolactin and the immune response. *Lancet* 2, 106-107.

Maslar, I.A. and D. H. Riddick (1979) Prolactin production by human endometrium during the normal menstrual cycle. *Amer. J. Obstet. Gynecol.* 135, 751-754.

Moriyama, I., T. Sugawa (1972) Progesterone facilitates implantation of xenogeneic cultured cells in hamster uterus. *Nature (New Biol.)* 236, 150-152.
Payne, J.M. and S. Payne (1961) Placental grafts in rats. *J. Embryol. Exp. Morph.* 9, 106-116.
Siiteri, P.K., F. Febres, L.E. Clemens, R.J. Chang, B. Gondos, D. Stites (1977) Progesterone and maintenance of pregnancy: Is progesterone nature's immunosuppressant? *Ann. N.Y. Acad. Sci.* 286, 384-397.
Siiteri, P.K. and D.P. Stites (1982) Immunologic and endocrine interrelationships in pregnancy. *Biol. Reprod.* 26, 1-14.
Sternberger, L.A. (1978) *Immunocytochemistry.* N.J. Englewood, Cliffs, 2nd Ed. Prentice Hall, Inc. pp. 104-169.
Stimson, W.H. (1980) Are pregnancy associated serum proteins responsible for the inhibition of lymphocyte transformation by pregnancy serum? *Clin. Exp. Immunol.* 401, 57-163.
Thorell, J.I., and B. Johansson (1971) Enzymatic iodination of polypeptides to high specific activity. *Biochem. Biophys. Acta* 251, 363-370.

Trophoblast Research 1:371-374, 1983

IMMUNOLOGY REPORTS

Chronic Habitual Abortion: Histocompatibility Polymorphism in Maternal Immune Reponses

(Beer and Quebbeman, 1982)

Alan Beer presented an indepth study of 125 couples who had repeated losses of pregnancy (three to twelve abortions). These couples were divided into two groups: the control group of known etiology and the experimental group of unknown etiology. There were between 37 and 40% of the couples with unknown etiology for habitual abortion. It was proposed that alterations in immune reactivity that occurs in the female as a result of exposure to maternally derived determinants during pregnancy can be associated with habitual abortion. These alterations also may have a role for major histocompatibility complex products in the reproductive process. These couples were evaluated in detail including uterine evaluation with Sector B Scan Ultrasonography and hysterosalpinography; a genetic evaluation of both individuals; a uterine tissue sampling for microbial patterns; an endocrine evaluation (progesterone measurements and a timed endometrial biopsy to test for luteal defects); an antigen antibody complex survey as well as both serum and cervical antibody testing. Other tests included HLA antigen testing, where 20 antigens were tested at the A locus, 22 at the B locus, 8 at the C locus and a variable number at the DR locus. Mixed lymphocyte cultures were examined between female and male, female and a third party and mixed cultures. In the experimental group (undiagnosed), the pregnancies were lost between 6.6 and 8.9 weeks. In this group, living children did appear and were the first born. It was consistently documented in this group of undiagnosed etiology that mixed antigens at multiple loci did appear which were not present in the control group with known etiology. There was also no leucocyte antigen responsiveness. In an attempt to modulate this lack of immunological responsiveness to paternal antigens, 18 women were immunized with 40 million paternal lymphocytes on two different occasions. It was noted in these women that there was an increased immune response as defined by cytotoxic antibody, blocking antibody as well as mixed lymphocyte culture testing. Of these 18 women, three women have given birth to full term infants. Thus, it appears that a documented lack of immunological responsiveness to paternal antigens during pregnancy is not conducive to continued trophoblast survival in the uterus.

In the discussion that followed, Robert Brent inquired about the use of progestational agents and whether they do have any suppressant activity to account for the effect on pregnancy outcome. In unpublished studies, Alan Beer indicated that 10 fold higher concentrations of progesterone were needed than was present at the choriodecidual junction to prevent graft rejection in a nonuterine site. Therefore, it appears that progesterone is an immunosuppressant but cannot totally account for the suppression seen during pregnancy.

Page Faulk indicated that there seems to be growing evidence that some of the glycoproteins of the trophobast membrane can be grouped into allotypic antigens.

Some of these antigens are indeed shared by lymphocytes. Thus, it appears essential that for a normal pregnancy, the mother must mount a healthy immune response to the blastocyst, and if the blastocyst contains antigens which are shared with the maternal lymphocytes, it makes it improbable that she would in fact mount the necessary protective immune response to prolong this implantation. One interesting point Page Faulk raised was the fact that one of the patients in the Beer study had a common father and two different wives who both were linked to spontaneous abortions. This could mean that they also share HLA antigens with the father and it makes the idea of a trophoblast lymphocyte cross reactive antigens rather more complex. Unfortunately, in this particular case, only one of the wives was examined in detail.

Thus, the resolution of both this paper and discussion was that a substantial number of undiagnosed pregnancies may be due to deficient immunologic responses. Data generated in both the previous Faulk studies and especially in this Beer study, do indicate that treatment with paternal lymphocytes may allow for successful pregnancies.

It has become clear that maternal sensitization to paternal major histocompatibility complex (MHC) antigens is a common event during successful pregnancies. The alterations in immune response reactivity that occur in the female as the result of exposure to paternally derived determinants during pregnancy raises the question of the role of major histocompatibility complex products in reproductive processes. The present study represents a comprehensive search for evidence of an association of reproductive differences with differing degrees of MHC antigen disparity between females and males and demonstrated alterations in one-way mixed lymphocyte culture immune responses between spouses and unrelated third party cells. Women with recurrent consecutive spontaneous abortions of unknown (experimental) etiology compared with those of recurrent spontaneous abortions of known (control) etiology had a significantly increased frequency of sharing HLA antigens at the A, B, and D/DR loci with their spouses. In addition, a number of females in the experimental group also demonstrated specific hyporesponsiveness to spouse antigens in one-way mixed lymphocyte culture. This hyporesponsiveness did not always correlate with HLA antigen sharing as might have been expected. More recently, preliminary findings in a couple where the female demonstrated hyporesponsiveness to paternal antigens raise the question as to the presence of a suppressor T lymphocyte present in the peripheral blood stream of females with recurrent pregnancy wastage. The presence of this suppressor could prevent the appropriate immunoreactivity known to be associated with successful pregnancies. A search for antileukocyte antipaternal antibodies showed them to be lacking in the experimental group but present with expected frequency in the control females. The results indicate that histocompatibility between mother and conceptus and documented lack of immunologic responses to paternal antigens during pregnancy are not conducive to continued trophoblast survival in the uterus, perhaps as a consequence of an inability on the part of the female to generate an antigen-specific protective immunologic response.

Classic and Partial Hydatidiform Moles: Their Origin and Relationship to Malignant Sequelae

(Szulman, 1982)

The conference was pleased to have Aron Szulman lead the workshop on Trophoblastic Neoplasia. During this workshop, Dr. Szulman presented his extensive work on the chromosomal constitution of hydatidiform moles and lead a stimulating discussion of molar pregnancies and choriocarcinoma. To summarize the work of Dr. Szulman in one paragraph, does not do it justice. But rather the reader should review his previously published works.

Hydatidiform moles have been usually divided into two categories based upon the presence or absence of embyro. Classical moles have no embryo, but do have a particular chromosomal constitution. There are two types, 46xx or 46xy, which result from a single spermatozoon or two spermatozoa fertilizing an "empty egg" devoid of maternal chromosomes. Dr. Szulman proposed that this allograft in the mother its homozygousity may partially account for the high incidence (5-10 percent) of choriocarcinoma by unmasking specific genes in these trophoblastic cells.

Partial moles do have a fetus, which -however- tends to die before 9 weeks menstrual age. The molar change is focal as is the trophoblastic hyperplasia. These moles are diandric triploids, i.e. the 69 chromosomes are derived from a single maternal set of 23X plus two sets from the father, usually due to fertilization by two sperms. Two maternal sets plus one paternal one (digyny) virtually never give rise to a partial mole.

The morphology gross and microscopic is distinct from complete and partial moles and they can be told apart by pathologists without recourse to cytogenetics in nearly 100 percent of cases.

Ovarian Pregnancy: Criteria for Diagnosis

(Campbell et al., 1982)

Ovarian pregnancy has been a difficult clinical issue because of the diagnostic criteria. Even 105 years after the original guidelines of Spiegelberg (1878), missed diagnoses and inappropriate grouping of ectopic pregnancies often occur masking the true incidence of ovarian pregnancies. James Campbell reviewed the history of ovarian pregnancy and especially its possible associations with IUD use, anti-coagulant therapy and induced ovulation. Such iatrogenic risks require careful epidemilogical studies with detailed protocols diagnosing the pregnancy. Dr. Campbell and his associates have developed such protocols (Campbell et al. 1977; 1981). The major points of Dr. Campbell's presentation were the criteria for diagnosis. Ovarian pregnancy is often misdiagnosed as idiopathic hemorrhage from corpora lutea (ovarian apoplexy). Ten cases were reviewed taking into account the need to 1.) examine the extravasated blood for abortuses released from the ovarian site and 2.) perform serial histopathologic sectioning of the ovarian implantation site to detect trophoblastic tissue. With these additions to Spiegelberg's criteria and improved epidemilogic technics, there may be a means to unmask iatrogenic problems of ovarian pregnancy. Perhaps with such intense screening and documentation, definitive associations between therapy and disease can be established.

REFERENCES

Beer, A.E., and Quebbeman, J.F. (1982) Histocompatibility Polymorphism and Maternal. Immune Responses in Chronic Habitual Abortion. *9th Rochester Trophoblast Conference* Abstracts p. 21.

Campbell, J.S., Krongold, I., Bell, M.E.A., and Fergusson, J.P. (1977) Tubal pregnancy in a low risk population: occasional association with follicular salpingitis. *Europe J. Obstet. Gynecol. Reprod. Biol.* 7, 287-291.

Campbell, J.S., Mikhael, N.Z., Napke, E. (1981) Evidence and Appraisal of adverse reactions to drugs and other preparations used in hospital practice. Detection, validation, outlook for the future. *Meth. Achiev. exp. Pathol.* 10, 221-243.

Campbell, J.S., Jolly, E., Zamah, N., Mikhael, N., Drouin, P., Tolnai, G., Crowley, J., Walters, J., and Hurteau, G. (1982) Ovarian pregnancy update: 104 years after Spiegelberg, *9th Rochester Trophoblast Conference* Abstracts, p. 37.

Spiegelberg, O. (1878) Zur Casuistik der Ovarialschwangerschaft. *Arch. Gynaekol.* 13, 73-79.

Szulman, A.E. (1982) The origin of classic and partial hydatidiform moles in a relationship to malignant sequelae, *9th Rochester Trophoblast Conference* Abstracts, p. 20.

LIST OF CONTRIBUTORS AND ATTENDEES

J.G. Aarnoudse
Dept. of Obstetrics
University Hospital
Groningen, The Netherlands

Abdel Ghaffar Ahmed
Dept. of Obstetrics and Gynecology
University of Aberdeen
Royal Infirmary
Aberdeen, AB9 2ZB, Scotland

Mahmoud S. Ahmed
Dept. of Biochemistry
UTCHS, College of Medicine
894 Union
Memphis, Tennessee 38163

Eliane Alsat
INSERM
75014 Paris, France

Virginia Anderson
Dept. of Pediatrics
SUNY Downstate
Staten Island Hospital
Staten Island, New York 10305

Hisham A. Arab
University of Manitoba
59 Emily Street
Winnipeg, Manitoba R3E OW3
Canada

Lavanya Ashok
I E P and T
Albany Medical College
47 New Scotland Avenue
Albany, New York 12208

Raymond B. Baggs
Dept. of Lab Animal
Medicine and Surgery
University of Rochester
Rochester, New York 14642

Jeffrey V. Baker
University of Cincinnati
School of Medicine
Cincinnati, Ohio 45267

Wadi A. Bardawil
University of Illinois
Dept. of Pathology
Chicago, Illinois 60672

Sara E. Bardsley
Div. of Perinatal Medicine
MRC, Clinical Research Centre
Watford Road, Harrow
HA1 3UJ Middlesex, United Kingdom

Stanley L. Barnwell
Dept. of Pharmacology
Vanderbilt University School of
Medicine
Nashville, Tennessee 37232

David Beckman
The Stein Research Center
Jefferson Medical College
920 Chancellor Street
Philadelphia, Pennsylvania 19107

Monique Bedin
INSERM
Materinité de Port-Royal
75014 Paris, France

Alan E. Beer
Dept. of Obstetrics and Gynecology
University of Michigan
Medical Center
Ann Arbor, Michigan 48109

Francis L. Bellino
Dept. of Biological Sciences
109 Cooke Hall
SUNY/Buffalo
Buffalo, New York 14260

Robert Benveniste
Gynecic Endocrinology Lab
Michael Reese Hospital
and Medical Center
504 E. 29th Place
Chicago, Illinois 60616

Paul Bischof
Dept. of Obstetrics and Gynecology
University of Geneva
Maternité, 1211
Geneva 4, Switzerland

Nica Borgese
University of Milan
20122 Milan, Italy

Robert L. Brent
The Stein Research Center
Jefferson Medical College
920 Chancellor Street
Philadelphia, Pennsylvania 19107

Carol M. Brownscheidle
Endocrine Biochemistry Dept.
Medical Foundation of Buffalo, Inc.
73 High Street
Buffalo, New York 14203

John D. Brunzell
Dept. of Medicine RG-20
University of Washington
Seattle, Washington 98195

James S. Campbell
Health and Welfare Canada
Toxicology Research Division
Ottawa, Ontario KIA OL2
Canada

Sean W. Carey
Dept. Animal Genetics U-39
University of Connecticut
Storrs, Connecticut 06268

Lise Cedard
Maternité de Port-Royal
U. 166 INSERM
123, Bld de Port-Royal
Paris, France 75014

Bojana Cemerikic
Dept. of Endocrinology
Immunology and Nutrition
INEP
Zemun, 11080, Yugoslavia

Curtis Cetrulo
Dept. of Medical Research
and Laboratories
St. Margaret's Hospital for Women
Tufts University School of Medicine
89 Cushing Avenue
Boston, Massachusetts 02125

Clare L. Chatot
University of Connecticut
Storrs, Connecticut 06268

H. C. Cheng
Dept. of Obstetrics and Gynecology
University of Kansas
College of Health Sciences
Kansas City, Kansas 66103

Carolyn B. Coulam
Mayo Clinic
200 1st Street SW
Rochester, Minnesota 55905

James Crowley
Toxicology Research Division
Health and Welfare Canada
Ottawa, Ontario KIA OL2
Canada

Violetta Cuenca
Upstate Medical Center
Dept. of Obstetrics and Gynecology
750 East Adams Street
Syracuse, New York 13210

Jeanne Cullinan
Dept. of Obstetrics and Gynecology
University of Rochester
Rochester, New York 14642

R. H. Curry
Dept. of Laboratory Medicine
Ottawa Civic Hospital
1053 Carling Avenue
Ottawa, Ontario K1Y 4E9
Canada

Milos Cvetkovic
INEP
Dept. of Endocrinology
Immunology and Nutrition
Zemun, 11080, Yugoslavia

Ivan Damjanov
The Stein Research Center
Jefferson Medical College
920 Chancellor Street
Philadelphia, Pennsylvania 19107

Joseph Dancis
New York University Medical Center
550 First Avenue
New York City, New York 10016

Giuseppe de Virgiliis
University of Milan
20122 Milan, Italy

Yoram Z. Diamant
Bikur Cholim Hospital
Jerusalem, Israel

P. Anthony di Sant' Agnese
Dept. of Pathology
University of Rochester
Rochester, New York 14642

Martha Elliott
Harvard Medical School
Southboro, Massachusetts 01772

Richard F. Endress
Upjohn Pharmaceutical Company
19550 Clement Road
Northville, Michigan 48167

Donna Lee Faletto
Division of Toxicology
University of Rochester
Rochester, New York 14642

W. Page Faulk
Faculté de Médecine
University of Nice
Avenue de Vallombrose
06304 Nice-Cedex, France

W. Timm Fredrickson
University of Washington
Seattle, Washington 98195

Risa A. Freedman
Division of Toxicology
University of Rochester
Rochester, New York 14642

Mary Fronckowiak
Medical Foundation of Buffalo, Inc.
110 Sweet Avenue
Buffalo, New York 14212

Antoine Geinoz
Dept. of Obstetrics and Gynecology
University of Geneva
Maternité, 1211
Geneva 4, Switzerland

Olga Genbacev
Dept. of Endocrinology
INEP
Immunology and Nutrition
Zemun, 11080, Yugoslavia

John M. Gibbons, Jr.
Director of Obstetrics and Gynecology
St. Francis Hospital
and Medical Center
Hartford, Connecticut 06105

Dorothy Goodwin
Dept. of Obstetrics
University of Aberdeen
Aberdeen, AB9 22B, Scotland

Robert M. Greenstein
University of Connecticut
Farmington, Connecticut 06032

Francesca Guidobono
University of Milan
20122 Milan, Italy

Mark E. Hahn
Division of Toxicology
University of Rochester
Rochester, New York 14642

J. W. A. Heeren
Erasmus University
Dept. of Chemical Pathology
3000 DR Rotterdam, The Netherlands

B. Frederick Helmkamp
Dept. of Obstetrics and Gynecology
University of Rochester
Rochester, New York 14642

Ellen C. Henry
Division of Toxicology
University of Rochester
Rochester, New York 14642

Robert O. Hussa
SUNY/Buffalo
Buffalo, New York 14260

John V. Ilekis
Dept. of Obstetrics and Gynecology
Michael Reese Hospital
and Medical Center
504 E. 29th Place
Dreyfuss Building - Room 814
Chicago, Illinois 60616

Nicholas Illsley
Division of Perinatal Medicine
Clinical Research Centre
Harrow, HA1 3UJ
United Kingdom

Patricia Jennings
Div. of Inherited Metabolic Diseases
MRC, Clinical Research Centre
Watford Road, Harrow
HA1 3UJ Middlesex, United Kingdom

Marcela Jensen
The Stein Research Center
Jefferson Medical College
920 Chancellor Street
Philadelphia, Pennsylvania 19107

Robert Kaufmann
Dept. of Obstetrics and Gynecology
Southern Illinois University
Springfield, Illinois 62708

Rita Kissilevitz
Dept. of Obstetrics and Gynecology
Bikur Cholim Hospital
Jerusalem, Israel

John R. Kelly
428 Canisteo Street
Hornell, New York 14843

Bruce J. Kelman
Biology Dept.
Battelle, Pacific Northwest Laboratories
Richland, Washington 99352

Robert Kilpper
Health/Safety
Xerox Corporation
Rochester, New York 14604

Norman W. Klein
Dept. of Animal Genetics U-39
University of Connecticut
Storrs, Connecticut 06268

Arnold Klopper
Dept. of Obstetrics and Gynecology
Royal Infirmary
University of Aberdeen
Aberdeen, AB9 2ZB, Scotland

Gail Koscinski
Medical Foundation of Buffalo, Inc.
73 High Street
Buffalo, New York 14203

Thomas R. Koszalka
The Stein Research Center
Jefferson Medical College
920 Chancellor Street
Philadelphia, Pennsylvania 19107

Anthony Labrum
Dept. of Obstetrics and Gynecology
University of Rochester
Rochester, New York 14642

S. A. Lederman
Columbia University
Inst. Human Nutrition
630 West 168th Street
New York, New York 10032

Marsha K. Leith
University of Manitoba
Winnigeg, Manitoba
R3E OW3 Canada

Steven A. Lerman
Division of Toxicology
University of Rochester
Rochester, New York 14642

Philip Levine
Ortho Research Foundation
Route 202
Raritan, New Jersey 08869

Juliet Lobo
Dept. of Biological Sciences
109 Cooke Hall
SUNY/Buffalo
Buffalo, New York 14260

Clara Lowy
St. Thomas' Hospital
London, SE1 7EH, United Kingdom

Dieter H. A. Maas
Frauenklinik, Medizinische
Hochschule
Podbielskistrasse 380
D-3000 Hannover, West Germany

Debabrata Maulik
Dept. of Obstetrics and Gynecology
University of Rochester
Rochester, New York 14642

John A. McCoshen
University of Manitoba
59 Emily Street
Winnipeg, Manitoba R3E OW3
Canada

John A. McIntrye
Southern Illinois University
School of Medicine
Dept. Obstetrics and Gynecology
P O Box 3926
Springfield, Illinois 62708

James A. Merrill
Dept. of Obstetrics and Gynecology
University of Oklahoma
College of Medicine
P O Box 26307
Oklahoma City, Oklahoma 73126

Kalliope Michael
Dept. of Obstetrics and Gynecology
University of Manchester
Manchester, M13 OJH, England

Leon Metlay
Dept. of Pathology
University of Rochester
Rochester, New York 14642

Richard K. Miller
Dept. of Obstetrics and Gynecology
University of Rochester
Rochester, New York 14642

John J. Moore
Newborn Division
Dept. of Pediatrics
Metropolitan General Hospital
3395 Scranton Road
Cleveland, Ohio 44109

Robert D. Moore
Dept. of Pharmacology
Vanderbilt University School of
Medicine
Nashville, Tennessee 37232

W. M. O. Moore
St. Mary's Hospital
Manchester, M13 OJH, England

Eberhard Muechler
Dept. of Obstetrics and Gynecology
University of Rochester
Rochester, New York 14642

N. V. A. Murthy
Dept. of Physiology
University of West Indies Mona
Kingston, 7, Jamaica
West Indies

Navin C. Nanda
Cardiology Unit
University of Rochester
Rochester, New York 14642

Wendy Ng
Dept. of Obstetrics and Gynecology
University of Rochester
Rochester, New York 14642

Umberto Nicolini
University of Milan
20122 Milan, Italy

Richard D. O'Brien
University of Rochester
Rochester, New York 14642

Yoshio Osawa
Endocrine Biochemistry Dept.
Medical Foundation of Buffalo, Inc.
73 High Street
Buffalo, New York 14203

Maurice Panigel
Biologie de la Reproduction
Université de Paris VI
75827 Paris Cedex 17
France

Paul Penfold
Division of Perinatal Medicine
Clinical Research Centre
Watford Road
Harrow HA1 3UJ
Middlesex, United Kingdom

Rogelio Perez
Centro General de Intoxicaciones
Apartado Postal 40,005
Caracas 1040-A, D.F. Venezula

Alan M. Poisner
Dept. of Pharmacology
University of Kansas
Medical Center
Kansas City, Kansas 66103

Roselle Poisner
Dept. of Pharmacology
University of Kansas
Medical Center
Kansas City, Kansas 66103

Paul Purkiss
Div. of Inherited Metabolic Diseases
MRC, Clinical Research Centre
Watford Road, Harrow
HA1 3UJ Middlesex, United Kingdom

Roberto Rainoldi
University of Milan
20122 Milan, Italy

Gianni Remotti
University of Milan
20122 Milan, Italy

Philip A. Rice
Dept. of Chemical Engineering
and Materials Science
Syracuse University
Syracuse, New York 13210

Gene P. Sackett
University of Washington
Seattle, Washington 98195

Vasant Saini
Dept. of Obstetrics and Gynecology
University of Rochester
Rochester, New York 14642

R. Jim St. Hillaire
GI Research Laboratory
Veterans Hospital
San Francisco, California

M. K. Sanyal
Dept. of Obstetrics and Gynecology
Yale University Medical School
333 Cedar Street
New Haven, Connecticut 06510

B. V. Rama Sastry
Dept. of Pharmacology
Vanderbilt University Medical Center
Nashville, Tennessee 37232

Anthony Sbarra
Dept. of Medical Research
and Laboratories
St. Margaret's Hospital for Women
Tufts University School of Medicine
89 Cushing Avenue
Boston, Massachusetts 02125

Anne Marie Schindler
Centre de Cytologie et de
Depistage du Cancer
51 bd de la Cluse
CH-1205 Geneva, Switzerland

Probat Sehgal
Harvard Medical School
Southboro, Massachusetts 01772

Lucia P. Sereni
University of Milan
20122 Milan, Italy

Shashi Sharma
Dept. of Obstetrics and Gynecology
University of Rochester
Rochester, New York 14642

Mario Sideri
Prima Clinica Ostetrica e Ginecologica
dell'Universita di Milano
via Commenda I2
20122 Milan, Italy

Melvin R. Sikov
Biology Dept.
Battelle, Pacific Northwest
Laboratories
Richland, Washington 99352

Roy D. Simmons
Dept. of Obstetrics and Gynecology
University of Rochester
Rochester, New York 14642

Thomas C. Spelsberg
Mayo Clinic
200 1st Street SW
Rochester, Minnesota 55905

Aron E. Szulman
Dept. of Pathology
Magee-Womens Hospital
Forbes and Halket Streets
Pittsburgh, Pennsylvania 15213

Gisele Tanguy
INSERM
Maternité de Port-Royal
75014 Paris, France

Francois Teasdale
Hospital Ste-Justine
3175 Chemin Ste-Catherine
Montreal H3T 1C5
Quebec, Canada

Henry A. Thiede
Dept. of Obstetrics and Gynecology
University of Rochester
Rochester, New York 14642

Christopher R. Thomas
Dept. of Medicine
St. Thomas' Hospital
London, England

Henri Thoumsin
Clinique Gynecologique
et Obstetricale
Liège, Belgium

Carlos Torres
Dept. of Pediatrics
University of Rochester
Rochester, New York 14642

Beryl M. Tracey
Div. of Inherited Metabolic Diseases
MRC, Clinical Research Centre
Watford Road, Harrow
HA1 3UJ Middlesex, United Kingdom

George Trombetta
Dept. of Obstetrics and Gynecology
University of Rochester
Rochester, New York 14642

John E. Tyson
University of Manitoba
59 Emily Street
Winnipeg, Manitoba
R3E OW3 Canada

J. P. van Dijk
Erasmus University
Dept. of Chemical Pathology
3000 DR Rotterdam, The Netherlands

B. K. van Kreel
Erasmus University
Dept. of Chemical Pathology
3000 DR Rotterdam, The Netherlands

Claude A. Villee
Harvard Medical School
45 Shattuck Street
Boston, Massachusetts 02115

Tzuneng Wang
Frauenklinik der Medizinischen
Hochschule Hannover
3000 Hannover 51
West Germany

Jeffrey A. Whitsett
Dept. of Pediatrics
University of Cincinnati
Cincinnati, Ohio 45267

Patrick J. Wier
Dept. of Obstetrics and Gynecology
University of Rochester
Rochester, New York 14642

Myron Winick
Institute of Human Nutrition
Columbia University
701 West 168th Street
New York, New York 10032

Agnes Wodzicki
University of Manitoba
Winipeg, Manitoba
R3E OW3 Canada

Gary W. Wood
Dept. of Pathology
University of Kansas
College of Health Sciences
Kansas City, Kansas 66103

Ralph M. Wynn
Ravenswood Hospital
Medical Center
4550 North Winchester
Chicago, Illinois 60640

Carol Yarborough
Endocrine Biochemistry Dept.
Medical Foundation of Buffalo, Inc.
73 High Street
Buffalo, New York 14203

INDEX

All page numbers listed below represent the first page of each chapter, where the subject is located.

Abortion, 271, 307, 315, 347, 371

Acetylcholine, 81

N-Acetylglucosaminidase, 301

Adenohypophysis, 197

Adenosine, 81

S-Adenosyl-L-homocysteine, 81

S-Adenosyl-L-methionine, 81

Alanine, 121

Alcohol, 7, 175

Amino acid,
- Metabolism, 27, 55, 81, 167
- Transfer, 27, 37, 55, 71, 209
- Uptake, 37, 71, 81, 101, 121

α-Aminoisobutyric acid (AIB), 37, 71, 81, 101, 121

Amniocentesis, 167

Amnion, 361

Androgen, 237, 249

Androstenedione, 237, 301

Anneploidies, 167

Anoxia, 27, 55, 121

Antibody,
- Blood groups, 271, 307, 315, 347
- Teratogenic, 335
- Yolk sac, 335
- Abortion, 271, 307, 315, 335, 347, 371
- Transcobalamin, II 121

Anticonvulsants, 167

Arachidonic acid, 289, 301

Aromatase I, 301

Aromatase II, 301

Arylhydrocarbon hydroxylase, 175

Aspartate, 27, 81, 101

Autoradiography, 185

Benzo(α)pyrene, 175

Benzoylethyltrimethyl-ammonium, 81, 101

Blood,
- Embryo culture, 347, 371
- Flow, 7, 149
- β-hCG, 271
- hPL, 223, 271
- IgG, 307, 347
- PAPP-A, 223, 271
- Progesterone, 223
- SP_1, 223
- $SP_1α$, 271
- $SP_1β$, 271
- Transcobalamin II, 121

Calcium, 81, 167, 185

Carbamazepine, 167

Carnitine acetyltransferase, 81

Chlormadinone acetate, 237

Cholesterol, 209

Choline acetyltransferase, 81

Choline chloride, 167

Cholinergic system, 81, 101

Chorion,
- Membrane, 159, 271, 279, 301
- Perfusion (Ussing), 279

Choriocarcinoma, 289, 301, 371

Chorionic gonadotropin, 175, 223, 279, 289, 301,361

Chromatin, 249

Circulation, 37, 149
Cobalamin, 121
Cocaine, 101
Coffee, 7
Colchicine 81
Complement (human), 323
Creatine, 121
Culture technics, 279, 289, 121, 301, 347
Cyclic nucleotides, 185, 301
Cytochrome P_{450}, 301
Cytoskeleton, 81

Decidua, 197,361
Dehydroepiandosterone sulfate, 237
Depolarization, 167
Dexamethasone, 249
Diabetes mellitus, 7, 209
  Gestational, 7, 209
  Insulin dependent, 209
Diethylstilbestrol, 7
Digitonin, 279
Dinitrophenol, 121
DNA, 7, 81, 175
Doppler, 149

EDTA, 323
Embryo culture, 167, 347
Enzymes, 135, 175, 185, 209, 301
Epidermal growth factor, 289
Erythro-9-(2-hydroxy-3-nonyl)-adenine, 81
Estradiol, 237, 249, 301
Estriol, 7, 301
Estrone, 237, 301
Estrogens, 7, 175, 237, 249, 301
Estrogen synthetase, 301

α-Fetoprotein, 167
Fetus,
  Brain, 7
  Capillary leak, 37
  Growth, 7
  Weight, 7, 223, 167
Flow impedance, 149

Gel electrophoresis, 185
Genetic engineering, 175
Genetics, 167, 371
Glucocorticoids, 249
Glucose, 27, 55, 209
Glucose-6-phosphate dehydrogenase, 209
Glutamate, 27
Glycine, 121
Graft, 361
Growth failure, 7, 237
Growth hormone, 301
β-Guanidinopropionic acid, 121
Guinea pig, 71, 135, 167

Hemin, 301
Hemorrhage (idiopathic), 371
Heparin, 323
Histocompatability complex, 371
HLA antigen testing, 371
Homocysteine-thiolactone, 81
Hydatiform moles, 371
Hyperplasia, 7

Imidazole, 289

Immunofluorescence, 279

Immunology, 209, 307, 315, 323, 371

Indomethacin, 289

Intrauterine growth retardation, 7, 167, 237

Inulin, 37, 121

Iodoacetate, 121

Iron, 167

Isoleucine, 81, 101

JEG-3 cells, 289

Labor, 301

Lactate, 27, 37, 55, 197

Latex particles, 301

Lecithin, 301

Leucine, 37, 197

Lipase (lipoprotein), 135

Lipids, 209

Lipoxygenase, 289

Lymphocyte culture (mixed), 371

Lysine, 81, 101

Lysolecithin, 301

Metabolism, 81, 175, 209
- Amino acid, 37, 81, 101, 121, 197
- Cholinergic, 81
- Estrogen, 175, 237
- Fatty acid, 135
- Glucose, 121, 209
- Gonadotropins, 289
- Lipids, 81, 135, 209
- Palmitate, 135
- VLDL, 135
- Xenobiotic, 7, 175

Methyl transferase I, 81

Methyl transferase II, 81

Morphine, 101

Morphometry, 167

Mother,
- Height, 223
- Weight, 223

α-Naphthoylethyltrimethyl-ammonium, 81

Narcotics, 101, 301

Nicotine, 101

Nordihydroguaiaretic acid, 289

Nuclear binding, 249

Nutrition, 7, 121, 167

Organic acids, 55

Osmolarity, 197

Ouabain, 37, 121, 197

Oxygen consumption, 27, 37, 55, 197

Palmitate, 135

PAPP-A, 223,323

Perfusion,
- Human, 27, 37, 55, 149, 237, 279
- Guinea pig, 7, 71, 135, 167

Phagocytosis, 301

Phenobarbital, 167

Phenytoin, 167

Phorbol myristate acetate, 289

Phosphocreatine, 121

Phospholipase A_2, 301

Phosphorylation, 185

Phospholipids, 81, 209

Phosphatidylcholine, 81

Phosphatidylethanolamine, 81

Pig, 167

Pinocytosis, 121, 335, 301

Polymorphism, 371

Placenta,
- Acetylcholine, 81
- N-Acetylglucosaminidase, 301
- Amino acids, 27, 37, 55, 71, 81, 101, 121
- Aromatase I and II, 301
- Calcium, 81, 185
- Capillary integrity, 37
- Cholesterol, 209
- Cholinergic system, 81
- Chorionic gonadotropin, 175, 223, 279, 289, 301
- Circulation, 37, 149
- Culture, 289,301
- Cytoskeleton, 81
- DNA, 7, 175, 209
- Enzymes, 135, 175, 185, 209, 237, 289, 301
- Estrogen, 237, 301
- Estrogen synthetase, 301
- Glucose, 27, 37, 55, 197, 209
- Glucose-6-phosphate dehydrogenase, 209
- Glycogen, 209
- Guinea pig, 71, 135, 167
- Human, 7, 27, 37, 135, 81, 101, 121, 149, 185, 197, 209, 223, 249, 279, 289, 301, 361
- Immunology, 323, 335
- Lactate, 27, 37, 55, 197
- Lactogen(human), 175, 223, 301
- Lipids, 81, 135, 209,
- Metabolism, 27, 37, 81, 101, 121, 135, 175, 209, 223, 289
- Methyl transferases, 81
- Morphology, 157, 159, 167
- Organic acids, 55
- Oxygen consumption, 27, 37, 55, 197
- Palmitate, 135
- Perfusions, 27, 37, 55, 71, 135, 167, 279

Placenta (continued)
- Phospholipase A_2, 301
- Phospholipids, 81, 209
- Progesterone, 289
- Proteins, 175, 197, 209, 223, 323
- Protein kinase, 185
- Rat, 7, 335
- Receptors, 159, 175, 249, 301
- Renin, 279
- Slices, 81, 101, 121, 197
- SP_1, 271
- Steroids, 175, 223, 237, 249, 279, 301
- Steroid sulfatase, 237
- Transport, 27, 37, 55, 223
- Viability, 37, 101
- VLDL, 135, 209
- Ultrastructure, 15, 37
- Weight, 7, 167, 209, 223

Plasma membranes, 15

Porcine, 167

Potassium, 167, 197

Potassium cyanide, 167

Pre-eclampsia, 223

Pregnancy,
- High-risk, 167, 223
- Molar, 371
- Ovarian, 371

Prenatal genetics, 167

Primate, 347

Progesterone, 223, 249, 279, 289, 371

Progestin, 237, 371

Prostaglandin E_1, 289

Protein,
- Calcium-dependent, 185
- Synthesis, 37, 101, 185, 197

Protein kinase, 185

R1881, 249

R5020, 249

Rat, 347, 167

Receptors, 121, 175, 249, 301
Androgen, 249
Estrogen, 249
Glucocorticoid, 249
Opiate, 301
Progesterone, 249

Reichart's membrane, 335

RNA, 175

Rochester trophoblast conference, 1

Serum, 167, 301

Skin, 361

SP_1, 223

Steroids, 249, 289, 301

Steroid sulfatase, 237

Sucrose, 81

Teratogenesis,
Antiserum, 335
Rat, 167, 347, 335

Testosterone, 237

Theophylline, 301

Thromboxane, 289

Toxicology, 37, 81, 101, 121, 175, 289

Transcobalamin II, 121

Transport,
AIB, 37, 71
Amino acid, 27, 37, 71
Leucine, 37

Transport (continued)
Lipids, 135
Palmitate, 135
VLDL, 135

Transferrin, 167
Human, 167
Guinea pig, 167

Triploides, 167

Umbilical flow, 149

Urea, 27

Ultrasound, 167

Ultrastructure, 15, 37, 159
Freeze fracture, 15
Human chorion, 159
Human placenta, 15, 37

Ussing chamber, 279

Valporic acid, 167

Vitamin supplementation, 167

Vitamin, 121, 323

VLDL, 135

Weight,
Fetal, 223
Maternal, 223

Yolk sac, 335
Teratogenic antiserum, 335

MIX
Papier aus verantwortungsvollen Quellen
Paper from responsible sources
FSC® C105338
FSC
www.fsc.org

If you have any concerns about our products,
you can contact us on
ProductSafety@springernature.com

In case Publisher is established outside the EU,
the EU authorized representative is:
Springer Nature Customer Service Center GmbH
Europaplatz 3, 69115 Heidelberg, Germany

Printed by Libri Plureos GmbH
in Hamburg, Germany